An Historiography of Twentieth-Century Women's Missionary Nursing Through the Lives of Two Sisters

This volume draws on a trove of unpublished original material from the pre-1940s to the present to offer a unique historiographic study of twentieth-century Methodist missionary work and women's active expression of faith practised at the critical confluence of historical and global changes.

The study focuses on two English Methodist missionary nursing sisters and siblings, Audrey and Muriel Chalkely, whose words and experiences are captured in detail, foregrounding tumultuous socio-political changes of the end of Empire and post-Independence in twentieth-century Kenya and South India. The work presents a timely revision to prevailing post-colonial critiques in placing the fundamental importance of human relationships centre stage. Offering a detailed (auto)biographical and reflective narrative, this 'herstory' pivots on three main thematic strands relating to *people*, *place* and *passion*, where socio-cultural details are vividly explored.

The book will appeal to a wide range of readers, both the interested public and the academic alike, where a lively, entertaining, literary style introduces readers to the politics of women's lives, and principle and professional service foreground ethno-class-caste oppression, emancipation, conflict, commitments and religious tensions. It reveals the human, vulnerable qualities of these women, illuminating their stories and courageous choices.

Sara Ashencaen Crabtree is Professor of Social and Cultural Diversity, Bournemouth University, UK, and Professor Emeritus, University of Stavanger, Norway. An internationally renowned social scientist, she publishes prolifically, on faith, gender, diversity, welfare and vulnerability.

Routledge Research in Gender and History

For more information about this series, please visit: https://www.routledge.com/
Routledge-Research-in-Gender-and-History/book-series/SE0422

An Historiography of Twentieth-Century Women's Missionary Nursing Through the Lives of Two Sisters

Doing the Lord's Work in Kenya and South India

Sara Ashencaen Crabtree

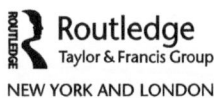
Routledge
Taylor & Francis Group

NEW YORK AND LONDON

First published 2024
by Routledge
605 Third Avenue, New York, NY 10158

and by Routledge
4 Park Square, Milton Park, Abingdon, Oxon, OX14 4RN

Routledge is an imprint of the Taylor & Francis Group, an informa business

ISBN: 978-1-032-41796-7 (hbk)
ISBN: 978-1-032-41795-0 (pbk)
ISBN: 978-1-003-35974-6 (ebk)

DOI: 10.4324/9781003359746

Typeset in Sabon LT Pro
by codeMantra

In loving and respectful remembrance of Muriel
and Audrey Chalkley, missionary nurses and sisters
in mission.

Contents

Figures

Acknowledgements

Many have assisted in the writing of this book to whom I extend a heartfelt thanks.

A big shout of gratitude goes first and foremost to Muriel Chalkely herself, a wonderful subject and participant. From Muriel, I received the sisters' photographs, especially for inclusion in this book. I would also like to recognise posthumously my dear colleague and friend, Professor Dr Fran Biley, who originally found and recruited the Chalkley sisters.

Hugely important were those who generously gave their time to help me understand the sisters' individual mission work in Maua and Ikkadu. My profound thanks go to Muriel's Kenyan 'family' of friends and colleagues, including Professor Dr Leah Marangu, Sister Florence Mutiga, Sister Margaret Aritho and son John, and Sister Barbara Dickinson. Through a chain of helpful introductions, I can warmly thank Reverend Dr Gnanavaram Masilaman, together with Reverend Ruth Wells, Reverend William Allberry, Dr Eleanor Jackson and Mr Sumanth Bommarthi. Of those who knew the sisters so well in England, my warmest thanks go to Susi, Kath and Beryl, Susan Dutton and Helen Cooper, among unnamed others.

Many thanks to the Bournemouth University (BU) Women's Academic Network for providing vital research funds to continue this work when other wells ran dry, not forgetting the colleagues of the BU Memories of Nursing oral history project. The librarians of the Special Collections at SOAS, University of London, the Cadbury Library, University of Birmingham and BU deserve a special mention.

Sincere thanks are due to the editorial teams of Max Novick, Louise Ingham and Emily Briggs at Routledge on both sides of the Atlantic for helping me bring this book to fruition.

Finally, I owe a huge debt of gratitude to the unwavering support, faith, encouragement and help of *mi alma mia*, my wonderful husband and scholarly 'critical friend', Professor Dr Jonathan Parker, as much of this story as anyone, as was Jack (Professor John Mark Crabtree) in his time. *Gracias hijas*, Isabel Crabtree Parker, for her excellent photography skills and tuition. Last but never least, 'baby' of the family, Miranda (Milly) Crabtree Parker, ever cheering me on.

1 Sketching the sacred

An introduction to a contemporary hagiography

Introduction: a mission

Muriel, as usual, is tracking the sun. She is seated in one of her reclining chairs in one or another of the cramped, fusty rooms of a small, sunny upstairs flat carved out of a large, shabby house run as lodgings by a religiously affiliated charitable housing association that, for want of the right custom, is now turning towards supporting a more secular clientele. The house has been so chopped about that its former elegant features are in something of a sorry state. Thieves came in the night and robbed the patrician portico of its lead tiles while Susi, the downstairs tenant lay awake, quaking and helpless. Now the precariously bulging, cracked and crudely repaired stained glass panels in the front door reveal how grand an abode this must once have been, while the external key safe, wheelchair-friendly slope and utilitarian handrails speak of what good purpose it now serves. A noble philanthropic gift it was donated years past to the cause of sheltering retired missionaries returning home after long years of service with big hearts and empty pockets, in need of a safe berth by the gentle sea of Bournemouth; a former convalescent and now university town, on the sunny English Dorset coast. Doughty in deed, hearty in hope and mild in manner, one imagines missionaries welcomed to this haven were a perfect amalgam of these two elderly sisters, Muriel and Audrey, for whom this book is dedicated and about whom it is concerned. From three missionaries who lived in the house of five individuals not long past, only one now remains, and the sisters are there no more.

Unseen histories

Oral histories and documents relating to the experiences of women missionaries working overseas, in the twentieth century and prior, remain a comparative rarity (Compton Bouwer, 1990). The missionary is more often captured in novels than in research, occupying an allegorical rather

DOI: 10.4324/9781003359746-1

than realistic significance in the plot. The scholarly neglect of inquiry into women's historical roles in the mission field (beyond or including that of wifedom) is argued to be peculiar to Britain, whereas the United States and Canada boast a strong history of women's overseas mission (Compton Bouwer, 1990; Spencer, 2016).

What autobiographical works can be found pertaining to British women missionaries are highly illuminating, such as Deaconess Carol Graham's (1980) who served faithfully in the Church of South India under Bishop Azariah of Dornakal. Missionary memoirs and diaries, often unpublished, like Dorothy Ross' serving in Nigeria before the Second World War, have their own fascination. The socio-historical details provided by these precious troves of miscellaneous writings, diaries, letters and memoirs report the minutiae of colonial lives, where spartan and sometimes grim accounts rub shoulders with the frivolities of polo, parties and *tiffin*. These, mostly found in university archives in Britain, like the University of London's School of Oriental and African Studies (SOAS), or the Nonconformist-endowed Cadbury Library of the University of Birmingham, are accessed by special permission only; forming vast, fascinating collections that the keen but bewildered researcher can lose themselves in for many a day.

In addition, of great interest, are some of the uncompromising, indignant polemics on the status and care of India's women, found in the medical missionary booklets written by Lilian A. Underhill (1932, 1935), who will reappear later. Furthermore, with the rise of the Internet and the monopoly of the Amazon empire, one can now find a small body of largely self-published memoirs from recent, mostly non-British, missionaries (Chapman, 2016; Michie, 2018; Watson, 2018). But this genre can be a dissatisfying read for the scholar, where insights and interpretations are often under-critical and overly naïve. Looking more widely, there are a few contemporary British biographies available, for example, *Africa Calling: A Medical Missionary in Kenya and Zambia*, Gerrard's (2001) account of his father, Dr Herbert Gerrard, a gung-ho exemplar of 'muscular Christianity' in pre-War colonies.

For the most part, the bulk of available information pertaining to the mission is connected to the wider topic of the British Empire, which is where sociological and historical inquiry coalesces. An essential historical context provides the backdrop against which mission is seen as both principle and practice; moreover, missionary enterprises are conventionally heavily critiqued as merely another arm of imperialism (Burton and Burton, 2007; Etherington, 1996; Nestel, 1998). Correspondingly, the wealth of information, autobiographical or scholarly, regarding foreign missionaries and their work dwindles significantly as we approach the mid-twentieth century, mirroring the decline in missionary work and its aspirants (Porter, 2004).

A historiography of twentieth century women missionaries

A history of lives lived true to a profoundly passionate faith, this research monograph draws on a rich collection of hitherto unpublished, original data to offer a historiographic study of twentieth-century Methodist missionary work and women's active expression of faith practised at the critical confluence of historical and global changes in Kenya and South India in the twentieth century. Two English Methodist sisters, by birth, by profession and by vocation, form the central, unifying motif foregrounding a grander historical backdrop marking the closing of British imperialism and the start of new journeys for independent post-colonial nation states. Muriel and Audrey born at the end of the First World War (the Great War), wove their own lives and experiences into these national and regional stories, albeit in ways that were unknown and unseen beyond the circle of those whose many lives they touched.

The wider context of the sisters' story is magnified among the vast mosaic of complex social, political and cultural historical events of nation states, the details of which threaten to overwhelm with unwieldy comparisons and confusing contrasts, signifying not a great deal. However, by drawing on the Chalkleys' accounts and scrutinising the relics they held dear, it affords readers the vistas and glimpses of what role and purpose they felt their lives served among 'people they came to love, and who, by all accounts, cared for them in return.

The study is contained within the wider context of mission and medicine in colonial and post-colonial contexts but offers a timely revision of aspects of post-colonial literature in placing the fundamental importance of human relationships centre stage. Thereby, it debunks prevalent myths decrying wholesale, western religious importation.

Two deaths and a beginning

Who were the Chalkley sisters? At the beginning, they were simply two anonymous participants recruited to an oral history project, developed at a provincial university in a pleasant town, where retired nurses came to enjoy their sunset years in residential care dedicated to the care of veterans of this respected public service. Nursing had a great advocate in Professor Dr Francis (Fran) Biley, a former qualified mental health nurse and the principal investigator of this nursing history project, as well as being a good colleague to me as he was to many. Fran was something of a maverick with the features and hair of a dog fox. A scholar and deeply committed family man, he otherwise presented as a typical old hippy in his dress, habits and inclinations. A talented woodsman, gardener, philosopher, writer and lover of the arts, Fran had a profound understanding of dis/ease, friendship and how to care for others through madness or dying. A great collector too of eclectic tastes, apart from his Tracey Emin limited editions and various esoterica, he treasured his covetable collection of antiquated, iron, nursing badges and medals. Most being so small and non-descript only a magnifying glass could reveal much of interest.

Unsurprisingly, Fran was completely intrigued by the possibilities offered by the ungarnered memories of the residents of the Retired Nurses National Home in Bournemouth. Having made friends there, he followed snowballing introductions to a pair of retired nurses who lived, as close, unmarried sisters may, in adjoining warrens, spending their days companionably together after having been separated by great geographical distances, and the demands of work for years on end. They were an interesting find, these sisters, he told me conversationally; although, as he viewed it, they were also aimable but anachronistic leftovers from an unsavoury period of British history that was replete with assumptions of innate superiority and moral authority, with the power of imposition and interference. In other words, the sisters had been missionaries. Fran's interests lay not with Christian missiology but with Western, 'allopathic'/'biomedicine' and its pretentions, and thus, he intended that the Chalkley sisters' medical missionary work would be subject to a post-colonial critique focusing on the suppression of indigenous forms of healing under an imported colonial health regime. I remember congratulating him on this genuinely fascinating research, but having spent long years studying psychiatry in post-colonial contexts myself (Ashencaen Crabtree, 2012), argued for a more nuanced position regarding the harm of colonialised medicine and the romance of indigenous healing practices.

What is known is that Fran began a co-authored paper, which no doubt would have been well received into the established research canon had he been able to complete it. He also presented a paper about the Chalkley sisters at a conference in 2010, at Royal Holloway, University of London, on International Perspectives on the History of Nursing, where frustratingly only a brief abstract seems to have survived, without reference to specific findings. Fran's work was interrupted when a short period of ill health ensued, and from feeling generally unwell to specifically and deeply ill, he made his peace with a tragic diagnosis, bid his family and friends goodbye to swiftly depart into a gentle death; exemplifying that acceptance of the inevitable that he had advocated for others in his time.

Fran's death left a huge gap for those who knew him, particularly for his widow left with two young children of the same ages as my dependent brood. I tried to fill a temporary vacuum by stepping in to help resuscitate the oral research project until it was picked up by colleagues far better qualified to understand the nursing profession. As for the Chalkley data, to my best knowledge, it was not included in the final oral history dissemination which regrouped around different priorities connected to the Nursing Home (Thomas and Rosser, 2017). Then, as well, while interesting, the Chalkey data was admittedly an awkward fit with the professional, secular focus, which seemed to have always been at its heart. Yet equally, for justice to be done with this inchoate and anomalous material, it also required a new beginning and a different steer. This meant starting afresh and it was no easy task. Fran died in November 2012 aged fifty-three and the year after Audrey Chalkley's declining health resulted in her death in June 2013, aged ninety-four, a bare three months, before I got to properly know her younger, grieving, sister, Muriel Chalkley, then aged ninety-one years.

Muriel, as she said, 'had the gift of the gab'. I knew her properly from the time we met in 2013 until the spring of 2020, when, one fall at home too many, she was sequestered in residential care and quickly disappeared from view under the draconian COVID-19 pandemic lockdowns, becoming as inaccessible to me as a walled-in nun. Against the odds she reached her centenary, but much had been lost, and it was doubtful that she still remembered me or the adventures of her former existence. She lived, contentedly (I hope), moored by the daily routines of care: the cleaning, wrapping, nurturing, cossetting and lulling her new state demanded, and which she herself was once so adept at, becoming quickly attached to her African keyworker. The longest lived of all her siblings by far, Muriel died on the evening of 9 March 2022 and was interred by her remaining relatives in a very private, 'family only', thereby a poorly attended ceremony. It seemed a poignant commendation of her mortal remains to the earth, contrasting with the charismatic, great-hearted, loving and lovable character she had been. Nonetheless, this did not prevent her friends from connecting with each other, where in Kenya, as well as in Britain, her life was celebrated rather than her death mourned.

Muriel, as I remember her, was one of the most gregarious, upbeat and cheerful people one could meet. Feminist epistemologies encourage egalitarianism and the removal of the researcher-subject hierarchy (Skeggs, 2009), while Bloom (1998) goes so far as to advocate intimacy in the fieldwork relationship. Both were easily achieved with Muriel, a delightfully talkative lady, full of laughter and bonhomie. Originally our chat began with a purpose in mind and that was to gather as many of Muriel's memories as possible, decanting them into safe storage for research purposes. It was agreed, to Muriel's self-depreciating wonder, that a book would be my gift to commemorate the service that she and Audrey gave themselves up to so selflessly. Throughout our friendship, which became close, Muriel was completely happy to continue participating, finding it a hilarious business, marvelling at my interest and encouraging it by passing on some items for inclusion. Not much given to introspection, she never seemed to realise that there could be any equivocation others might hold regarding the medical mission element of their remarkable careers. Instead, she held fast to missionary nursing as her dominant life's purpose, embodying in her enthusiasms, being a lover of contemporary hymnals, Daniel L. Schutte's (1981) rousing congregational verse:

Here I am, Lord, is it I, Lord?
I have heard you calling in the night.
I will go, Lord, if you lead me.
I will hold your people in my heart.

The collection of memories was completed long before her dementia took full hold and as time went on this repetition became an aide memoire, returning Muriel to herself, as mild and then increasing dementia took hold and our conversations went round in ever diminishing, but still cherished, circles. Over time our relationship evolved from an excellent working one to one of loving kindness, as Muriel now needed me to remind her of her own life and those she had known and spoken of so often. From raw data, the later sheltering of these memories became its own raison d'être.

Muriel, as both Fran and I found, was always extremely hospitable and generous with her time and information about her own life and what she knew of her sister's, about whom she always had the highest regard and respect. Yet that sounds too cool a statement, the reality was that Muriel loved and idolised Audrey. Her praises were sung on every possible occasion, with the differences and commonalities between the two of them carefully delineated: Audrey holding the upper berth of superior intellect and worth. Although she believed her sister 'safe in the arms of Jesus', Muriel missed her with an intensity equal to her devotion, tempered with faithful hopes of an eternal reunion.

Muriel was not inured to loneliness and it affected her deeply, despite the fleeting daily visits provided by professionally cheerful, efficient home carers, her nieces' regular phone calls, those of her devoted, wheelchair-bound neighbour, Susi, downstairs, plus the distractions of the odd visitor like me. For someone once immersed in the most hectic work schedules and responsibilities imaginable, the solitude and stillness were extremely hard to endure, especially as Muriel became increasingly housebound. The little landing outside her flat was ill-lit with a few darkly yellowing light bulbs and a once lovely stained-glass skylight was blackened, the stairs perilously steep for anyone, let alone someone who relied on a walking frame. It became apparent that Muriel would never be able to leave her flat again save by ambulance or undertaker. Muriel longed for death, as she frequently said, but with the most positive spirit imaginable. She earnestly wanted to 'see the Lord', to be with Audrey again and just wished

He would hurry up about it. But this matter of the disposing of her life was according to His will and in His good time. I do not think that for one moment, Muriel would ever have entertained the notion of assisted dying, were it even possible in Britain. At least, as she said with thankfulness, she suffered little physical pain, despite trouble with her heart, breathing and plumbing, along with severe anxiety attacks in the night and wobbliness on her feet. Despite all, somehow her strong constitution kept her going long after she wanted or could appreciate its stubborn stamina. When I began to write this first chapter, Muriel was still alive but by the time I had completed a draft of Chapter 3, she was no longer so; but at least, this book, Muriel's book and Audrey's as well, celebratory, commemoratory and critical, is now finished.

Aims, approaches and the significance of the study

Deep immersion

The story of missions and missionaries has been to date the domain predominantly of historians who have brought their own professional, disciplinary methodological approaches to these inquiries. Although non-historians have occasionally attempted to stake their own unique claim in the missionary territory, the social science approach has yet to convince scholars like Etherington (2012), arguing that such studies require a longitudinal, interdisciplinary approach, coupled with strong skills in archival research and religious history. Point taken, to a degree. Potentially, therefore, a scholar like myself stands at something of a disadvantage, as a feminist social scientist, neither historian nor theologian, but one whose research approaches are informed by qualitative, comparative social scientific methodologies rather than conventional historical methods. Direct face-to-face fieldwork, the forging of fieldwork relationships and the generation of primary, normally ethnographic, data are the traditions I use within a feminist epistemological framework, where gender is the analytical framework engaged with. As such, it offers a methodological toolkit appropriate to the study of women's lives. Social scientists also work with secondary data as well, where research literature, demographics, statistics, policy documents and written records of all kinds are commonly accessed. Thus, a historiography in the social sciences may well be composed of a compilation of both primary and secondary data (Ashencaen Crabtree, 2012), and such is the case here.

The approach I take challenges the form of academic writing to offer an innovative, involved rational-emotive feminist biography. It adopts a deeply immersed, reflexive biography, using Caetano (2015) comprehensible definition of the reflexive as grounded in personal and subjective reflections upon social circumstances. Following van Stapele (2014: 14) self-reflexivity is proposed as a common device in feminist epistemology as an analytical tool recalibrating bias and leanings towards potential normative givens/assumptions, enabling alternative readings to emerge (Harding, 1987). Such epistemological strategies permit researchers to insert their own subjective reflections, particularly at junctures of apparent certainties, as well as the ambivalent or inchoate.

The Chalkley narratives, forming the foundation of this study, are treated as partial, fragmentary, ambiguous, contradictory and fluid in iteration. We can neither gain, nor should attempt, complete mastery over these narratives. Likewise, we cannot configure each sister into one unchanging subjective, essential entity, immutable and unambiguous, an endeavour Bloom (1998) identifies as a humanist and masculinist fallacy. In reference to the historiographic process, Glenn (2000, p. 389) jettisons the dualities of an objective 'truth' or 'falsity', to focus on questions of knowledge, ethics and power in historiographies; how these are represented and for whom; with greater responsibility demanded in the representation of women and other 'disenfranchised' groups in history.

In terms of the narratives, the appropriateness of oral history to capture the biographical is well established in nursing studies (Beidermann, 2001; Boschma et al., 2008). Narrative inquiry can accommodate a range of different methodological approaches (Kohler-Riessman, 2008; Riley and Hawe, 2003). Narratives are treated here as socially constructed, storied accounts subject to qualitative thematic analysis. Yet because the Chalkey narratives were derived from distinct but overlapping data sets conducted at specific temporal points with two individuals, one of whom had since died, this could not always permit the experiences, perspectives and interpretations of the sisters to be fully drawn out (Sherman Heyl, 2009). Instead, productive gaps were revealed, enabling omissions to be 'felt' as experienced exercises of tactile, immersive reflexivity. My own histories have spontaneously arisen through this process as a natural condition of my encounters, proving so relevant they demanded interweaving into this story.

Significance of the study

'Playing devil's advocate, why should anyone be interested in two old, colonial missionaries?' This comment was put to me by a sceptical colleague gatekeeping my application for a prestigious research fellowship in connection with the completion of this book. Possibly a fair question, it was also a strong reminder of how the combination of religion, as faith experience, coupled with the topic of women, particularly old women, is a subject little respected compared to other academic areas of inquiry. This despite the tentative but emboldening interest from largely feminist scholars in the '"feminisation" of faith' (Gaitskell, 2010, p. 74) and where Hempton (2005) argues that the influence women have had on the shaping of Methodism has yet to be fully understood.

Throughout my career, I have written about faith and vocation, making what many would regard as a strong, international academic reputation based on my work on Islam and social work (Ashencaen Crabtree et al., 2016; Ashencaen Crabtree, 2022). I am rightly proud of that corpus, but more latterly have started scholarly excavation into faiths that include Christianity and gender (Ashencaen Crabtree, 2021). In so doing, I cannot help but be aware that this kind of scholarly inquiry is one that is less encouraged.

In the UK, at least it would seem that serious interest in religion tends to be viewed as not only a minority interest but as an interest *of* minorities (Ashencaen Crabtree, 2022). Faiths associated with minority ethnic (ME) communities are often received with dutiful respect, particularly in academia, in a way that is somewhat reminiscent of the anthropologically inclined, paternalistic fascination for the 'Other'.

When it comes to Christianity, this interest markedly declines, where it occupies a very different status, being inevitably viewed in secular or post-Christian thinking as loaded with oppressive and exploitative assumptions, an embarrassing anachronism, associated with heel-dragging on certain progressive, liberal agendas and child sex abuse scandals. Equally, Christianity's gravitational, global importance to countries beyond the West is conveniently ignored or potentially linked to the ongoing ills of imperialism as religious hoodwinking (Parker et al., 2018).

Since now incorporating Christianity in my scholarly work and practice, I have experienced this chilling effect in ways that have been personally bruising and intellectually dismissive. It would be easy to see this as a case of sour grapes or alternatively, perhaps a whiff of gas-lighting, but other scholars also comment on the freezing out of an intellectual engagement regarding matters of Christian faith, where the closure or merging of established theology departments with other disciplines speaks tellingly of institutional priorities (British Academy, 2019). Billington Harper goes further in her biography of Bishop Azariah of South India, denouncing a zeitgeist of cynicism coupled with a failure of imagination regarding the whole concept of sincere piety in the 'critical-modern analytical mind' and where:

> most modern biographies take religion seriously only when debunking its many pretensions, hypocritical postures, and false illusions. Religious rhetoric is rarely believed, if it is considered at all.
>
> (Billington Harper, 2000, p. 3)

The intellectual play of the deconstruction of concepts can occupy overlapping territory with the sport of spotting feet of clay among idols.

It is also one that by its very nature sets up oppositional binaries. But if compelling lucidity and rigour can be found in reasoning and concepts, professed belief and principles may also arise from luminous, profoundly sincere conviction.

For feminists, such as myself, the question of religion among women has proved challenging. While acknowledging early feminist activism as connected to their spiritual principles, women's adherence to apparent patriarchal religions has tended to be viewed as the remaining chains of gendered oppression to which feminist consciousness-raising pedagogy is the cure. Accordingly, Braidotti (2008) argues that in the Global North, the feminist terrain of struggle is civic rather than theistic, although elsewhere 'feminist' or pro-women polemics take aim at the patriarchal parasitism that has wormed itself into otherwise gender-liberatory faiths (Ashencaen Crabtree et al., 2016). Yet, even if secular, civic rights are a notable feature of Second Wave feminism, this has nonetheless provided the intellectual context wherein feminist theologies in the 1980s grew, in particular, the rise of Christian and Jewish women's critiques, as well as reclaimed Goddess-orientated pathways (Ashencaen Crabtree, 2021). For Llewellyn (2015, p. 4), Third Wave feminism has the potential to bridge the ongoing discontinuities between 'feminist studies and religious feminism' through the seeking of commonalities between women.

Given, this contentious and inhospitable climate implicating academia, feminism and public perception, it can come as little surprise that white, women missionaries are regarded as a questionable choice of topic. To be fair, it is a moot point and one that encourages reflection upon the potential obsolescence, insignificance and the much critiqued, potential harmfulness of missionary work and its proponents. My response to this challenge is found in the pages of this book, where, although one cannot obviate the smallness of individual lives, the greatness of intention and aspiration such individuals demonstrated in deeds as well as words, demand recognition, interest and respect too. What good was achieved and what legacies remain is for the reader to decide.

The sisters

The Chalkley sisters were born at a time when missionary service, whether Anglican or Nonconformist, was dwindling, but it was still a respected vocation in the popular mind. One, moreover, imbued with the romance of adventure, and, significantly, *even* open to women. It diverged from a time when missionary work was a male preserve only, where, as Charlotte Brönte's Jane Eyre learns from St John Rivers, what missions required were subordinate, helpful wives, not equal female pastors. Yet the sense of vocation to serve in a bigger world beyond the local parish church could not be denied, particularly where women missionaries were seen to have access to minds, hearts and places that male colleagues were prevented from entering (Kent, 1999). Thus, mission overseas promised opportunities far beyond the possibilities of most women, particularly those without independent means and freedom from ties and obligations at home. Missionary work offered a potential road for the hardy, determined and Bible-inspired woman to step far beyond the walls of her home, the employers' or the factory into a sharply contrasting life, whether to encounter unaccustomed luxuries or unexpected hardships or an odd mixture of both.

Missionary work was often a family calling across generations, where children of missionaries were born in the countries their parents were stationed, as in the case of Dr Lilian Underhill born in India to mission parents stationed on the North-West Frontier, or Handley Douglas Hooper, the Kenyan-born son of generations of missionaries. Neither circumstance applied to Audrey and Muriel Chalkley, whose parents were solidly North of England, Cheshire born, bred and rooted, and whose missionary zeal was aimed more at neighbourhood advocation rather than action in the foreign missional field; although on their own, home turf ministry was sovereign. What inspiration or persuasion did the sisters experience to make them leave their family and homeland to serve in countries so far away and unknown to them is a question we may ask. Perhaps of more importance is what motivated them to continue walking this path for so many decades, where altogether they served a total of fifty-four years as missionary nurses (Biley, 2010).

Documenting lives

The Chalkley narrative interview data fall into five parts: the earliest are two separate sets of interviews dated 1994. The second set is dated 2012–2013 and the last set dated 2014–2016, with supplementary data added in 2021–2022. Data falls into three neat camps: first, earlier secondary data comprising interviews; second, secondary data including writings from the sisters; and the latter, my primary data. The earliest interviews formed part of a collection of missionary narratives that Audrey and Muriel participated in in 1994 for the Methodist Church's Overseas Division, and many of Audrey's words are sourced from this resource. These recordings were donated to SOAS, copies of which are now held in the British Library as part of the British Library's 'Sounds Interesting' project.

None of the interview secondary data, so far as I can discern from extensive searches, has been subject to publication, although Muriel contributed some limited data on female genital mutilation for a paper and book on reproduction in Kenya (Thomas, 2001, 2003). Of the writings produced by the sisters, these comprise an unpublished, short autobiography by Muriel;

a booklet of co-authored verse and two nursing textbooks by Audrey. The latter may seem an unlikely choice of secondary data but working on the premise that all such compositions reveal much about the author's choices, priorities and biases, I have included them.

The story of creating and compiling the narratives is best told diachronically. The data I inherited from Fran following his death was unsurprisingly incomplete, for while there was a folder awaiting information there is no record of any interviews he undertook with Audrey, whose health was also beginning to fail around that time. Happily, Fran was able to carry out some useful interviews with Muriel from 2012, although these tended to concentrate on Muriel's nursing training and nursing practice in the UK (the main focus of the oral history project) with less solicited about her mission years.

In the development of this historiographic study, the threads of the original study had to be picked up again, but to consolidate fragments of lives into a continuing history has required considerably more investigation. Thus, from 2015 onwards, I conducted several new interviews with Muriel, later supplementing this information in 2021–2022 with those who knew the sisters or their work in the South Indian and Kenyan Methodist context.

There can be little more pleasurable to a scholar, apart from spending time talking to delightful and informative people than digging around in the quiet vaults of archives. This study required such joyful periods of immersive 'timeless time' (Ylijoki & Mäntylä, 2003, p. 62), to borrow a term referring to those very rare monastic hours when the world is shut out and word is splendidly immanent. Lack of research funds and the mutating plague years of the COVID-19 pandemic, which thrice infected me and mine, made travel to see the mission hospitals of Ikkadu and Maua, very difficult to achieve, a deficit partly met by Zoom and Skype. Then too the hospitals and local area had been subject to much change since the sisters' time there. Island-bound in Britain I had to 'reach out' to anyone who knew the sisters in Maua and Ikkadu, a hunt that returned interesting results some of the time and exasperated me much of the rest. My main strategy was to locate gatekeepers to the sisters' contacts. In Muriel's case, this was Professor Dr Leah Marangu, the eloquent and elegant, retired vice-chancellor of the Africa Nazarene University in Kenya, once one of Muriel's first student nurse trainees in Maua, and of whom she was very proud. Professor Marangu, Leah, introduced me to a number of other of Muriel's old friends, all of whom were very happy to talk to me and made me feel that I now had a brand-new friendship network in Kenya.

Lulled into a false sense of security following this success, Audrey's case proved a far harder nut to crack. Over a period of increasingly frustrating months, I wrote more than once to the Methodist Missionary Society, the Church of South India (CSI), the Church Mission Society and the CSI Wesley Church in Ikkadu. Replies were either not very hopeful or non-existent. In Britain, the housing charity was unable to help me with information. Only one person in the congregation of the Methodist Churches she worshipped in post-retirement volunteered to speak to me; perhaps because, as a vicar said, they knew so little about her.

The CSI Mission Hospital where Audrey had worked and attached CSI School of Nursing in Ikkadu, I had high hopes of as an obvious source of information, but they never replied to my mailed letters; indeed, without emails either, they observed the kind of cut-off remoteness I otherwise enjoyed in the archives. The CSI Boys' Home that Audrey supported did not seem to exist anymore, nor could I find information about any corresponding Girls' Home that I was told by her surviving relatives she had assisted. My dislike of Facebook and its ilk was temporarily put to one side to see if I could find anyone who knew Audrey in India. Unfamiliar with and rather appalled by social media I was at first intrigued that seemingly hundreds of people seemed so keen to get to know me, but it transpired absolutely none at all knew Audrey. I got nowhere with the publishing house in India still producing Audrey's textbooks. I began to despair until finally, I got a bite on my forlornly dangling hook. A chaplain colleague of mine put me in touch with a Methodist connexion network which then directed me to a semi-retired Anglian clergyman, Reverend William Alberry, who was involved in a group called 'Friends of the Church of South India', of which Audrey had once been a member – not that William actually knew her himself. He later mentioned that one of his good colleagues might know of Audrey, and so it was, which is how I got to know Reverend Dr Gnanavaram Masilamani, former principal of the Tamil Nadu Theological Seminary. A miracle! For Gnanavaram knew Audrey during her healthy, energetic retired years when he was a doctoral student in Oxford with his young family. Finally, just prior to deleting my nightmarishly proliferating Facebook account, I sent a message off to Ellesmere Methodist Church, hoping to find a Susan Dutton who had written Audrey's obituary for the *Methodist Recorder* in August 2013. Soon after, Susan, a Methodist lay preacher on the Shropshire and Marshes circuit, and her younger sister, Helen Cooper contacted me. They turned out to be older versions of the two animated young girls in a tennis court, smiling at the camera alongside their mother, Mary Rathbone. These were none other than Muriel's old family friends, whose photograph she kept close by.

Otherwise, the sisters' miscellaneous memorabilia entrusted to me by Muriel did not seem to amount to a great deal. Of greater value than all else, was the company of the living, vibrant Muriel to talk to, although over the details of her stories became flattened in detail and texture. Audrey was inevitably more of an enigma, a thinker rather than a talker in life, she left few mementoes. Among these keepsakes were old, jumbled photographic slides, a few letters of farewell from friends in Ikkadu, and a curious collection of 1920s correspondence from a former Brahmin turned Methodist clergyman – to be unsealed in Chapter 6.

Slowly a more comprehensive picture of both sisters was built, mapped against the wider context of events influencing attitudes and behaviour. While some gaps in our knowledge of the Chalkleys remain and where lost details may never be retrieved, this does not detract from a wider story of women's contemporary Christian mission, as represented by these sisters. They lived at a time of great social changes that affected their lives in specific ways: war, welfare and work formed the macro structures framing expectations and possibilities. However, their histories, as examples of female, professional, caring vocations and religiously inspired philanthropy, make a distinctive contribution to a broad church of reader interests: gender and feminism, nursing studies, contemporary religion, community and development studies, and finally, empire and nation. For those seeking an in-depth, historical or socio-politico-cultural understanding of Kenya and South India, this book will disappoint. Such a vastly complex exercise would, by its very scale, erase memories of two people as unutterably insignificant in comparison. But when magnified, these lives provide a better understanding of the wider context, as Miller explains in respect of oral histories:

> Adopting a biographical perspective leads by definition to an overview of the whole life course and hence to the historical events that have shaped a life.
>
> (Miller, 2000, p. 21)

The motifs of the sisters' narratives link together three thematic strands resting on the concepts of people, passion and place. In respect of *people*, in addition to the sisters, it embraces those they knew as colleagues, cared for as patients, joined in fellowship and loved. *Passion* emerges strongly as well. It was passion we may assume that induced these professional women to leave England, inhaling new-found peace and enjoying increasing security in the post-war period and to exchange that to serve wheresoever the need was deemed to be the greatest in the last years of the British Empire. Finally, in reference to *place*, Ikkadu in the state of Tamil Nadu (formerly the Madras State) and Maua in the Meru County of Kenya may have seemed remote and rural outposts in one sense, but they were far from removed from the tumultuous historical shifts shaping the contours of new nation states.

In adopting a self-reflexive approach, I have gone further by weaving in not only myself (Aull Davies, 1999) but also those dear to me, whose lives intersected at times with the histories of these sisters, whose own lives were closely intertwined. In this way, personalised and fresh information is presented, grounded in the psychosocial. While engaging with postcolonial theorisation, a more nuanced discussion of lives lived in post-imperial and post-colonial missionary contexts provides a dialectical tension between religiously inspired philanthropy, professional, feminine caring vocations and the politics of power. By drawing on both primary and secondary data concerning the sisters' work and reflections thereof, this historiographical account weaves together the following narrative strands.

The importance of women's contribution to mission service and qualified women's employment is a recurring theme across the chapters. The skills and authority women brought to their overseas postings are presented, challenging the gendered, subaltern status of female mission workers as primarily wives or ineffective handmaids, placing them as central to colonial mission enterprise. Equally, women missionaries' initiative, leadership and capabilities served as important progressive examples of their abilities, forming an overt challenge to gender-based, exclusionary tactics and bigotry prevalent back home.

The magnitude and exactitude of missionary nursing and midwifery as experienced in Tamil Nadu, India, and Maua, Kenya are discussed in Chapters 5–8. The contexts of sickness, care and healing form a dominant strand throughout the book, implicating issues of gender and ethnic normativity as well as bodily integrity.

Colonial and post-colonial relations are critically discussed as moulding the socio-cultural background to politicised changes and resultant turbulence in the wake of the Second World War, duly discussed in Chapters 3, 5, 7 and 8. These social constructions were implicated in the rapid decline of the British Raj, the move to Home Rule, *swaraj* in India, as well as the Mau Mau uprising and *Uhuru* in Kenya; but cannot in turn be disconnected from the development of indigenous religious forms there.

The interpersonal relationships between expatriates and indigenous populations are clearly important and these are reviewed in terms of imposed, negotiated, hierarchical and egalitarian social positions. The imprinted, clustered contexts of class and colonialism in Britain, Kenya and India foreground textured social realities in Chapters 7 and 9.

A theorised distinction is drawn throughout the work between internalised levels of oppression at the localised level of colonialism, and the global rationalisations of imperialism, in which we see how these served to intersect, overlap and influence one another. Additionally, self-reflexivity enables biographical information to be treated as directly intersecting with history, drawn from insights gained from these narratives. I also offer my own reflective signature to deliberate more deeply upon the meanings emerging from the narratives as resonating with my own historically and culturally located understanding as a contemporary woman of faith (Ashencaen Crabtree, 2021).

Offering revisionary scholarship into Methodist missionary endeavour, this proposed monograph generates important insights into Methodism's servant ethos. It moves us from the position of service within local communities to the *diaconic* promotion and undertaking of 'women's work' in the wider world, considered across this historiography in respect of vocation, professionalisation, globalisation, women's religious leadership, community welfare and gendered liberation.

The final strand interrogates the potential legacy of Methodist mission as a global, post-imperial phenomenon. This employs the motif of the Chalkley sisters, their excavated experiences and the interplay of reflexivity through the integration of themes, overlaid with plural perspectives.

Structure and organisation

This book is divided into ten chapters, of which this forms the first. In Chapter 2 the foundations of Wesleyan Methodism are examined, providing a literary overview of a theology welding heart and spirit together. Here we uncover the theological foundations of a tradition into which the Chalkey sisters were born. An overview of mission work, particularly women's mission, in India and Africa, provides the historical context to their service overseas.

The early lives of the sisters and their family form Chapter 3, where their formative years in the North of England are explored, indicating how Methodism ideals were woven into birth, death, together with wider social expectations of a responsible and respectable life.

Chapter 4 picks up on the narrative thread spun in the previous chapter to examine the development and professionalisation of nursing, a vocation into which the sisters entered at the commencement of the Second World War. Accounts of pre-Beverage health care are compared with the Chalkley experiences of post-war universal healthcare.

The religious 'call' to mission forms the topic of Chapter 5. This draws on personal correspondence to consider the psychosocial drivers impelling single women of faith to volunteer, including how potential mission recruits were viewed, evaluated and selected (see also Chapter 7). The perceived priorities for and demands of Methodist Mission work in India in the 1940s are discussed with respect to women mission workers, social positioning, expressed authority and external ambivalence towards communities of need.

Chapter 6 – the year is 1947 in South India where we find tumultuous social and political events arising, which Audrey Chalkley, newly arrived at Ikkadu Hospital, will personally witness. This is the year of the Independence in India (*swaraj*), along with the portentous rise of the Church of South India and the melding of Methodism into ecumenicalism.

The action moves from post-war Beverage Britain and midwifery to Maua in Kenya in Chapter 7. Here the steps of Muriel Chalkey, now a qualified nurse and midwife, are traced from religious crisis to Christian obedience and adventure. This chapter begins to explore the early years at Maua Methodist Hospital and the task set before our reluctant missionary.

Further unpublished biographical data and interviews provide the content for Chapter 8 where mission midwifery in Kenya is examined, together with an analysis of the politics of indigeneity, national identity and gender. This incorporates compelling anecdotal information regarding maternal and child mortality in the Maua region, implicating the ethno-national politics of female genital mutilation and the Mau Mau uprising of the dispossessed.

Chapter 9 forms the penultimate chapter and is divided into two dominant themes. The first focuses on the triumvirate of Methodist mission aims that overseas missionaries were expected to demonstrate, as illustrated by the sisters' work. The wider ramifications of international health agendas, influencing mission nursing, are further discussed. The second theme pivots on the personal. Here we gain additional insights from those who knew Muriel and Audrey Chalkley, delving deeper into their professional relationships, friendships, pleasures, joys, losses and intimacies.

Chapter 10 concludes the Chalkley history. The theme of people, place and passion is revisited in consideration of a *post* post-colonial position to reflect upon the legacies and meanings arising from women's twentieth-century mission.

References

Ashencaen Crabtree, S. (2022) Islamic perspectives, inclusivity and revitalisation in conceptual frameworks for European social work. In Hansjörg Schmid and Amir Sheikhzadegan (Eds.), *Islamic Social Work. From Community Services to Commitment to the Common Good*. Cham, Switzerland: Springer Nature Switzerland AG., pp. 249–264.

Ashencaen Crabtree, S. (2021) *Women of Faith and the Quest for Spiritual Authenticity: Comparative Perspectives from Malaysia and Britain*. London: Routledge.

Ashencaen Crabtree, S. (2012) *A Rainforest Asylum: The enduring legacy of colonial psychiatric care in Malaysia*. London: Whiting & Birch.

Ashencaen Crabtree, S., Husain, F. and Spalek, B. (2016) *Islam & Social Work: Islam and Social Work: Culturally Sensitive Practice in a Diverse World*. 2nd ed. Bristol: Policy Press.

Aull Davies, C. *Reflexive Ethnography*. London: Routledge

Beidermann, N. (2001) The voices of days gone by: Advocating the use of oral history in nursing. *Nursing Inquiry*, 8, 61–62.

Biley, F. (2010) A tale of two sisters: Deconstructing missionary nursing and midwifery in the British post-colonial era. Paper presented at the *International Perspectives in the History of Nursing*, 14–16 September 2010. Royal Holloway, University of London, Egham, Surrey.

Billington Harper, S. (2000) *In the Shadow of the Mahatma: Bishop V.S. Azariah and the Travails of Christianity in British India*. London/New York: Routledge.

Bloom, L.R. (1998) *Under the Sign of Hope: Feminist Methodology and Narrative Interpretation*. Albany, NY: SUNY Press.

Boschma, G., Scaia, M., Bonifacio, N. and Roberts, E. (2008) Oral history research. In Sandra B. Lewenson and Eleanor Krohn Herrmann (Eds.), *Capturing Nursing History: A Guide to Historical Methods in Research*. New York: Springer, pp. 99–102.

Braidotti, R. (2008) In spite of the times: The postsecular turn in Feminism. *Theory Culture & Society*, 25(6), 1–24.

British Academy (2019) Theology and religious studies risks disappearing from our universities, says the British Academy. Available at xhttps://www.thebritishacademy.ac.uk/news/theology-and-religious-studies-risk-disappearing-our-universities-says-british-academy/ [Accessed 7 February 2022].

Burton, J. and Burton, O.A. (2007) Some reflections on anthropology's missionary positions. *Journal of the Royal Anthropological Institute*, 13, 209–217.

Caetano, A. (2015) Personal reflexivity and biography: Methodological challenges and strategies. *International Journal of Social Research Methodology*, 18(2), 227–242. https://doi.org/10.1080/13645579.2014.88515

Chapman, C. (2016) *The Night the Angels Came*. Grand Rapids, MI: Monarch Books.

Compton Bouwer, R. (1990) *New Women for God: Canadian Presbyterian Women and India Missions, 1876–14*. Toronto: University of Toronto Press.

Etherington, N. (2012) Social theory and the study of Christians in Africa: A South African case study. *Africa*, 47(1), 31–40.

Etherington, N. (1996) Recent trends in the historiography of Christians in Southern Africa. *Journal of South African Studies*, 22(2), 201–219.

Gaitskell, D. (2010) Feminising faith: A reflection on personal and academic journeys. *Journal for the Study of Religion*, 23(1/2), 71–103.

Gerrard, J.W. (2001) *Africa Calling: A Medical Missionary in Kenya and Zambia*. London: The Radcliffe Press.

Glenn, C. (2000) Truth, Lies, and Method: Revisiting Feminist Historiography. *College English*, 62(3), 387–389. https://doi.org/10.2307/378937.

Graham, C. (1980) *Between Two Worlds*. Madras: Selly Oak College.

Harding, S. (1987) The method question. *Hypatia*, 2(3), 19–35. https://doi.org/10.1111/j.1527-2001.1987.tb01339

Hempton, D. (2005) *Methodism: Empire of the Spirit*. New Haven, CT.

Kent, E.F. (1999) Tamil Bible women and the zenana mission of colonial South India. *History of Religions*, 39(2), 117–149.

Kohler Riessman, C. (2008) *Narrative Methods for the Human Sciences*. Newbury Park, CA: Sage.

Llewellyn, D. (2015) *Reading, Feminism and Spirituality: Troubling the Waves*. Houndsmill, Basingstoke: Palgrave Macmillan.

Michie, S. (2018) *God's Patchwork: Stories of a Missionary Nurse in Rural Zambia*. Watford, Herts: Instant Apostle.

Miller, R.L. (2000) *Researching Life Stories and Family Histories*. London: Sage.

Nestel, S. (1998) Administering angels: Colonial nursing and the extension of empire in Africa. *Journal of Medical Humanities*, 19(4), 257–277.

Parker, J., Ashencaen Crabtree, S., Reeks, E., Marsh, D. and Vasif, C. (2018) 'River! that in silence windest' The place of religion and spirituality in social work assessment: Sociological reflections and practical implications. In Christian Spatscheck, Sara Ashencaen Crabtree and Jonathan Parker, J. (Eds.), *Methods & Methodologies of Social Work: Reflecting Professional Intervention*. Erasmus SocNet, Vol III. London: Whiting & Birch, pp. 94–114.

Porter, A. (2004) *Religion versus Empire? British Protestant Missionaries and Overseas Expansion, 1700–1914*. Manchester: Manchester University Press.

Riley, T. and Hawes, P. (2003) Researching practice: The methodological case for narrative inquiry. *Health Education Research*, 20(2), 226–236.

Schutte, D.L. 1981. OCP Worship. Available at: https://www.ocp.org/en-us/songs/1523/here-i-am-lord [Accessed: 10 November 2020].

Sherman Heyl, B. (2009) Ethnographic interviewing. In Paul Atkinson, Amanda Coffey, Sara Delamont, John Lofland and Lyn Lofland (Eds.), *Handbook of Ethnography*. Showalter, CA: Sage, pp. 369–383.

Skeggs, B. (2009) Feminist ethnography. In Paul Atkinson, Amanda Coffey, Sara Delamont, John Lofland and Lyn Lofland (Eds.), *Handbook of Ethnography*. Showalter, CA: Sage, pp. 426–442.

Spencer, B.B. (2016) *'Ours is a Great Work': British Women Medical Missionaries in Twentieth-Century Colonial India*. PhD. Dissertation. Georgia State University.

Thomas, L. (2003). *Politics of the Womb: Women, reproduction and thee Sate in Kenya*. Berkeley: University of California Press.

Thomas, B.G. and Rosser, E. (2017) Memories of nursing: Research findings from an oral history study. *British Journal of Nursing*, 26(4), 210–216.

Underhill, Lillian. A. (1935) *Extremes Meet: Some Acts about India's Women*. London: Highway Press.

Underhill, Lillian. A. (1932) *Liberty for India*. Farnham, Surrey: E.W. Langham.

Van Stapele, N. (2014) Intersubjectivity, self-reflexivity and agency: Narrative about 'self' and 'other' in feminist research. *Women's Studies International Forum*, 43, 13–21.

Watson, J. 2018) *Born For Life: Midwife in Africa*. New Zealand: Cherry Hinton Limited.

Ylijoki, O.-H. and Mäntylä, H. (2003) Conflicting time perspectives in academic work. *Time & Society*, 12(1), 55–78.

2 Methodism

People, passion and piety

Methodism – the yearning soul

Given a background in the sociology of religion, I came to Methodism late and had I not met Muriel would have been not much wiser now than I was then. Although to avoid raising readers' expectations I will say, without any excess of modesty, that I do not know a great deal more today. Two main sources have been extremely helpful in the writing of this chapter: for a thorough and thoroughly entertaining examination of the life and character of John Wesley, one cannot improve on Roy Hattersley's (2014) biography. For an elegant, witty overview of Methodism as an expansive global panorama, David Hempton (2005) cannot be beaten. I make no apologies for referencing their work, as well as the great literary canon of nineteenth-century English literature, particularly George Eliot's novel, *Adam Bede*. Drawn from the female side of Eliot's family connection with Methodism it illuminates the mission, mystique and political transitions within Methodism through the character of the young, female, Methodist lay preacher, Dinah Morris. Yet, despite this sympathetic portrayal, the sincere luminosity of Methodism has failed to catch the imagination of novelists:

> It seems that, despite George Eliot's best efforts, Methodism has become, in English fiction since 1900, a convenient cipher for repressive religious hypocrisy.
>
> (Dickinson, 2012, p. 321)

This seems a shame as such an adoringly ardent faith of the heart offers a strangely apposite wellspring for aspiring writers to draw from; but where fiction falls short, scholarship must suffice. Travelling from dark ignorance to dawning insight is bound to change one's perspective considerably, and having lived with Methodism through Muriel for some years,

DOI: 10.4324/9781003359746-2

I found I could not easily recapture my own early assumptions regarding the faith or its followers. So, I casually asked Jonathan, my right-hand man, someone far more theologically knowledgeable than me, and who had himself grown up in a Nonconformist tradition, what he felt was the popular attitude towards Methodism, receiving the brisk retort of: 'upper-working class, self-righteous prigs'.

Following in Christ's footsteps

Prigs or otherwise, Methodism has been phenomenally successful as a modern denomination where Hempton (2005) states that by 1880, there were twenty-five million Methodists across the world. Wilson (2001) places the current number of devotees as considerably higher, claiming there are seventy-five million Methodists living across 130 countries. Whatever the figure, both agree that this is an extraordinary achievement, given how recently in modern history Methodism stepped upon the English stage of religious identity, dominated by the Established Anglican Church, the Church of England.

Methodism is the offshoot of the tumultuous Protestant Reformation in Europe and its local manifestation of the English Civil War in the seventeenth century (Bragg, 2011), continuing its reverberations well into the next two centuries. Sparked by Martin Luther's defiance against the authority of the Pope, and articulated in his *Ninety-Five Theses* of 1517 attacking Papal indulgence, Luther's obstinate independence earned him Papal excommunication but helped to light the fuse of the anti-Rome Northern European, Protestant revolution. Erasmus, although opposing Luther, mocked reverence for the exoteric symbols of popular faith encouraged by Rome, including relics and pilgrimages (Wilson, 2011). It is an interesting point of reflection that, bereft of religious certainties, insecure and angst-ridden, the twenty-first century enthusiastically rediscovers the spiritual pilgrimage (Mayhew-Smith and Haywood, 2020). Furthermore, Christian retreats, far from dying out, still draw those in need of God's peace, contemplation and solace.

Erasmus, having earlier taken an open pot-shot at the esotericism of the professional theologian, the complexities of philosophical gymnastics were eschewed in favour of the right disposition, spirit and conduct. Erasmus subverted socio-religious hierarchies in proposing that if such virtues were embodied in the humblest labourer or weaver, such had the making of being an equally good, and perhaps more authentic, theologian (Dickens, 1974). This position would later resonate strongly in Methodism with its advocacy of lay preaching from the lower echelons of society: the grassroots 'aristocracy of labour', to coin a Marxism (Kerswell, 2019; Strayer, 1978).

Luther also became preoccupied with the genuine, rather than fraudulent man of faith

> In the scriptures it is best to distinguish between the Spirit and the latter, for it is this that makes a true theologian'. Eberling clarifies, 'For the Holy Spirit is present and life-giving, by contrast to the letter which owes everything to the past and consequently speaks of the past.
>
> (Eberling, 1970, pp. 98–99)

Moreover, Luther, in his opposition to Papal authority, advocated that a genuine 'man of faith could act with energy and joyfulness in serving the community, and by so doing, be a "'little Christ'" to his followers (Dickens, 1974, p. 64); again, not unlike the way John Wesley was viewed by his followers and popularly sanctified later.

These traditions of counter-ecclesiastical authority, in addition to a continuing proliferation of Protestant sectarian splinters, budded to form their own branches of theological distinctiveness. Such movements and developments would give rise to Methodism and *he* most associated with early Methodism, John Wesley, a prolific reader and inveterate magpie when it came to delving into the scriptures, doctrine, theological sources, arguments and debates (Hattersley, 2014). A multiplicity of Christian traditions, too numerous to consider in detail, acknowledge syncretism in Methodism carrying Catholic, Orthodox, Anglican, Protestant and Nonconformist traditions (Wilson, 2011). This suggests an eclectic or syncretic theology, rather than an original contribution to Christian thinking; although none the worse for that, judging from Methodism's extraordinary socio-religious future impact.

Methodism's starting point, although certainly this was not recognised at the time as being so, was generated in the domestic, marital dissent within the parental home of John and Charles Wesley, in two highly intelligent, opinionated, uncompromising and politically and maritally combative parents: Susanna and Samuel Wesley. Susanna, in modern parlance, a 'strong woman', despite the enormous brood of children she bore, was a strict disciplinarian regarding childrearing. She held enlightened views towards the demanding education of daughters as well as that of sons, offering formidable parenting approaches designed to break down the obduracy of the childish will and guide it towards dutiful paths (Cragg, 1977). Her influence over John would continue throughout her life and he frequently consulted her respectfully during his adult years.

A scholarly auto-didact Susanna was also a huge admirer of the anti-Papist philosopher John Locke; furthermore, a supporter of the Jacobite uprising, attempting to return the Catholic 'Old Pretender', James Stuart, to the throne usurped by the new Protestant monarchs, William of Orange and his wife Queen Anne, James' sister. Samuel, however, was loyal to the House of Orange and to the Church of England (Heitzenrater, 2013).

Craig (1977, p. 141) describes Samuel Wesley as 'ardent, opinionated, impractical; a poet as well as an irrepressible controversialist, an unbending churchman, and an unyielding Tory'. Coming from a difficult family history of conflict with authority, Samuel's grandfather and father had held Cromwellian Commonwealth sympathies, a troublesome inheritance once the Stuarts returned to power, resulting in his father's imprisonment on the charge of treason and Nonconformist unorthodoxies, until later rehabilitation as an Anglican cleric. As Hattersley (2004, p. 8) remarks, it says much about his character that Samuel disapproved of and disliked Dissenters as 'frivolous', although others found them equally tiresome for their opposite tendencies. However, Samuel's limpet-like adherence to the Church of England would form a legacy generating paradoxical crises bedevilling Methodism later.

The start of the theological movement known as Methodism and its founding 'oligarchy', as Vidler (1977, p. 42) describes the familial cabal of its leadership, is subject to much hagiography. At any rate, their unconventional upbringing of contested views and independent stances left its mark upon Methodism's founders, the brothers John and Charles Wesley. By the time John, something of a prodigy, had been made a Fellow of Christ Church, Oxford and Charles Wesley's first year at the University had witnessed a certain amount of undergraduate hedonism, a more earnest pathway was being established. Turning over a new leaf in his second year in 1729, Charles and his friend, William Morgan began a Bible reading Fellowship group, the 'Holy Club', soon labelled the 'Methodists', as well as other less flattering names (Hattersley, 2014). The urge for 'do-gooding' grew and a year later, after John Wesley had joined the group, at Morgan's instigation the group began making prison visits to offer solace to the wretched prisoners of Oxford's debtor jails (Heitzenrater, 2013). From this wellspring 'the Holy Club' turned their attention to the needs of others in need and want.

Heitzenrater's (1995) view is that Methodism was an organic development of sympathetic minds and motivations. Yet, without question, it is John Wesley, rather than Charles, who appears to have coalesced the movement and sparked it into a newly imagined community. It is John that ultimately, if most reluctantly, accepted the Methodist movement peeling slowly away from the Church of England. This owing to irreconcilable differences of principles, mostly constructed by John Wesley himself, revolving around Methodism's priority mission of the saving of souls through conversion achieved by preaching, and crucially, to whom the prerogative of this serious duty would fall. For the Church of England, this was decidedly the province of the ordained clergy and they alone were permitted to conduct the Eucharist. This position grated with Wesley, a veritable glutton for the holy wine and wafer of Communion for himself and his followers. Although Wesley tried to avoid a complete break with the Church of England, as demanded by some followers, Methodism's momentum was fundamentally driven by its mission and that to be delivered by its itinerant preachers, of both sexes, many being illiterate and of the labouring classes, whose qualifications and authority were much at odds with the Established Church's conventional hierarchy. In the years to come a split from the Church of England would become inevitable, much to Wesley's sorrow; and, as Wilson (2011) notes, while many attempts have been made to reunite, the gulf has remained unbridged. Although Methodism would eventually become independently Nonconformist, more disunity would emerge from within the ranks of Methodism itself, leading to schisms.

Charles Wesley, a more circumspect, contained man than his brother, remained faithful to Anglicanism his entire life. His particular contribution to Methodism and later Anglicanism, as well as to the wider world of spiritual music, was psalmody. This was largely a Methodist innovation of capturing the dynamic voice of the congregation, moving heart and spirit in uplifting devotional song. Charles' compositional output was prodigious, writing literately thousands of hymns. The Church of England eventually adopted the use of hymnals as an effective means of engaging a passive, bored congregation and where today the Anglican collections of hymns carry the gifts of many of Charles' compositions. Audrey and Muriel Chalkley were enthusiastic songsters themselves, and in fact, while writing this chapter, I had occasion to sing with renewed interest one of Charles Wesley's hymns. This is a melodically demanding but rousing affair, commencing with the somewhat disconcerting first line: '*And can it be that I should gain an interest in the Saviour's blood!*' Indeed Adamthwaite (2016) in his contextualised and annotated round-the-Christian-year-with-Charles-Wesley hymnody compilation argues that it is this Wesley brother who now attracts the greater interest.

The Established Church certainly needed a little livening up during this time of complacent, privileged stultification following the excesses of the religious conflagrations of the turbulent seventeenth century. The evangelical revival of the period, from which Methodism arose, was a direct challenge to the self-satisfied laxity of the Hanoverian Established Church, which, at worst, was indolently corrupt (Hattersley, 2014) and cravenly flaccid (Hempton, 2005). Too often considered merely a suitable living for the gentry's superfluous sons, rather than an inspirational calling from God, it was unlikely to capture the devotion of the congregation, or inspire virtue, or indeed spiritual interest. Grassroots evangelism by contrast was a stirring and energising experience speaking directly to the ordinary working person and their experiences of hardship and suffering, together with a yearning for something better; a higher than animal existence, particularly when the vehicle of grace was a preacher identifiable as *for* or *of* the common people.

Although the term 'Methodist' was derogatively applied to the Holy Group's Fellowship, prior to John Wesley joining it, and well before

Methodism was recognised as a distinctive theological movement, it was apt; particularly when applied to Wesley's quotidian regime of strict personal accountability of time and deed. From 1702 to 1703, he was devising for his daily usage and prescribing for others, a devised 'Exactor Diary'. In this every hour of every day were set out in detail not only visits and appointments but also resolutions, met or otherwise, with measurements of Wesley's own 'state of devotion' and 'simplicity' (Hattersley, 2014, p. 75).

Such a no-nonsense regime of exactitude is reminiscent of Charlotte Brontë's depiction in *Jane Eyre* of the mentally and emotionally desiccated, judgemental, self-cloistering, Miss Eliza Reed's rigid, daily regime

> Take one day; share it into sections; to each section apportion its task: leave no stray unemployed quarters of an hour, ten minutes, five minutes – include all; do each piece of business in its turn with method, with rigid regularity.
>
> (1847, 1984, p. 264)

A Roman Catholic (a highly distrusted breed in England), rather than a Methodist, Eliza Reed, Jane's cousin, is completely devoid of any real awareness of God's love, unlike John Wesley, welding together a routine designed to fill her privileged, empty hours and separate her from others.

The coincidence of this methodical, indeed obsessive habit of organising an entire waking life, one in fact and the other in fiction, may be partially explained by the influence of Methodism on Charlotte Brontë's work, which emerges with closer scrutiny. For the Brontë children, Maria, Elizabeth, Charlotte, Emily, Ann and ne'er-do-well brother Branwell were the offspring of a union between an Ulster Irish, Anglican heritage on the father's side and Cornish Methodism on the mother's (Wright, 2020).

The Methodist resonances continue in *Jane Eyre*, where in contrast with Miss Eliza Reed's nihilistic self-entombment, and beneath her plain, Quaker grey and the iron constraints of her circumstances, Jane's passionate spiritual yearning is barely contained, erupting violently when she cries out to Rochester,

> I am not talking to you now through the medium of custom, conventionalities nor even of mortal flesh: it is my spirit that addressed your spirit; just as if we both had passed through the grave, and we stood at God's feet, equal – as we are!
>
> (Brontë, 1847, 1984, p. 281)

The spirit is both upon Jane and within her. The vitality of Methodism was in this emphasis on the Holy Spirit, following St Paul's affirmation of this grace lying within the Children of God, and where 'The witness of the spirit is justification by faith and the assurance of God's presence' (Wilson, 2011, p. 71). Thus, Jane's spirit meets in disembodied dialogue with Rochester, and their spirits too are witnesses of the power of the Living God.

Yet religious 'enthusiasm', as Vidler (1977) states, did not sit well with aloof, Enlightenment reason and the culture of prosaic, unemotive, introverted clericism in England. This culture would be shaken by the new spirit of evangelism and the power of preaching was the medium by which it would be spread. At the vanguard, naturally, was John Wesley and a good friend from the 'Holy Club', the roving Anglican minister, Dr George Whitefield. Although Wesley attracted a good deal of unwanted mob attention in his time, the success of Methodist preaching among the working classes and particularly, the miners of Cornwall, Shropshire and Bristol was undeniable.

At the centre of numerous setbacks and crises in managing and progressing the Methodist Connexion, these kinds of hiatus continued after Wesley's death, when Methodism splintered into three different groups led by different factions, to become the Wesleyan Methodists, the United Methodists and the Primitive Methodist; the latter, seeking some earlier, purer form of Methodism, a pull to primal purity that we see in other religions too, such as Islam (Ashencaen Crabtree et al., 2016). In the meantime, Methodist theology was a continual work-in-progress, where Wesley was ever tinkering with the developing doctrine as new ideas and issues occurred to him.

Orderly in his habits to the point of compulsion, egocentric in his preoccupations, autocratic in his communications, obsessive in his doctrinal examinations, zealous and demanding, unafraid of courting controversy, but tactless to the point of offence, frequently naïve in his interactions, often infatuated with women but unsuccessful in adult intimacy (Hattersley, 2014; Heitzenrater, 2013), John Wesley, by contemporary standards, would probably be thought to sit squarely on the autistic spectrum.

Under his demanding leadership, however, Wesley's natal respect for female piety and wisdom enabled women to play a far more significant part than was conventionally permitted in religious circles. Women in turn were drawn to both Wesley and Methodism in significant numbers, particularly single and widowed women (Hempton, 2005). This is perhaps not surprising when we apply intersectional theorisation, which, although originating in US Black feminist critical race, legal studies (Crenshaw, 1991), has proved superbly adaptive to analysing women's wider positionalities in respect of the 'triple oppressions' of race/ethnicity, gender and class (Yuval-Davies, 2006, p. 199); and wider subaltern aspects, such as faith, disability and sexuality (Anthias, 2012; Ashencaen Crabtree, 2021). Intersectionality provides clues to the phenomenon of working-class women's evangelism and how Methodism, almost uniquely at the time, enabled oppressed people to experience and be affirmed in their vocalisations of psychologically intense, spiritually ecstatic expressions of the deepest pain and most joyous praise (Hempton, 2005). The profound nature of salvation through conversion lifted suffering to the sacred light to be healed.

> They (the people) wanted hope, salvation, a lifting of the burdens of life: and some joy, some song, some acclamation with a place for the public ecstasy of the ignored and the powerless: some pride: and a place in the Kingdom of Heaven.
>
> (Bragg, 2011, p. 103)

Thus, not only was Methodism popular among lowly women but also some, like Sarah Crosby, Mary Bosanquet and Elizabeth Ritchie, were recognised by Wesley as gifted preachers in their own right; a gift that lay within Muriel Chalkley as well. Methodist women, being respected and entrusted to travel and preach, must have felt they had embarked on an extraordinarily cathartic spiritual journey of liberation. This was literally a God-sent opportunity, offering a brief but important respite from the intersectional burdens of gender, class and poverty; where illiteracy appeared no barrier to the authority of the Word when issued from the mouths of passionate working women.

Thus, by the time of Wesley's death, the West Riding of Yorkshire had beheld and Leeds, in particular, had become a centre of the 'Female Brethren' preacher sorority of Methodist revivalism (Dews, 1986). Maison (1986) draws our attention to how Nonconformism in its dissent from the orthodox overturned to a degree gendered conventions, bestowing greater levels of liberty and equality upon dissenter women. Accordingly in the urbanised, industrialising Midlands and the North of England, Primitive Methodism attracted brave, spiritually ardent and thereby subversive women.

> Primitive Methodism, youthful and energetic, with a rough, unthought-out but practical theology, in which conversion of the sinner was all-important and order and respectability almost totally irrelevant, became a natural home for women preachers.
>
> (Dews, 1986, p. 84)

The labouring classes of early industrialisation were ripe for conversion to a vivid and emotionally invigorating faith, where Eliot depicts Dinah visiting bucolic 'Loamshire', where life is gentler but the spirit decidedly lacking, compared to the greater religious thirst in industrialised conurbations like Leeds 'of low-pitched gables up dingy streets' (Eliot, 1859, 1994, p. 43).

Yet despite their success at saving souls, the autonomy and power of these 'Female Brethren' would be attacked and brought to heel by Methodist male leadership over time. From 1835, a hardening line was being taken against women preachers, otherwise a force of compelling feminine energy in their organisation, preaching and conversion, through their liturgical writings and, like Charles Wesley, their compositional works of praise too (Maison, 1986). Indeed, 200 years later in an obscure corner of South India, a quiet English missionary nurse would also be turning her musical hand to psalmody. Harnessing the energies of women equipped with such skills and talents, enabled the appeal of Methodism to travel much further, more swiftly and with greater accessibility to marginalised people than would otherwise have been possible.

The clamp-down on Wesleyan Methodism on women's itinerary preaching is commented on at the end of *Adam Bede*. The year is 1807, only a few years since Wesley's death, and the annual Methodist conference has decided to suppress women preachers. A decision Dinah meekly complies with, giving up her preaching entirely, much to her Methodist brother-in-law, Seth's disgust, who thinks they should both have left the Wesleyans for 'a body tht'ud put no bonds on Christian liberty'. Adam, Seth's superior brother, long schooled on woman's place as instructed by his misogynistic old tutor, Bartle Massey, passes his authoritative judgement to Seth:

> 'Nay, lad, nay', said Adam, 'she was right and thee wast wrong. There's no rule so wise but what it's a pity for somebody or other. Most o' the women do more harm nor good with their preaching – they've not got Dinah's gift nor her sperrit'.
>
> (Eliot, 1859, 1994, 2005, p. 589)

Dinah *is* one of those extraordinary women that even the Methodist Conference would presumably endorse, but instead sets an example of woman's duty to her fellow preachers, confining herself to the home; unlike Eliot's actual Methodist aunt, Elizabeth Evans, who responded to these restrictions by joining the freer Primitive Methodists.

Methodist portrayals of the character, vision and leadership of John Wesley have a strongly hagiographic quality, which Vickers (2012s) traces back to early nineteenth-century roots, commencing often with his miraculous early childhood escape from a burning house. Indeed, a brief portrait of Wesley is found in George Elliot's (1859, 2008, p.19) *Adam Bede*, by the inspired young preacher, Dinah,

> I remember his face well: he was a very old man, and had very long white hair; his voice was very soft and beautiful, not like any voice I had ever heard before... such a different sort of man from anybody I

had ever seen before, that I thought he had perhaps come down from the sky to preach to us.

(Eliot, 1859, 1994, 2005, p. 19)

Here the naïve, childish intertwining of Wesley as saint and Messiah is deliberate, it is a misapprehension, as Dinah recognises, but one, it is implied, that given the peerless and exemplary nature of this remarkable man is understandable.

Vickers (2012, p. 143) regards the 'embellishments' of Wesley as basically poor history, the real-life Wesley, appears to have been a somewhat contradictory and more fallible person than these adoring accounts suggest. Although Wesley's respect for his formidable mother, Susanna, is viewed by Heitzenrater (2019) and Hattersley (2014) as having been foundational in his support of women in the Methodist movement, his inability to form stable intimate relationships with women is regarded as a puzzle by the former. By contrast, Hattersley regards the perverseness of his lifelong attraction to women and yet his inability to sustain honest ties of integrity, as a sign of deep immaturity, and 'emotional irresponsibility' (2014, p. 66). Hattersley goes so far as to wonder whether sexual intimacy ever existed in Wesley's late and disastrous marriage, where, following some poorly hidden emotional if not physical infidelity, the combustible Mary Wesley was said to have dragged her husband around by his hair in apoplectic rage. Wesley was released with much relief back to a bachelor's life upon the eventual death of his wife, and to managing the complexities of the Methodist connexion which swung regularly from crisis to trial to ordeal and back again, for 'women were his weakness, doctrinal promiscuity his abiding sin' (Hattersley, 2014, p. 4).

Wesley continued his leadership undaunted with an exhausting regime of itinerant preaching covering hundreds of miles on horseback over the years, his physician and fellow preacher, Dr John Whitehead (1797) claiming in his epitaph that Wesley travelled 225,000 miles as an itinerant preacher and preached 40,560 sermons in his lifetime. Undeterred by criticism, and

denounced by ecclesiastic authorities Wesleyan preachers took to the streets and fields, drawing thousands to hear their impromptu sermons. Their messages of salvation, we are told, transported audiences from despair to bliss

(Comaroff and Comaroff, 1991, p. 47)

Wesley died in 1791 after several days of relapsing into unconsciousness to be rallied back into lifetime and again with the help of his fixated followers, the gentle succumbing to death being earnestly punctuated with prayers and interrogations into the state of Wesley's grace, his last orders and messages, where rousing himself he sang one final hymn, 'I'll Praise My Maker While I've Breath'. A good Methodist death was an essential part of the Methodist life and Wesley's death without question fully exemplified that. Some decades later, the artist son of a Methodist Minister, Marshall Claxton, underlined this point heavily in a sanctifying depiction of the passing of the great man with the accompanying title (in case the point was missed): 'The Holy Triumph of John Wesley in His Dying'.

Whatever anomalies Methodism sported in terms of the Establishment, it was in step with the Enlightenment spirit of individual self-improvement (Tholfsen, 2019, p. 203), spiritually, morally and materially, in foretelling a future where brute labour would be superseded by the demand for the educated 'man'. Elsewhere this drive to remake society resulted in the French Revolution; Methodism, fulminates Thompson (1963) in his seminal work on the working classes, was culpable for damping down and re-channelling the working classes' emotive energy away from glorious revolution. Instead, Methodism involved the inner reconstruction of self, manifested externally through Christian virtues of religious observance, neighbourliness, simplicity, thrift, abstemiousness, sexual continence, responsibility and hard work. If religious Revivalism was an English revolution of a kind, it was certainty not of the bloodier 'à la lanterne!' variety.

Methodism's original followers were drawn from the artisan and labouring classes, but over time would take on the trappings of the respected bourgeoisie. This is illustrated in a useful, chronological social geographic mapping of class, occupation and location (Field, 1997), where from 1800 to 1837, conversions are common among miners in Cornwall, Devon and Durham; and among bricklayers and weavers from Dorset and Oxford. The richer centres of industrialisation and commerce, Manchester and Liverpool, compared to poorer Norwich, offer a different Methodist demographic; and by the early to mid-Victorian period, Methodism, although still retaining impoverished followers, particularly in West Dorset, was becoming a denomination of the respectable middle classes in areas like Manchester and Newcastle-upon-Tyne. By 1932, the year when the three Methodist factions united as the Methodist Church, Methodism had consolidated the embourgeoisement of its social position in the white-collar sector further (Field, 1997).

Evangelism and empire

The growth of Methodism globally was, if not entirely foreseen, at least absolutely aspired to, virtually from the very nascence of the faith.

> Methodism had a mobile laity before it had missionaries, it had missionaries before it had a missionary society.
>
> (Hempton, 2005, p. 30)

Christian conversion, today regarded as somewhat suspect, was generally considered essential for salvation, which the great majority of sincere Christians accepted. D'Costa et al. (2011), reminding us that the mission of Christianity is to evangelise:

> John 14.6 'I am the way, and the truth, and the life: no one man cometh unto the Father, but by me'.

Conversely then, to refrain from mission, as a central tenet of one's faith, could be a crime of omission against humanity, not merely in this lifetime but for all eternity. Wesley's example of preaching peregrinations formed not only a strictly observed practice throughout his life, but the blueprint for Methodist evangelism, in which no divide existed between the pastor and the evangelist (Comaroff and Comaroff, 1991).

While Methodism was being taken to Ireland to convert the population, John and Charles Wesley went to the crown colonies of America to enthusiastically do the same there in 1735, firstly, for the heathen indigenous population, and secondly, more reluctantly, to shepherd the Christian settlers. The transportation of wretched, neglected inmates from debtors' prisons to the new Georgia colony of America was regarded as both a benign and practical opportunity, becoming home to not only former convicts but also displaced Scots and persecuted Protestant religious minority groups from Germany (Hattersley, 2014). The sea crossing enabled Wesley to witness at first hand the great power of absolute faith, when the German Moravian sect passengers withstood a ferocious storm threatening to sink the entire ship with fearless, pious equanimity from man to child. For Wesley, this was a 'glorious' revelation. Unfortunately, the Wesley brothers' venture was far from successful. Beset by problems on all sides Charles Wesley lasted six months in Georgia. John Wesley, inflammatory and over-zealous, distrusted and disliked, persisted for a further two years, despite aggravating and offending the entire community, in addition to personal problems caused by an advance-retreat cyclical embroilment in an absurdly awkward, ambivalent indiscretion with an unhappily engaged woman (Hattersley, 2014). In turn, George Whitefield made several visits to America when sea travel was, as the Wesleys knew, a dangerous, frightening and squalid experience. By contrast, his American sermons were hugely popular being heard by thousands of people to thunderous acclaim (Bragg, 2011).

The idea of a Methodist society dedicated specifically to spreading the gospel was proposed to the ageing, intellectually diminishing Wesley by Dr Thomas Coke, a Welsh dynamo from Powys, who went on to become not only Wesley's 'main man' but a co-supervisor of the Methodist mission in the now triumphantly independent America. Subsequently American Methodist would be entirely autonomous from the British Connexion. Coke careered on becoming one of American Methodism's bishops, a most establishment status to aspire to for a dissenter, as well as being something of a snub to post-defeat Georgian England.

Coke in England had ever been focused on overseas missions and had tried to get the increasingly weary Wesley to agree to a mission to Africa in 1777, following this by petitioning for the 'Society for the Establishment of Missions among the Heathen', neither of which Wesley thought feasible. By 1786, the insuppressibly opportunistic Coke was formally proposing missions to places as close to home as Scotland and the Channel Islands, and as afield as the West Indies and Nova Scotia. Mission did not come cheap and those to Ireland, Antigua and St Kitts under Coke's poor administration had become extremely expensive by 1805, incurring the wrath of the Connexion (Porter, 2004). Undeterred Coke made a number of personal visits to the West Indies, resulting in the establishment of a Methodist Missionary Society there.

The strongly abolitionist position of Wesleyan Methodists in Britain was established early and where in the West Indies by 1833, when Britain abolished slavery, there were now seventy Methodist missionaries (Worthington Smith, 1950). In these British colonies, the anti-slavery pro-Wilberforce position of Methodism no doubt helped in terms of conversions of black communities and the rise of black sectarian churches.

However, the Methodist Road to the evangelism of slaves and others in the West Indies was continually blocked by the white slaving-owning communities. Commensurately, Grant (2012) describes the closure of Jamaican Methodist chapels and the explicitly aggressive intimidation of the Methodists. More widely in the colonies, a trend had become well-established towards a strong spiritual appetite for homespun Methodism as a liberatory theology. Although Wesleyan missionaries set foot in Cape Town as early as 1813, albeit forbidden to preach (Comaroff and Comaroff, 1991), by 1815, as Hempton (2005) calculates, there were 40,000 black Methodists in the US and 15,000 in the Caribbean.

Pentecostalism, frequently regarded as Methodism's spiritual heir (Hempton, 2005), has since superseded the latter's incredible sprint forward, making deep inroads into Africa, Latin America and Asia. The origins of the Pentecostal revival in the US are divided between, William Seymour, the black preacher of Azusa Street in Los Angeles, and the white theologian Charles Fox Parham (Gooren, 2004). The dynamism of Pentecostalism, whether as a specific denomination or as a syncretic faith practice, is strongly integral to the African American black Holiness religious experience (Yong and Alexander, 2011)

Christianity, mission and India

India, a vast subcontinent of diverse peoples of strange faiths, a Babel of many tongues and customs, has long sparked the missionary imagination.

The aristocratic novelist, Sydney Owenson (1811) captivated Romantic poet Percy Bysshe Shelley with her passionate, baroque novel of an India of the imagination concerning impossible love between the noble, Portuguese Roman Catholic missionary, Hilarion, and Luxima the lovely, Brahmin vestal virgin priestess. More prosaically, it is India that lies in St John Rivers' sights. This hard, driven, ambitious creature, of Brontë's pen, speaking of God's greatness, but as 'cold as an iceberg' towards others (Brontë, 1984, p. 468), regards India as offering both the greatest scope and the deepest challenge to his formidable talents, where the mission-ary's path is the road towards heathen salvation. Bending his despotic will towards forcing Jane into accepting a convenient but frigid marriage, his plans for an uxorial 'useful tool' are to work among the Indian women they will encounter.

The wives of missionaries were expected to conduct themselves unstint-ingly as both wives and subaltern mission helpers under the supervision of their husbands. By the mid-nineteenth century change was afoot, where, as the Methodist Missionary Society's (WWS) *Handbook for Women's Work* outlines, missionary wives' labours are saluted, with a reminder to readers of these wives' ultimate sacrifice: the worn-out, untimely death far from home, that Jane fears for herself.

> We cannot but praise the wives of the early missionaries of our Methodist Church....these women went willingly with their husbands to the far places of the world. ...Many lonely, and in some places, for-gotten graves mark the devotion of these truly noble women.
> (MMS *Handbook for Women*, no date, p. 5)

Indeed, in reality and increasingly so, the mission of a 'Jane' might have been viewed as just as important as that of a 'St John's', and possibly under certain circumstances even more so, for Protestant missions in India had marked caste Indian women and girls as forming the main bul-wark against Christianity in assumptions of their ignorant and stubborn allegiance to native religions to which they conformed unquestioningly and raised their children to do likewise. Whereas, such work fell to the unpaid spousal work of women married to missionaries, opportunities were opening up for unmarried women missionaries to labour in desig-nated gender-specific 'women's work', where, by virtue of their gender, such roles were less appropriate or indeed not open at all to male mis-sionaries (Prevost, 2010). This carved out a whole new area of mission as exclusively Protestant women's terrain, leading to the rise of a number of new societies catering for the demand, including the Wesleyan Mission Society's Ladies Auxiliary in 1859, the Baptist Zenana Society nine years later and in 1880, the Church of England Zenana Missionary Society (Pass, 2011).

The focus of this Protestant sorority attention was their Indian 'zenana' sisters, those Indian women subject to the religio-domestic geography of gendered seclusion from the public eye in high caste or affluent Hindu and Muslim households (Kent, 1999). In *purdah*, a custom adopted from the Muslim Moghuls, such women were removed from outsider male 'gaze', but not that of foreign women evangelists (MacMillan, 1998). Access could be achieved surreptitiously under the excuse of teaching literacy and some graceful distaff arts, with religion introduced covertly with clandestine cunning, as disapprovingly critiqued:

> These women, proto-feminists of a particular virulent Christian variety, gained entrance to the inner compartments where they did some teaching and a great deal of observing.
>
> (Forbes, 1994, p. 158)

Although *purdah* was regarded in colonial discourse as a miserable, stultifying confinement in a literally darkened and darkly enforced sequestration, Kent (1999) argues that this overstated matters. Yet Lilian Underhill (1935), a practising missionary doctor, and the child of missionaries in India, was characteristically decisive in her condemnation of *purdah* as a harmful practice imposed on the prepubescent female child in preparation for marriage, leading to physical debilitations imposed by lack of light, air and exercise, creating susceptibility towards tuberculosis, anaemia and crippling softening of the bones. Medically justified or exaggerated, *purdah* resonates with the historically connected harem, which Fatima Mernissi's (1975) the celebrated, late Moroccan feminist, born in a harem herself, argues to be a site of both socio-sexual gendered control and women's resistance. Irrespective colonial women undertaking Anglican *zenana* mission work were certainly not expected to display feminist *Wave Zero* subversiveness (Llewellyn, 2015), but instead to exemplify 'the sweet womanly graces of quietness, patience, carefulness, undistractedness and simplicity' (MacMillan, 1998, p. 210). Regardless of the tactfulness of *zenana* workers, this enterprise did not seemingly produce any particular conversion successes, argues Fitzgerald (1997). The perceived great needs of India required other approaches.

Not dissimilar to other colonised 'heathen' nations, India, like Africa, attracted a full palette of denominational missions, not all, however, had found themselves equally welcome by the local authorities. In India, the powerful British East India Company had been unwelcoming to mission ventures as potentially destabilising the religious hierarchies of local communities, thereby risking the Company's profiteering. Unable to resist some incursions by the Church of England, they had taken a hard line against Nonconformist missionaries (Blair, 2008). Now, under Queen

Victoria, with the demise of this 'quasi-sovereign power' (Neill, 1964, 1979, p. 323), missionaries in theory had some greater access to the millions in need of salvation to a degree unknown since St Thomas, the Apostle in the first century. As legend tells, Thomas, he of the famous doubts, as the Scriptures (John 20:24–29) relate, was enslaved to an Indian merchant, and built not the monument he was tasked to erect in India but a far greater edifice of enduring Christian spirit. Reputedly imprisoned, castrated and martyred by furious Brahmins in India, the ancient Church of the Thomas Syrians Christians in the South-west of India was established and remains (Forrester, 1980; Neil, 1979).

The mission momentum would continue through the nineteenth to the twentieth centuries. Methodist missions forming a global vanguard, where by 1932, the Methodist Ladies' Auxiliary was relabelled 'Women's Work of the Methodist Missionary Society' (Pritchard, 2014) (WWMMS); hardly a progressive sounding title and yet, it was an acknowledgement of the skills educated Christian women were able to offer to unmet spiritual, social and physical needs in Crown colonies. The Methodist committee developed from this initiative appeared administratively efficient in respect of information collation and dissemination as well as in missionary recruitment.

Like other British missionary societies, India absorbed the greatest number of their missionaries, male and female (Pritchard, 2014). Pass (2011) notes that by the end of the nineteenth century, 62% of British Protestant missionaries in South Asia were women. However, following the Great War, Compton Brouwer (1990) states that British missionaries to India had dwindled, with the slack taken up primarily by Canadian missionaries, where, as previously, there was a demand for teaching and medically qualified individuals. By the twentieth century, qualified medics were in high demand in India and China as well as Africa; and by 1916, in India alone, Christian missions were treating 1.25 million patients annually across 183 mission-run hospitals and 376 dispensaries (Fitzgerald, 1997).

However, it would be an injustice to suggest that women medics were purely a twentieth-century phenomenon. In 1870, Dr Clara Swain, an American Methodist, became the first female missionary doctor in India establishing the first mission hospital for women in Bareilly in the State of Uttar Pradesh, with a health-crushing workload (Hardiman, 2008).

With the aim of becoming a medical missionary, Anglican Londoner, Dr Fanny Butler, qualified with a medical degree in 1880 from Dublin, writing to her family to announce the good news with wry humour

I can now put L.K.Q.C.P.I. after my name, which means Licentiate of the King's and Queen's College of Physicians, Ireland, or if you prefer it, Licensed to Kill, Qualified to Cure, Patients Invited!

(Tonge, 1930, p. 14)

Shortly afterwards, she sailed for India to eventually become a medical practitioner at the Zenana Mission House in Bhagalpur in the State of Bihar, busily practising general medicine, surgery and running dispensaries until her early death in 1889. In the cases of Butler and Swain, Etherington (2005, p. 272) reminds us that a call to mission work in tropical countries was quite often a 'death sentence'. This, I poignantly saw when wandering through the semi-abandoned but beautiful, and mosquito enlivened, Protestant Cemetery in Penang, where the old tombs of the untimely dead missionaries, wives and little children, proliferate.

A pioneering path was opened by Victorian missionary women, where Hardiman (2008) notes that by 1900, the British Medical Register held 258 women on its register, of which 72 were medical missionaries; and where once again, the greatest demand was for India. By 1910, the demand for excellent and well-qualified missionary nurses has outstripped the demand for doctors, where in both cases, the training of local staff was now a pressing priority to meet local needs (Fitzgerald, 1997). The colonial neglect of the sick owing to severe nursing scarcities offered E.M. Forster (1924, p. 14) ammunition of merciless parody on the presumed tender care of colonial nurses:

> 'I really do know the truth about Indians. A most unsuitable position for any Englishwoman – I was a nurse in a Native State. One's only hope was to hold sternly aloof'.
> 'Even from one's patients?'
> 'Why, the kindest thing one can do to a native is to let him die', said Mrs Callendar.

By the 1920s, in Madras alone, Beach and Fahs (1925) list eight different American and Canadian mission societies along with five British ones, including the Church Missionary Society (CMS), the London Missionary Society (LMS) (to which Livingstone had offered his African-bound services), the Salvation Army, the Society for the Propagation of the Gospel (SPG) and the Wesleyan Methodist Missionary Society (WMMS).

Madras became something of a shining example regarding the progress of colonial medicine in India, particularly in respect to women's reproductive health in the form of lying-in hospitals and midwifery training. Lang points to the efforts in Madras focusing on women's health, later emulated in Bombay and Bengal, as intriguing in undermining post-colonial arguments regarding the merely self-interested colonial medicine practices of the British Raj:

> Unlike cholera or typhoid, it was not likely to affect the European population, nor could it be laid fairly at the door of government. Unlike

infanticide there was no intent to kill, and as birthing took place behind closed doors, mothers who died in childbirth did not make front-page news in the popular press in the way that the very public deaths through sati did. Government resources were limited, and its medical priorities were always epidemic disease and public health. Why, therefore, did Madras channel so much energy and money?

(Lang, 2005, p. 376)

Lang believes the answer lies in the authorities' indignation towards the needless human wastage of women's lives, congruent with the Raj's discourse concerning the cultural oppression of Indian women. However, if women's health was not specifically self-serving to the colonial government, much else has been written about the Raj's impositions on childbirth beliefs and practices in India with a particular focus on the demonisation of the traditional birth attendant, the *dai*, an issue we will revisit in Chapter 6. Suffice to say here, the nineteenth-century mortality rate of Indian women in childbirth was considered to be high and their ordeals great, and where conventional skilled midwifery practices, as they were understood in Anglo-European society, were lacking, and subject to alternative role and caste constructions, according to Hindu religious purification beliefs (Pinto, 2008). The colonial propaganda surrounding the dreadful suffering of Indian women at the hands of ignorant and brutal attendants was so notorious it was personally brought to the attention of a concerned Queen Victoria via the vice-reine, Lady Dufferin. No stranger to the travails of childbirth, dismayed Victoria expressed her wish to 'relieve the suffering of the women of India', resulting in the 1885 'The Countess of Dufferin's Fund', designed to train Indian women as doctors and to attract European women to practise medicine in India (Forbes, 1994, p. 161). This galvanised the campaign back in the motherland for women physicians to be recognised on the Medical Register (Moulds, 2012) and where finally, between 1874 and 1890, four women's medical training institutions were founded in Britain (Hardiman, 2006). The Indianisation of medical provision through the training and recruitment of local people, women as well as men, was viewed as essential in order to meet the needs of such a gigantic population, where even under the most strenuous colonial efforts, whether by state, or independent missions, could reach only a fraction of those that needed care.

Mission and Africa

The majority of missionaries, particularly women, were diverted to Asia rather than Africa (Prevost, 2008), as beyond colonised coastal areas, the great interior of Africa was still terra incognita. That is, until David

Livingstone began to draw attention to his particular brand of adventurous Victorian Christianity: the Bible, the medical bag and the machete, through which the unknown interior began to be revealed (Pakenham, 2002). Projecting an individualistic but publicly compelling conceptualisation of the missionary, and Christian mission, Livingstone presumed the Messiah to be *the*, medical missionary *par excellence* to a suffering world.

Although Livingstone's repute is that of a nineteenth-century explorer of central Africa, rather than missionary doctor or fierce opponent to the Arab-African slave trade, his example proved inspirational. The romance of the 'jungle doctor' medical missionary was an alluring one, a combination of the thrillingly 'intrepid' and the nobly 'altruistic' argues Hardiman (2006, p. 5) following Vaughan (1991). One choosing to follow in Livingstone's footsteps was Dr Herbert Gerrard, an English Primitive Methodist medical missionary, setting out for Zambia in 1915.

However, although Methodism made a significant contribution to medical missionary work, Nonconformism and medicine were not easy bedfellows beyond mission work, owing to a socio-cultural divide fractured by the intersections of religion, philanthropy, ethics, class, professional boundaries and protected esoteric knowledge. Dissenters and Nonconformists of the Hanoverian and early Victorian period were deeply distrustful of physicians, generally regarding them as mercenary, overprivileged Establishments quacks pandering to the hypochondriac foibles of the rich. Indeed, this was not an altogether unfair assessment of the skills of doctors of the time or their favoured clientele; bolstering further Nonconformist concerns for the unmet health needs of the poor (Hardiman, 2008). These polarised positions are described in George Eliot's (1871) *Middlemarch*, where the idealistic young doctor, Tertius Lydgate, takes a fatal fork in the road, finding himself entrapped in a materially affluent life of disappointed failure 'wide is the gate, and broad is the way, that leadeth to destruction' (Matthew 7:13–14).

John Wesley was interested in health issues and promoted a sensible regime of hygiene, temperance and ordered living to his followers; along with a number of rather more idiosyncratic health beliefs, prescribed in his writings, *Primitive Physick*. Being a self-help guide of free, folk remedies, the advice probably did no more harm than most of the official cures of the day, but equally was unlikely to do much more good either, short of avoiding expense.

Following Comaroff and Comaroff, Fitzgerald (1997, p. 66) comments on medical missionaries' concern to cure both the sick body as the corporeal tomb of the 'sin-sick soul'. Yet of course such an association is but part of a Christian understanding of health in its widest sense, for as the Anglican morning penitential prayer for God's mercy states, as sinners 'there is no health in us'.

Yet, Livingstone was also of the mind that in general the Central African people enjoyed overall better physical health and easier births than many in Britain (Etherington, 2005). Nevertheless, the extent of the wretched slave caravans of the pernicious Swahili-Arab slave trade (Good, 1991) convinced Livingstone that the problem could not be legislated away effectively, given the lack of legal infrastructure. His belief in greater rather than less benign European incursion than the odd philanthropist explorer led him to formulate his famous message of the '3 cs': commerce, Christianity and civilisation (Walls, 1987). The British public campaign against slavery was also bolstered by missionary reports from Nyasaland (later Malawi) and those across wider British East Africa (Good, 1991). Beneficially, the response to the Indian Ocean (Swahili-Arab) slave trade generated philanthropic responses in which European women missionaries were prominent, such as the Universities' Mission to Central Africa (UMCA) in British East Africa. This took in the hapless female booty rescued from the trade (Pritchard, 2017); from which eventually the UMCA would establish a precarious mission hospital in Nyasaland.

However, the unassailed remoteness of Central Africa was now also visible as resources to be exploited, generating the European 'scramble for Africa'. Carving up the continent for unequal bites across six voracious nations opened up enormous territories for development, delivering millions of bewildered indigenous peoples into different and oppositional, imperialist hands (Pakenham, 2002). Livingstone's call to 'practical Christianity' was equally heard by multiple missionary agencies seeking to stake their own territorial claims, with Roman Catholic missionaries gravitating towards areas controlled by France, Belgium, Portugal and the Spanish slivers of Africa (Good, 1991). In the meantime, reports circulated of the horrifying murder of the CMS missionary bishop James Hannington and several young local Christians, many of them mere children, by the dangerously erratic and lately succeeded, King of Buganda, Mwanga in East Africa (later Uganda), (Pakenham, 2005). These terrible murders, along with human sacrifice and the rampant slave trade, proved to Europeans, if needs be, that Christianity brought the light that Africa was sorely in need of.

Commensurately, Etherington (2012) refers to the mass proliferation of mid-nineteenth-century Christian missions, particularly in Zululand, Natal and Pondoland of which the Protestant denominations were represented by Anglicans, Congregationalists, Lutherans, Presbyterians and Methodists from the British Isles, the Scandinavian countries, Germany and the United States. The anti-imperialist Americans, together with the Germans and Norwegians, avoided British-controlled territories, nurturing naïve imperialist ambitions of their own, where Americans wished local Africans to adopt a US-type, value-based republic; the Germans wished to recreate a medieval

Saxony peregrinating, monastic model; and the Norwegians supported Zulu independence, provided Lutherism was embraced. The British clergy in Natal in contrast promoted a tolerant 'Broad Church approach' of acceptance of local African customs and scholarly studies of their healing practices and mythology (Etherington, 2012, p. 33).

The invasion of the African centre and the trappings of 'civilisation' further exposed local people to European-borne diseases (Nestel, 1998), providing a challenge as well as a rationale for colonial medical services via missions or the State. Advances in public health, antisepsis, and antibiotics lagged behind infectious diseases advancing rapidly across land cleared for cash cropping, new railways lines and labour migration (Etherington, 2005, p. 278)

The new Uganda Railway was a classic example of how industrialised power was opening up European colonisation of East Africa, where Britain and Germany vied for territory, which they finally agreed to share in 1886 (Van der Bilj, 2017). Ultimately, Germany would lose their East African possessions to Britain following the 1918 defeat. However, despite European sabre-rattling in Africa, the Great War lay some time into the future. In the meantime, the Africa 'scramble' was accelerated by the building of transportation links. Thus, prior to the end of the nineteenth century, the Uganda Railway, begun in the British East Africa (BEA) Protectorate, was not completed until the beginning of the new century, and at a huge cost.

BEA covered much of future Kenya, part of Uganda, abutting the British colony of Zanzibar, where in the latter case a substantial Indian presence was already well established (Kyle, 1999). The tremendous logistical power of the British Empire meant that migrant populations could be moved from one Crown colony to another in the construction of new infrastructures and to meet perceived colonial needs for labour, bureaucracy, trade and policing, as seen in the Indian diaspora to Malaya for example, as well as that to Hong Kong (Ashencaen Crabtree, 2012; Hew and Ashencaen Crabtree, 2012). In East Africa, 25,000 indentured Indian labourers were brought in to build the Uganda Railway; in their wake came Indian builders, artisans, clerks, administrators and traders. So populous was this Indian diaspora, that this part of Africa was pronounced an Indian enclave where 'the Indian rupee and the criminal code was that of India' (Kyle, 1999, p. 5).

Yet this state-driven imperial focus on territory, infrastructure, commerce and defence was an aggressively boisterous and disruptive later addition to an earlier, quieter colonisation by missionaries in East Africa. Stuart (2011) points to the foothold established by the Anglican CMS under the recruited German missionary, Johann Krapf and his wife Rosine in 1844; where by 1914, the start of the Great War, it grew to sixteen missions. With this key historical date in mind, Good (1991) observes that up to 1914, it was missions like the Church of Scotland that provided any colonial medical services, to the African communities in the future Kenyan territory.

Professional women missionaries had not delayed their work in Africa either, where Uganda witnessed the first group of Anglican women missionaries arrive in the 1890s, Madagascar having beheld their arrival some twenty years earlier (Prevost, 2008). Methodism, although a lesser presence, also kept a close eye on African missions. By 1916, in a privately circulated communique within the Wesley Methodist connexion, F.P. Wigfield (2016), commented on how the impact of the Great War had generated interest towards denominational medical missionary work, which if so, troubles Compton Brouwer's (1990) point regarding missionary interest in Britain; unless the war delayed translating potential interest into able bodies, as seems likely.

The need in Africa however was balanced equally by the differing problems of infrastructure, colonial policy and, to use contemporary jargon (apology, readers), a 'skills gap' in the various Crown colonies. The solution, Wigfield (2016) writes, was to foster an indigenous, self-sustaining Church, one where male and female Africans were medically trained to meet local needs. This had become a generally accepted ideological position among missionaries, where learning of Livingstone's experiences, the Reverend William Monk was duly convinced that Africans are indeed 'bone of our bone...flesh of our flesh' (Porter, 2004, p. 283). A noble sentiment indeed, overlooking, perhaps, the unfortunate corollary that such is Eve unto Adam in the Bible, intact with an implicit patriarchal hierarchy of dominance and subservience. That aside, the general Enlightenment idea of fraternity and egality for Africans and other colonised peoples, prevalent among Christian missions, had begun to erode towards the end of the century under new race theorisations (Strayer, 1978). Nonetheless, the Methodist fidelity to an autonomous, African-led Christian Church chimed harmoniously with the views of young Handley Hooper, newly married, who took up his CMS missionary appointment in BEA in 1916 with Cecily his bride; for Handley, this was effectively a return home to his native land (Cassons, 1998). His conviction was that African potential needed to be recognised, as possibly latent but powerful, making the impassioned plea against colonial dehumanisation, for

> no theory of incapacity can justify the refusal of opportunity....The Negro must be allowed the hope of a fully equipped and unfettered manhood for his race.
>
> (Cassons, 1998, p. 393)

The brutality meted out to Africans by many Europeans, who appeared to regard the former as no more than dumb animals, appalled and outraged Christian missionaries (Porter, 2011). Missions could at least offer something of an antidote to this oppression in creating some opportunities for local people. Writing to the Vicar of Holton, Suffolk, in 1916, Hooper described the beneficial patronage from missions that a typical African Highland lad might receive in BEA

> He comes with a letter of introduction to the missionary in charge of Nairobi; in his spare time he continues his education at the mission school, he comes to the mission church, he gets to know the mission native circle, and plays football on the mission ground, and very often the missionary is the means of getting him good employment. There is the inevitable danger of a low motive underlying his attachment to the mission, but the missionary is constantly combating that in his teaching, and all the time the boy is getting a solid foundation of a knowledge of the Gospel to counteract his selfish tendencies. It is amazing to see the movement in the native spiritual life in Nairobi as contrasted with the coast life.[1]

In 1920, the BEA became the British colony of Kenya. It was another step in the fortunes of a territory whose boundaries had been drawn, named and renamed within an imperial system where a future independence was not seriously questioned, but only the *when*, *who* and *how*. It would continue to be unclear for the next few decades, embroiling Christians both African and European in the coming ferment.

Mission as imperialism

Stuart (2008) comments that colonial Kenyan history has been subjected to greater intensity of academic interest than neighbouring African colonies with fierce debate regarding missionaries' embroilment with colonial governments. Postcolonial discourses tend to dismiss Christian mission as merely another prong of the imperial fork composed of militia, administration and medicine (Ashencaen Crabtree, 2012). Such critiques have long formed a tension regarding missionary work in colonies as either so steeped in imperial discourses and agendas to be utterly compromised, or alternatively potentially redeemable (Etherington, 2006). Porter (2011), however, questions the 'given' assumptions of an implicitly embroiled relationship between mission and imperialism. As Comaroff (1991) also observes, Nonconformist traditions, like Methodism, stood in tension with the Establishment, creating the paradox that while foregrounding certain conditions of colonialism (most obviously through a European pastoral presence and resources), Nonconformist discourse was one that directly contested colonial dominion.

> Missionaries rarely regarded the interventionist, omnicompetent imperial state with anything other than suspicion.
>
> (Stuart, 2011, p. 17)

Acknowledging in apologist tones that mission has been implicated in racist ideas and is now generally viewed as both arrogant and passé, Ucko (2011, p. 37) offers the plea

> that mission has also contributed to human dignity, literacy, health and all that we usually say is part of the good life.

A casual and lazy equation that Christian evangelism in colonised countries equals bad, full stop, closes down a closer scrutiny of the relationship between European missionaries and local people in histories of the indigenisation of churches. As Etherington (1996) says, the heavy weight of academic scrutiny has been on the evangelised, rather than the evangeliser, for obvious and good reasons, but the balance requires some redressing if we are to gain a more informed and nuanced understandings of missionary lives and mission as legacy. It is here that the Chalkley story begins to illuminate the mothballed mysteries of a life of devotional service in foreign fields. None more so, perhaps than the enigmatic presence of the recently beatified Roman Catholic Saint Teresa of Calcutta, whose charity 'The Missionaries of Charity' has recently been blocked by the Indian government from receiving foreign funds on the grounds of offence to Hindu religious sentiments (Ellis-Peterson, 2021).

In the next chapter, the early influences on the lives of the Chalkley sisters will begin to be traced, for theirs is a story of uncommon commitment to Christian love and service. The mission path would unfold in time, first would come the childhood anointment where Methodism provided both the cultural milieu and the cradle of convenance.

Note

1 Handley Douglas Hooper, C.M.S. Kahuhia, Fort Hall, B.E.A 30/3/1916. Hooper Family papers. Cadbury Library, University of Birmingham. CMS/ACC85, Accession 85.

References

Adamthwaite, M.R. (2016) *Through the Christian Year with Charles Wesley*. Eugene, OR: Wipf & Stock.

Anthias, F. (2012) Hierarchies of social location, class and intersectionality: Towards a translocational frame. *International Sociology,* 28(1), 121–138.

Ashencaen Crabtree, S. (2021) *Women of Faith and the Quest for Spiritual Authenticity: Comparative Perspectives from Malaysia and Britain*. London/New York: Routledge.

Ashencaen Crabtree, S., Husain, F. and Spalek, B. (2016) *Islam & Social Work: Islam and Social Work: Culturally Sensitive Practice in a Diverse World*. 2nd ed. Bristol: Policy Press.

Beach, H.P. and Fahs, C.H. (1925). *World Missionary Atlas*. New York: Institute of Social & Religious Research.

Blair, C.F. (2008) *Christian mission in India: Contributions to some missions to social change*. Unpublished. PhD. Simon Fraser University.

Bragg, M. (2011) *The Book of Books: The Radical Impact of the King James Bible, 1611–2011*. London: Hodden & Stoughton.

Brönte, C. (1847, 1984) *Jane Eyre*. London: Penguin.

Cassons, J. (1998) 'To plant a garden city in the slums of Paganism....': Handley Hooper, the Kikuyu and the future of Africa. *Journal of Religion in Africa*, XXVIII, 387–410.

Comaroff, J. and Comaroff, J. (1991) *Of Revelation and Revolution: Christianity, Colonialism and Consciousness in South Africa*, Vol. 1. Chicago, IL: The University of Chicago Press.

Compton Brouwer, R. (1990) *New Women for God: Canadian Presbyterian Women and India Missions, 1876–14*. Toronto: University of Toronto Press.

Cragg, G.R. (1977) *The Church & the Age of Reason 1648–1789*. Harmondsworth, Middlesex: Penguin.

Crenshaw, K. (1991) Mapping the margins: Intersectionality, identity politics, and violence against women of color. *Stanford Law Review*, 43(6), 1241–1299.

D'Costa, G., Knitter, P. and Strange, D. (2011) Christianity and the world's religions: A theological appraisal. In Gavin d'Costa, Paul Knitter and Daniel Strange (Eds.), *Only One Way? Three Christian Responses to the Uniqueness of Christ in a Pluralist World*. London: SCN Press. pp. 3–46.

Dews, D.C. (1986) Ann Carr and the female revivalists of leeds. In Gail Malsmgreen (Ed.), *Religion in the Lives of English Women, 1760–1930*. Kent: Croom Helm Ltd. pp. 68–88.

Dickens, A.G. (1974) *The German Nation and Luther*. Glasgow: William Collins Sons & Co. Ltd.

Dickinson. D. (2012) Methodism in English fiction. *International Journal for the Study of the Christian Church*, 12(3–4), 309–323. https:/doi.org/10.1080/1474 225X.2012.722909

Eberling, G. (1970) *Luther: An Introduction to His Thought*. Philadelphia, PA: Fortress Press.

Eliot, G. (1859, 2008) *Adam Bede*. London: Penguin.

Eliot, G. (1871, 2003) *Middlemarch*. London: Penguin.

Eliot, G. (1859, 1994). *Adam Bede*. London: Penguin Popular Classics.

Ellis-Peterson, H. (2021) India bans Mother Teresa charity from receiving funds abroad. *Guardian*, 28 December 2021. Available from: https://www.theguardian.com/news/2021/dec/28/india-bans-mother-teresa-charity-from-receiving-funds-from-abroad [Accessed 2 March 2022].

Etherington, N. (2012) Social theory and the study of Christians in Africa: A South African case study. *Africa*, 47(1), 31–40.

Etherington, N. (2005) Education and medicine. In Norman Etherington (Ed.), *Missions and Empire*. Oxford: Oxford University Press, pp. 261–284.

Etherington, N. (1996) Recent trends in the historiography of Christians in Southern Africa. *Journal of South African Studies*, 22(2), 201–219.

Fitzgerald, R. (1997) Rescue and redemption: the rise of female medical missions in colonial India during the late nineteenth and early twentieth centuries. In Anne Marie Rafferty, Jane Robinson and Ruth Elkan (Eds.), *Nursing History and the Politics of Welfare*. London & New York: Routledge, pp. 88–136.

Field, C.D. (1997) The social structure of English Methodism: Eighteenth-Twentieth centuries. *British Journal of Sociology*, 28(2), 199–225.

Forbes, G. (1994) Managing Midwifery in India. In Dagmar Engels and Shula Marks (Eds.), *Contesting Colonial Hegemony: State and Society in Africa and India*. London: British Academic Press, pp. 152–172.

Forrester, D.B. (1980) *Caste and Christianity*. London: Curzon Press.

Forster, E.M. (1924, 2005) *A Passage to India*. Penguin Classics.

Good, C.M. (1991) Pioneer medical missions in colonial Africa. *Social Science & Medicine*, 32(1), 1–10.

Gooren, H. (2004) An introduction to Pentecostalism: Global Charismatic Christianity. *Ars Disputandi*, 4(1), 206–209. https://doi.org/10.1080/1566539 9.2004.10819846

Grant, S. (2012) The Reverend Thomas Pennock, Wesleyan Methodist Missionary in Nineteenth Century Jamaica: A case study of acculturation, enculturation, or something else? *Wesley and Methodist Studies*, 4, 117–128.

Hardiman, D. (2008) *Missionaries and Their Medicine: A Christian Modernity for Tribal India*. Manchester: Manchester University Press.

Hardiman, D. (2006) Introduction. In David Hardiman (Ed.), *Healing Bodies, Saving Soul: Medical Missions in Asia and Africa*. Amsterdam: Brill, pp. 5–58.

Hattersley, R. (2014) *John Wesley A Brand from the Burning*. London: Abacus.

Heitzenrater, R.P. (1995, 2013) *Wesley and the People Called Methodists*, 2nd ed. Nashville: Abingdon Press.

Hempton, D. (2005) *Methodism: Empire of the Spirit*. New Haven, CT: Yale.

HEW Cheng Sim and Ashencaen Crabtree, S. (2012) The Islamic resurgence in Malaysia and the implications for multiculturalism. In Sara Ashencaen Crabtree, Jonathan Parker and Azlinda Azman (Eds.), *The Cup, The Gun and the Crescent: Social Welfare and Civil Unrest in Muslim Societies*. London: Whiting & Birch, pp. 82–100.

Kent, Eliza, F. (1999) Tamil Bible women and the zenana mission of colonial South India. *History of Religions*, 39(2), 117–149.

Kerswell, T. (2019) A conceptual history of the labour aristocracy: A critical review. *Socialism and Democracy*, 33(1), 70–87. https://doi.org/10.1080/0885 4300.2018.1512816

Kyle, K. 1999. *The Politics of the Independence of Kenya*. Houndsmill, Basingstoke: Palgrave Macmillan.

Lang, S. (2005) Drop the demon dai: Maternal morality and the State in colonial Madras, 1840–1875. *Social History of Medicine*, 18(3), 357–377.

Llewellyn, D. (2015) *Reading, Feminism and Spirituality: Troubling the Waves*. Houndsmill, Basingstoke: Palgrave Macmillan.

MacMillan, M. (1998) *Women of the Raj*. German Democratic Republic: Thames and Hudson.

Maison, M. (1986) 'Thine, Only Thine!' Women hymn writers in Britain, 1760–1835. 1986) In Gail Malsmgreen (Ed.), *Religion in the Lives of English Women, 1760–1930*. Kent: Croom Helm Ltd, pp. 11–40.

Mayhew-Smith, N. and Hayward, G. (2020) *Britain's Pilgrim Places*. London: Lifestyle Press Ltd.

Mernissi, F. (1975) *Beyond the Veil*. Cambridge, MA: Schenkman Publishing Company.

Moulds, A. (2017) Medical women: Perspectives from the Victorian medical professions. Bulletin of the Royal College of Surgeons of England. Available at: https://publishing.rcseng.ac.uk/doi/pdf/10.1308/rcsbull.2017.255 [Accessed 16 February 2022].

Neill, S. (1964, 1979) *A History of Christian Missions*. Harmondsworth, Middx: Penguin.

Nestel, S. (1998) Administering angels: Colonial nursing and the extension of empire in Africa. *Journal of Medical Humanities*, 19(4), 257–277.

Owenson, S. (1811, 2002) *The Missionary*. Peterborough, Ontario: Broadview Press.

Pakenham, T. (2002) *The Scramble for Africa*. London: Abacus.

Pass, A. (2011) *British Women Missionaries in India c. 1917–1950*. PhD Dissertation. University of Oxford.

Pinto, S. (2008) *Where There Is No Midwife: Birth and Loss in Rural India*. New York: Berghahn Books.

Porter, A. (2004) *Religion versus Empire? British Protestant Missionaries and Overseas Expansion, 1700–1914*. Manchester: Manchester University Press.

Prevost, E. (2008) Married to the mission field: Gender, Christianity and professionalization in Britain and Colonial Africa, 1865–1914. *Journal of British Studies*, 47(4), 796–826.

Prevost, E.E. (2010). *The Communion of Women: Missions and gender in colonial Africa and the British metropole*. Oxford: Oxford University Press.

Prichard, J. (2014). *Methodists and their Missionary Societies, 1900-1996*. London: Routledge

Pritchard, A.C. (2017) *Sisters in Spirit: Christianity, Affect and Community Building in East Africa, 1860–1970*. East Lansing: Michigan State University Press.

Strayer, R.W. (1978) *The Making of Mission Communities in East Africa: Anglicans and Africans in Colonial Kenya, 1875–1935*. London: Heinemann.

Stuart, J. (2008) Overseas mission: Voluntary service and aid in Africa: Max Warren. The Christian Mission Society and Kenya, 1945–63. *The Journal of Imperial and Commonwealth History*, 36(3), 527–543.

Stuart, J. (2011). *British Missionaries and the End of Empire: East, Central and Southern Africa, 1939-64*. Grand Rapids, Michigan/Cambridge: Wm. B. Berdsman Publishing Group.

Tholfsen, T. (1976, 2019) *Working Class Radicalism in Mid-Victorian England*. London: Routledge.

Thompson, E.P. (1963) *The Making of the English Working Classes*. New York: Vintage Books.

Tonge, E.M. (1930) *Fanny Jane Butler: Pioneer Medical Missionary*. London: Church of England Zenana Missionary Society.

Ucko, H. (2011) Protestant perspective: Christian mission among other faiths. In Lal Sangkima Pachuau and Knud Jorgensen (Eds.), *Witnessing to Christ in a Pluralistic Age*. Oxford: Regnum Books International, pp. 37–44.

Underhill, L.A. (1935) *Extremes Meet: Some Acts about India's Women*. London: Highway Press.

Van der Bijl, N. (2017). *Mau Mau Rebellion: The Emergency in Kenya, 1952–1956*. Barnsley, South Yorkshire: Pen and Sword Military.

Vaughan, M. (1991) *Curing Their Ills: Colonial Power and African Illness*. Stanford, CA: Stanford University Press.

Vickers, J.E. (2012) The Wesleys of blessed memory: Hagiography, missions, and the study of world Methodism. *International Bulletin of Missionary Research*, 36(3), 143–147.

Vidler, A.R. (1977) *The Church in an Age of Revolution*. Harmondsworth: Penguin.

Walls, A.F. (1987). The legacy of David Livingstone. *International Bulletin of Missionary Research*, 11(3), 125–129. https://doi.org/10.1177/239693938701100306

Whitehead, J. (1797) The Late Rev. John Wesley'. *Derby Mercury*, Thursday, 14 September 1797.

Wilson, K. (2011) *Methodist Theology*. London: T&T Clark International.

Worthington Smith, R. (1950) Slavery and Christianity in the British West Indies. *Church History*, 19(3), 171–186.

Wright, S. (2020) *The Mother of the Brontës*. Yorkshire, Pen & Sword Books.

Yong, A. and Alexander, E.Y. (2011) Introduction: Black tongues of fire: Afro-Pentecostalism shifting strategies and changing discourses. In Amos Yong and Estreleda Y. Alexander (Eds.), *Afro-Pentecostalism*. New York: New York University Press, pp. 1–20.

Yuval-Davies, N. (2006) Intersectionality and feminist politics. *European Journal of Women's Studies*, 13(3), 193–209.

3 The foundations of faith

A methodist girlhood

Memory, mythology and the known unknown

All family histories are evolving stories in the making, intertwined inchoate and conflicting mythologies of layered meaning, facets recalled, unremembered and reconstructed. Even across degrees of congruence in family accounts, such histories are rarely ever straightforward; and this is true of Muriel and Audrey's story, populated with details in one place and gaps elsewhere, loquacity here and silences there. It is a veritable *broderie anglaise*, opening reflexive, resonant spaces to interstices of my own family's history. This is not mine directly but mine by choice, through Jack, and then through Jonathan, Wirral men sharing geographically historicised cultural footprints, emerging from histories made reckless by social circumstances. One, Jack, was the older husband of my youth and Jonathan, the companion of my mature years. Muriel knew one but not the other, and yet their lives intersected with hers.

Encapsulations of oral narratives reconstruct 'messy lives' into ordered architectures of continuity and meaning (Henson, 2017, p. 224). Autobiographical or biographical these create scripted narratives of meaning-making (Abrams, 2012). Inconsistencies, re-sculpted and reframed in authorial narrative exercise that shoe-horn individual narratives to master narratives of great social and cultural events as transformations of the time should be resisted (Maslen, 2013). The two World Wars, post-war welfarism and sharpening secular trends form obvious monolithic markers against which to pin the Chalkley lives. Yet, the small-scaled, domestic, seemingly trivial points that narratives throw up require attention. For otherwise an apophatic authorial defining of lives as meaning *this* or standing for *that* may overwrite the actual significance and meanings by which lives were self-measured (Henson, 2017).

The responsibility of writing the histories of others as truthfully and thoughtfully as they deserve to be is an inhibiting burden. These are real lives and reputations that we are dealing with, after all. One version

DOI: 10.4324/9781003359746-3

of a truth must be balanced at times with that of another. Ambiguities, contradictions and uncertainties need grappling with and setting against what is 'known'. The social, cultural and historical structures of the time moulding social realities add some weight to the plausibility or otherwise of views and beliefs.

As someone who knew them observed of our two sisters, 'the world had moved on but they hadn't'. If that is the case, we may ask where were Audrey and Muriel? How do they position themselves in their own histories? Moreover, how do we reach back to that vacuum of insularity where, it is implied, they dwelt? If they were indeed suspended in an impenetrable amber of fixed time and place, which I would say is much open to question.

Beginnings: Bertha and Frank

Throughout her life, Muriel openly idolised her father, Frank Chalkley, referring to him even into her nineties as 'Daddy'. Of all his children, I doubt if any felt or were closer to him. Muriel herself attributed this attachment mainly to the fact that she was the youngest as well as the only child born after Frank was demobbed from the Great War; and was present to help care for her in infancy. No such adulation was felt towards her mother, Bertha, who was perhaps perceived as merely fulfilling an expected gendered role. Frank made Muriel feel special and lovely. A plain child with big, inharmonious features and prominent teeth, Muriel was an endearingly ugly duckling all her life. Yet her face softened with smiles when she recalled how, as a small child, she bloomed under the sunshine of her father's love as he mopped her baby face with a flannel, carolling 'Oh, what a beautiful little face'. It was a moment of such unconditional, joyful affirmation that she never forgot it. This was perhaps all the more important as Muriel knew she had come as a disappointment to her mother, who had hoped, after three daughters, to give birth to a son, already naming the unborn child in her womb, 'Kenneth'. Bertha had dedicated the quickening Kenneth to God upon his arrival, that bargain stuck fast when another baby girl made her quick and easy entrance to the world.

Frank was born on 9 April 1890, his birth recorded in the England & Wales Civil Registration Birth Index under this single diminutive. Perhaps after producing so many older sons, William Seabrook and his wife Eliza(beth) (official records truncating her name) had run out of imagination by the time the sixth arrived. Furthermore, there are no records to indicate that Frank was ever baptised. His future wife, Bertha Elizabeth Fitzgerald, was born on 13 June 1891 and baptised on 5 July 1891 at St Mary's Church in Birkenhead, an impressive Anglican church with a short lifespan, being newly built in 1822 and demolished owing to disrepair in 1975.

The Population Census of 1911 records Frank as an unmarried youth of twenty-one, living with his parents and younger sisters in a cheek-to-jowl neighbourhood of cramped terraces: 17 Eldon Road, Rock Ferry in Birkenhead on the Mersey, then busy docks. At this time, Bertha was living with her parents, John Joseph and Elizabeth Fitzgerald, and four siblings at 3 Colden Place, Tranmere, a subdistrict of Birkenhead, and today a missing address; perhaps municipally renamed, or given the pasting Liverpool received from the Luftwaffe during the Second World War, bombed out of existence. Two of her siblings were still at school in 1911, with the elder brothers being recorded on the Population Census as apprentice plumber and grocer's assistant.

By marrying Bertha on the eve of the Great War, Frank would have ensured that in the event of his death, she would have received some financial compensation through the 1916 war widows' pension; the first non-contributory and women-specific pension. However, widows were closely monitored by the Ministry of Pensions for moral purity thereafter: enjoying a 'fancy man' or 'the bottle' was sufficient for widows' pensions to be reduced or removed entirely (Parker, 2023; Smith, 2010a). Bertha was instead quickly occupied by pregnancy.

The couple's daughters were a wartime generation, just as Jack would be in turn. Arriving within a few years of each other, prior to, during, and after the Great War, the eldest child, born in October 1915, was duly christened Bertha Elizabeth after her mother. She was followed by Dorothy Lilian in March 1917, swiftly followed by Audrey Margaret in September 1918; and finally, Muriel Mercy, the youngest, her aunt's namesake, was born in January 1922 (Figure 3.1).

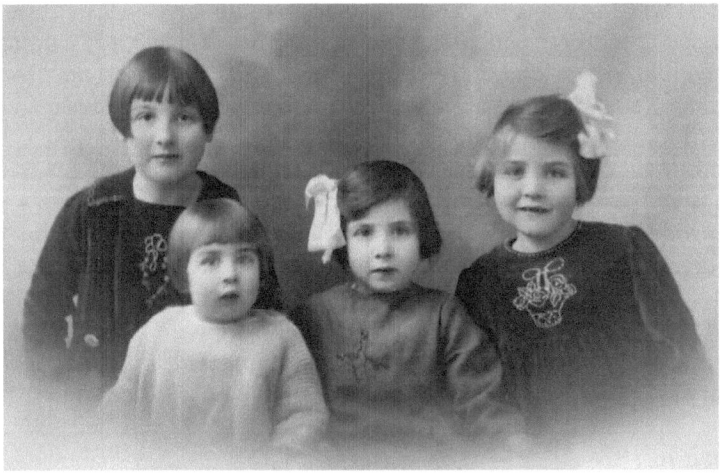

Figure 3.1 Four Sisters. Courtesy of Muriel Chalkley.

Of two photographs that Muriel had of her youthful parents, one shows Bertha as a well-built, round-faced young woman dressed sedately in Edwardian formality, a suggestion of lace collars and pearl necklaces, smiling sweetly beneath the brim of an enormous and stylish, dark hat. Frank in khaki, confident but ungainly poses in a wartime studio, his head tilted back, the Chalkley nose like a ship's prow in a long face, he gives an uncompromising, challenging stare at the camera. The photographs, taken singly, do not fit together easily, visually, or in terms of occasion or mood. Perhaps they were well-suited to this couple. Or perhaps their union was one of those awkward, intimate social accidents in a comedy of manners, resulting in a marriage surprising to all.

Socially, Bertha's marriage to Frank may have taken her down the social ladder a peg or more. Having no recorded occupation in the Census of 1911, Bertha shared the same status as the teenage daughters of her father-in-law, the rather classily named William Seabrook Chalkley, born in Liverpool in 1850. Eliza was a supported housewife, as was Bertha's mother. Yet Bertha's father had worked his way up from ordinary railway guard to the established professional classes of 'Railway Inspector', thereby becoming solidly entrenched in the middle-classes. William, by contrast, was a working-class joiner of dubious background. In a later record relating to his daughter, Mercy, William is ambiguously but discreetly described as a 'railway servant'. These wood-working skills may have taken William into railway work and therefore may have been instrumental to the couple meeting across the lines somehow, for it is doubtful that there would have been much social mixing between the families.

Joinery and carpentry skills were vitally important to the railways that bore the great steam engines, which today are cherished as heritage treasures, but that then sootily chugged and chuffed their way inexhaustibly across a complex of competing, interlocking and sometimes incompatible railway arteries sprouting across Britain. These linked great cities to towns, small villages and obscure country holts in ways we can only dream of wistfully, after Dr Beeching took his axe of vandalism to sever the veins of British public transport in 1963 to make way for the motor car.

Whether our couple, Frank and Bertha, met through tea dances, the bandstand or some other chance encounter in Birkenhead, William's son was fortunate to walk out with his lady friend, unless the Fitzgeralds were unusually high-minded. For William's background was far from salubrious: he had been no less than a convicted, if precocious, child criminal, having been sentenced in 1861 for a tariff of fifteen years by the age of eleven for the forgery of 'promisery notes': in other words, fraud.

We know very little about William's parents or his upbringing. His father was born in Suffolk, his trade that of a joiner and builder, migrating for work, for his wife and subsequent life was in Liverpool, an epicentre of industry. William appears to have been an only child and evidently could read, write and calculate, if only for nefarious activities. He may have been a grammar school boy, if his parents could have afforded the fee. It is far less likely that he received private tuition, a commodity of more affluent families than we assume were his, unless his fall from respectability had been spectacularly downward. More likely he was educated at one of the denominational church schools, which by 1833 were the fruits of a modest state grant for the building of schools. Although, as Timmins (2017, p. 67) states, the government at that time were 'still spending more on the Queen's stables than on educating its children'. Such schools, Anglican, Roman Catholic or Nonconformist, tended to regard education as vehicles for imparting their own religious principles to children, particularly in Liverpool (Liverpool Schools). However, if he was the beneficiary of church school education, we may draw some sobering conclusions about how successful a moral education was in young William's case. We might also guess that his brief formal education was not altogether interrupted by incarceration, for the State provided lessons for child soldiers and their prison and workhouse compatriots (Fraser, 2009, p. 96).

The Law is often, and justifiably, accused of valuing property over people. Even if those forerunners of probation workers, the Police Court 'missionaries' (of the Church of England Temperance Society), had intervened (Parker, 2023), William's crime was viewed as very serious, for among the list of convictions in the England & Wales, Criminal Register, 1791–1892, listing his name, the sentences for burglary ranged from two to six years; a sentence for manslaughter receiving the same fifteen-year tariff as his. By 1884, a freed man, working as a joiner, he married Eliza Samuels, one year his junior. Born in Wales in Montgomeryshire, her family gravitated to Liverpool as probably economic migrants. They proved a fecund union producing nine children in sixteen years of which Frank, born in 1890, was the seventh, with two sisters, Mercy and Margaret following him.

Muriel never alluded to her paternal grandfather's background and therefore was probably carefully concealed by Frank, and, if she knew of it, by Bertha as well. Conceivably he may have been ignorant of his father's early felonies, but this stretches credulity, for Frank was set upon a path that was entirely distanced from his father's example. He was not the only one bent on self-improvement, for some of his brothers and sisters also 'made good' in life, becoming gainfully employed and staying within the Law, where records list certain of their occupations as pipe fitters and ship painters, all skilled occupations. Of all of them though it was Frank's younger sister, Mercy, who rose to enter the professional echelons.

Frank proved himself a devoted, life-long Methodist of energy, zeal and charisma. I assumed, wrongly, that Muriel's parents were both 'birth-right' Methodists and it was this bond that brought them together. My original assumption was bolstered by discovering that Mercy was also recorded on her professional records as being 'Nonconformist'. However, official records suggest otherwise in the light of William Seabrook Chalkley's earlier life and where he was lately described to me by a family member as a 'very heavy drinker'. This hardly fits the image of Methodists as keen followers of the Temperance movement. I now believe that Frank was a Methodist convert (duly influencing Bertha); a redemptive act from a disreputable family background, which would explain Frank's exemplary religious zeal as a fresh convert.

Thus, at some point in his youth, Frank 'signed the pledge' demanded from the 'Band of Hope', vowing never to touch alcohol and expecting his later family to obediently follow suit. Muriel said this was because Frank had seen so many families torn apart by the ravages of alcohol dependency. Maybe Frank was referring to his own parental degradation, as William cannot have found it easy to support such a big, growing family or be an easy person to live with drowned in his cups. No doubt he had been both hardened and damaged by a traumatic childhood of penal servitude of many years.

Soap, service and safety

Frank did not follow in his father's manual labouring footsteps but moved quietly and diligently from a blue-collar background to the white collar of the lower-middle classes via the Cheshire soap empire. That modest ascent had already begun; the 1911 Population Census records twenty-one-year-old Frank as a 'soap manufacturer'. Being no entrepreneur that anyone knew of, this must have referred to Frank's status as factory employee. The biggest soap manufacturing industry by far was that of William Hesketh Lever's – the Lever Bros., which would eventually morph into a colossus, the multinational Unilever. Lever, a Bolton, Lancashire man, started his commercial empire with a soap product called 'Sunlight' in 1884. This made his fortune and that of the local Cheshire community, providing the bread-and-butter livelihood for the growing Chalkley family.

A larger-than-life character in all ways, no one could doubt Lever's business acumen. Originally rather ornately packaged, before eventually simplifying to an eye-caching yellow wrapping, Sunlight was a laundry soap with superior credentials. It caught the consumer imagination, coming in colourful wrapped bars advertising the manufacturers, and accompanied by the snappy slogan: 'Less Labour Greater Comfort'. Assuring buyers that it was 'Free from Adulteration' in the form of an absence of silicate of soda, it replaced much of the conventional tallow used with pleasanter vegetable fats. The advertising hype was refreshingly accompanied by actually enhanced performance, for it lathered well and gave a good wash, hence living up to the claim of lower effort for greater rewards (Hubbard and Shippobottom, 2003).

A very big organisation in the area, by 1907, Lever Bros. employed thousands of local people, accommodating many of them at the Lever corporation village, 'Port Sunlight', founded in 1888. By 1911, when Frank was still living at home at Rock Ferry, so successful had Lever become that he was elevated in society to become Viscount Leverhulme, and was now able to indulge his passion for art, philanthropy and politics in grand style (Rowan, 2003). Later, patriotism to the fore, the Viscount became an enthusiastic supporter of Lord Kitchener's call to arms. E.P. Thompson (1963) might well rail against Methodism as serving to historically subvert a glorious Anglicised French Revolution, with not even a Russian-type revolution forthcoming either; but the Great War towed Methodists, like Frank Chalkley, into its maw.

Apart from fathering children in brief interludes from active service, Frank's time in the army is vague owing to missing service records, a casualty of later Wehrmacht bombing raids. What partial records are available briefly note that Frank was a Staff Sergeant in the Army Service Corps in 1914, the year of his marriage to Bertha. Given that conscription had not yet begun at that point in the conflict, he must have volunteered for Army service at the outbreak of hostilities. He was part of a massing male vanguard thrilling to the call to arms, which included Jack's father, who to the fury of his own hard-headed, mercantile, Lancastrian father, to whom he was never reconciled thereafter, rode grandly to the recruiting offices on his white stallion 'Albert'.

Neither 'Walter' nor Frank, although occupying different social classes, came from the very poorest of backgrounds. The democratisation of the trenches would overturn class distinctions where they would rub shoulders with those drawn from the city slums and the fields (Smith, 2010a). Cowering under fire, stunted soldier 'bantams' would dine better on army rations in the body-fouled, treacherous mud of the trenches than ever before (Blythe, 1969).

More than likely Frank was probably one of the 700 volunteers from Port Sunlight who signed up in August 2014 in one of the splendid assembly rooms, Gladstone Hall, now turned into a temporary Army recruiting post. Large enough to form their own infantry unit, these 700 'Sunlighters' achieved their own local nomenclature, becoming known as the 'Port Sunlight Pals' (McQueen, 2011, p. 217). They were marched with strutting hubris by Lever himself down to General Henry McKinnon in Chester, with the band of the Sunlight Boys' Brigade leading the procession. After an amateurish period of combat training without uniforms or weapons, the Pals were shipped to the Front to be scythed down on the Somme, the graveyard of so many young men (McQueen, 2011).

The record is partial and the information incomplete. We know that like Jack's father, Frank survived and was eventually demobbed on an Army disability pension. Being sent to the Front with the other 'Sunlighters' seems an obvious conclusion to draw concerning his injuries and if so, he was decidedly lucky. Yet Muriel never said anything like this to me, for when asked about her father's service record, she stated that he had served in the 'Catering Corps', inadvertently conjuring up the image of an ill-tempered, aproned cook doling out unappetising slops to hungry and impatient troops. Nor did she ever mention any injury sustained. The strong impression provided was that Frank's served in the Army according to the dictates of his Methodist conscience and that excluded armed combat. He may have been in the kitchens, for he seems to have been a domesticated kind of man, judging from photographs of him by the sink of a modest, suburban kitchen in retirement with rolled up sleeves, holding a tea towel; but he was also an indifferent cook, which would not have disbarred him from the Forces' kitchens. Or maybe his role was more linked to the clerical work that he did on civvy street for Lever Bros., for the Army Service Corps was responsible for the administration of supplies of food rations, fuel, hospital supplies as well as ammunition, together with the transportation of these resources to front-line troops.

Frank returned home in one piece to pick up his job at Port Sunlight and there he stayed until retirement. Rowan (2003) exploring the capitalist drivers of Lever's corporate paternalism, argues of designed control over worker loyalties and thereby labour production: a contented man made for a better, more amenable worker. Frank's working life reflected the functionality of this ethos, for he showed no signs of wanting to change his employment. Maybe the harrowing attrition of the Great War and the aftermath of the Depression knocked that ambition out of him. Or more charitably, perhaps he found satisfaction in his work under good employment conditions, Lever and his ilk, if all canny, self-made men, hardly conformed to Dickensian mill-ogres; and Methodists were self-disciplinarians in shaping themselves to industrial capitalism, as Thompson (1963) disapprovingly notes. In his 'job for life', Frank's path was a respectable if undistinguished one, remaining a clerk of various grades in the Repairs Dept, ultimately controlling the departmental phone to answer callers with the authoritative greeting of 'Chalkely Repairs!' or perhaps the most tentative, 'Chalkey (full stop, comma or dash) Repairs'. It is not unreasonable to suppose that Frank's experiences in the Army paved the path he ultimately chose: the orderliness of clerical organisation of parts; the blessings of a quiet, regulated life, a peaceful marriage to a nice woman, children – and the counting of one's considerable blessings.

A village in a town 'by a city wall'

The Chalkey family for some years lived in Lever's Port Sunlight set in thirty-two acres of green land. Renowned architects, like William Owen, had been commissioned to build the first rows of attractive artisan houses, most of which today are 'Grade II' listed buildings, referring to their special interest as National Heritage conservation buildings. Prior to such listings, they were much admired as excellent housing. At Port Sunlight, there were numerous and novel amenities for the body, mind and soul, the entire area being designed as a sharp contrast to comparable housing elsewhere. The 'village' followed in a grand tradition of Victorian philanthropic social enterprise, aimed at lifting the worker from the degradation of a bare animal existence in dank slums kennelling the working poor.

Such grand social enterprises, so typical of late Victorian dissenter social consciousness, required deep pockets and stern resolution by these corporate philanthropists, where concern for the profit margin was directly linked to fostering a healthy, contented and grateful workforce. The implications of a 'health and efficiency' agenda was already apparent to these visionary entrepreneurs. Notable examples of this kind of corporate familialisation include Robert Owen's New Lanark tenements in Scotland with its strong focus on a broad, lifelong education of workers beginning from the earliest childhood (Davidson, 2010). In Bradford, Sir Titus Salt, the wool magnate created the corporation village of 'Saltaire' in 1883, equipped with household lavatories and running water (MacQueen, 2011). Let us not overlook the Quaker, George Cadbury's 'Bourneville' chocolate workers' village, with its focus on the salutary effect of gardening, vegetarianism, temperance and sexual restraint (Vallely, 2020). The domestic Eden was central to the vision of Sir James Reckitt's Garden Village in Hull where every worker's garden had two fruit trees to foster a love of healthy, outdoor husbandry. The 'Garden Village' concept, conceived of at the turn of the century, embraced the vision of the Quaker, Joseph Rowntree New Earswick in York together with the 'Garden Cities' of Ebenezer Howard's early twentieth-century ventures in Letchworth and Welwyn Garden City in Hertfordshire, 'marrying town and country' (Parker, 2023, p. 75).

Letchworth, the first of Howard's two garden cities, premised on the notion of social justice and equality (Ward, 1990), I knew well. The Letchworth I remember from the 1980s and 1890s was a very desirable, neat conurbation shielded by countryside, providing a pastoral oasis of quaint houses, lining broad tree-lined avenues divided by tidy parks. The whole scene merely missing a uniformed, prim Nanny pushing a Spanish galleon of a stately pram to evoke an English Toy Town timelessness, topped off by the defunct but splendid Art Deco Spirella Company corset manufacturing building (McEvoy, 2010).

Port Sunlight was built on an even more generous scale in respect of houses, gardens, pavements, roads, common grounds, public buildings like the Gladstone and Hulme Hall assembly spaces and art galleries, as well as municipal facilities: post offices and the United Reform Church, where no facility was squalidly cramped or prioritised the machine over the person (McQueen, 2011). This was no mean feat given that 3,600 employees and their dependents were housed there by 1907 (Jeremy, 1991). The diversity of house designs was much admired at the time and still is; no Stalinist Brutalism or Corbusier 'machines for living in' are seen here (Le Corbusier, 2007). Instead, all is English suburban and country nostalgia. Each row of homes adding its own statement to the diverse vocabulary of a charming architectural vernacular for the ordinary worker and their family. This was an almost unimaginable luxury compared to the heavily industrialised, under-latrined and over-crowded slums found elsewhere, and almost within a stone's throw locally.

At Port Sunlight, clerical staff, like Frank, were normally allocated the 'parlour cottages' rather than the blue-collar 'kitchen cottages'; but either type were a great advance on the dwellings that George Orwell described in his polemical/semi-ethnographic account of miners' lives in the 1930s, *The Road to Wigan Pier*. Orwell compares the Wigan slums versus the Wigan 'Corporation' (Council) houses superseding the slums as improved housing stock. Corporation houses were built to a standard specification of little variation on land available at the edges of conurbations, glumly surveyed by Orwell:

> Certainty most Corporation estates are pretty bleak in winter. Some I have been through, perched on treeless clayey hillsides and swept by icy winds, would be horrible places to live in.
>
> (Orwell, 2001, p. 65)

The alternative, 'slums', teemed with human life but equally were unfit for human habitation: 'Quite often you have eight or ten people living in a three-roomed house' (Orwell, 2001, p. 52), with an outside shared lavatory anything up to 200 yards (183 metres) away and no proper refuse storage either.

In Wigton, the Cumbrian town of Melvyn Bragg's (1999) semi-autobiography, *The Soldier's Return*, the social conditions in Northern England by the end of the Second World War were little improved, if at all

> the privy was at the corner of the alley next to the tap. As Ellen had anticipated, it was much used by the overspill from Scott's Yard where several big families shared the one lavatory, proudly declared to be 'always warm'.
>
> (Bragg, 1999, p. 118)

Unlike the Corporation houses, there was wider variation at Port Sunlight in terms of house style and ornamentation, in addition to being drawn along blue/white collar distinctions of 'parlour cottages' and the 'kitchen cottages. The latter had kitchens big enough for the family to cook and sit comfortably with a separate scullery for washing chores, a food larder as well as three upstairs bedrooms, in addition to the wonderful novelty of an indoor toilet and bathroom. It was not uncommon to find neither in some British houses even into the 1970s (Jonathan's first purchased Hull home had no bathroom whatsoever). The 'parlour cottages' were additionally equipped with a sitting room and in some houses a fourth bedroom. Sadly, we do not know which house Frank and Bertha Chalkley lived in, perhaps it was one of the Dutch-style or Swiss cottage-types, mock Tudor, a Scottish mini-baronial castle or a Jacobean terrace. Whichever it was, it was a more fortunate start in life than many children of the time could ever have hoped for.

Apart from the great attraction of affordable, comfortable, dignified and aesthetic housing, Port Sunlight was also a Nonconformist paradise, where the first minister for the 'village' church was a Wesleyan Methodist and a Christian Socialist (Hubbard and Shippobottom, 2003). Christian Socialism, a mid-nineteenth-century movement, brought together politics and Christianity. This was not the comfortable Christian lip service of the Establishment but an understanding of the radical egalitarianism of Christ's mission, as drawn out in the New Testament, of equating poverty of spirit with social inequalities and authoritarian venality. The figure of Christ was constructed as embodying the original socialist, overturning the tables of corruption and unfairness (Bragg, 2011). Christian socialism did not tend to sit comfortably with jingoism and the call to arms, so perhaps the rallying of the Sunlighters' recruitment to the Great War by a flag-waving Lever occasioned simmering, dissenting lather in the soap empire's kingdom.

Nevertheless, whether Wigton or Wigan, social conditions for working-class people had yet to match the splendid standards offered to the workers at Port Sunlight. It was a worker's Utopia of aesthetic and tasteful amenities, but one that also operated within a corporate Benthamite Panopticon (1789) of observed and visible social expectations, where a Foucauldian (1977) freedom for self-expression in feckless, irresponsible and antisocial behaviour was strictly denied. Contemporary neighbourhoods are much less subject to corporate, top-down surveillance, and socio-religious peer-group pressures have weakened, yet Port Sunlight is just as popular with residents and visitors today as then. It remains a litter and graffiti-free zone of urban decorum with little to mar its continuing charm. Moreover, community life in most towns and villages revolved around the gravitational pull of pubs and Parish churches, both offering contrasting but time-hallowed forms of fellowship and solace. While Lever and his dissenter philanthropists welcomed the latter, the former was definitely shunned.

Gravitating to Bournemouth in retirement was particularly appropriate for Audrey and Muriel. Modern Bournemouth was born through the sudden accidental death of an infant on his baptism day. To comfort his grief-stricken wife, Henrietta neé Portman, Captain Lewis Tregonwell, built a castle-crenelated mansion circa 1812 (Miller, 1996), on the picturesque, coastal, gorse-ridden wilderness where the Bourne river meets the sea. De-peopled through the anti-Commoner[1] Enclosures Act, 1801, it was a smuggler's haven, implicating high-living Tregonwell himself. By 1850, the year before the remarkable author Mary Shelley was buried in now fashionable, literary Bournemouth; two heiress sisters, Georgina Charlotte and Marianne Talbot lived on these seaside clifftops almost 150 years before it became my home too, where Jack would die, Jonathan would eventually live and our daughters grow. The Talbot wealth was used for the creation of the 465-acre 'Talbot village' to the wooded north of today's town, where model peasantry were provided with ample new cottages set in an acre of land for sober husbandry, plus Almshouses, a school, an Anglican Church and graveyard where those sisters now rest (Gillett, 1978). Bournemouth expanded from its splendid clifftop vantage points to absorb older communities and farm estates that preserved and used their traditional watering holes, but the original town was elevated by te conspicuous omission of that useful geographical and social landmark, the local pub.

Muriel happily signed up to lifelong temperance as a young girl of ten or so. She stuck to this pledge throughout her life, disliking Communion wine and annoying her family later with her rigid adherence to Frank's moral purity rules. Anonymously supplied family anecdotes illustrate Muriel's complete opposition to the 'demon drink': the 'swiping' of a small glass of champagne out of her widowed mother's hand to wet her baby granddaughter's newly christened head, with Muriel uttering the strident reproach 'What would Daddy think?!'

Poor Bertha in her old age, Frank long buried, was said to hide the occasional tiny bottle of Babycham at the back of her wardrobe whenever Muriel was visiting on her infrequent furloughs from Africa. The staunch evangelist got her unwitting comeuppance one day though, when instead of enjoying what she believed to be a sherry-flavoured jelly in a trifle, a naughty young relative substituted it for the wickedly real thing. Muriel smacking her lips later pronounced it the best trifle she'd ever eaten.

Muriel was so untutored that I am quite certain she had little idea that alcohol could ever be consumed regularly without any apparent ill effects or abuse; certainly, it was not associated in her mind with either pleasure or epicureanism, the latter of which she had no experience of anyway.

Her vice was tea-drinking, and how that would have shocked the sainted John Wesley, who condemned tea as the devil's brew (Hattersley, 2014). Muriel, no busy-bodying moral puritan, was not one for interrogating others about their tipples, and in truth she had little interest in either good food or drink, showing only the occasional weakness for milk chocolate buttons.

A methodist upbringing

The childhood that Muriel recalled was probably typical to many a scrimped and frugal upbringing, a make-do-and-mend of passed down, patched up, repainted and cherished goods. There was nothing remarkable in that, and she always described her upbringing as very happy and lucky. Gratitude was showered on her parents who provided their four little girls with a very sound, loving and godly upbringing. With only one breadwinner to support six people, money was tight, but with thrift basic daily necessities were always met. Mother holding the strings as firmly as she could to make ends meet, even managed a week's summer holiday annually: a trip to the Isle of Man was remembered. If Bertha was the scrimper-and-saver where 'charity begins at home', Frank was the big-hearted, sympathy-wrung spender.

MURIEL:[2] We weren't rich, we were quite poor. Mother would look after the money and save very carefully. Father would be too generous and give it away to other people who would beg for it – poor people.

A comfortable home and summer holidays – this hardly sounds like the *Road to Nabb End*, William Woodruff's (2002) fondly grim autobiography of a contemporaneous, impoverished Northern childhood in the grinding poverty of mill-working Lancashire in the twenties. Nor indeed much like Jack's poverty-stricken Merseyside childhood of the forties. The Chalkley children by contrast were thriving, loved and guided by conscientious, tolerant parents trying to do their best.

Bertha was a good but plain cook, Muriel said approvingly, disliking anything 'fancy' on her plate and there was always enough to eat. A cooked breakfast of bacon and eggs started the day, with Frank eating up the bacon rinds that the children left behind; his downfall, said Muriel sadly, certain that the added cholesterol accelerated his later ill health.

Frank, Muriel said, aware of how hard it must have been for Bertha to birth and raise their family alone during the war, in gratitude regularly brought his wife breakfast in bed to reward her for past privations. Frank must have been the one cooking breakfast then, his army skills of a fry-up put to good use on civvy street. After breakfast, before setting off for work, Frank conducted morning prayers upstairs with the family arranged kneeling around recumbent Bertha, as though for a death bed scene.

High tea was the main family meal of the day and not recalled as being anything particular, although Muriel had a fond memory of rabbit pie. Cake was a great treat and Sunday might see Bertha baking a family cake. Muriel recalled one such 'cake' her mother made, which was known in the family as a 'johnny cake' – composed of pastry with dried currants, sounding similar to an 'Eccles Cake', known in Jonathan's family as 'fly-cake': dried fruit resembling squashed insects. It would be interesting to know if Bertha's bore any relation to the Caribbean 'Johnny Cake', an unleavened, buttery fried bread treat, for the busy Liverpool ports and their multicultural populations were close by. Packed lunches were sandwiches with a scrimped, frugal filling and an apple; and Saturday saw a halfpenny for pocket money, quickly and merrily spent.

MURIEL:[3]   We would go to the sweetshop and gaze through the windows to see what we would get. We could get a piece of liquorish or a small stick of rock or a few sweets or a lollipop. I think I liked anything.

Christmas was a particularly happy occasion where Bertha and Frank put much thought into delighting their children.

MURIEL: On Christmas Eve we used to have a pillow case and put it in the front room on each chair in the siting room and the door would always be locked and then we'd go to bed. I can remember Daddy dressing up as Father Christmas and hearing him say, 'Have they been good girls?' and Mother saying 'Yes, Father Christmas'. We had wonderful Christmases, and we used to go into Mother and Daddy's bedroom and sing 'Christians Awake'. ...We always got one big present. ...We'd often have the same, like new bedroom slippers. I will never forget the year I got a bicycle, a second-hand sit-up-and-beg (bicycle). I was thrilled! They had painted it up. Audrey got a doll's house. We'd get lots of little presents, apple, orange and a penny or very often there would be a sweet mouse. They were a great treat.

The prudent and patient frugality of these parents was rewarded yearly with a family Christmas that seems as nostalgically charming as anything Charles Dickens could delight his readers with. Christmas in the Chalkley household was a truly wonderful time, unspoilt by excess, jaded palates or entitled demands. Not for them, the ubiquitous annual appearance in

Church for the once-a-year Christmas Eve Service (the only time in Britain when it is genuinely hard to find an empty church pew). The Chalkleys were steeped and fully dyed in the blood of the Lord: faith was not ornamental, optional or arbitrary, it was the Bread of Life itself.

Audrey spoke little of her childhood. She remembered[4] her Confirmation pride aged twelve and an early memory of being roped into collecting for mission charities aged five; shamefacedly having to jingle to her collection box under the noses of the neighbours, until she advanced to a more discreet notebook and pencil inventory. The Methodist Mission Society proved incredibly successful at raising millions of pounds for overseas missions via extensive networks of local associations collecting subscriptions large and small throughout the neighbourhoods (Prochaska, 2006). Moreover, Church missions were fully aware of how children's enthusiasms could be usefully harnessed for alms raising across denominations. An entire missionary publishing industry grew, aimed at tutoring British children into engaging with and supporting such missions based on morality tales of the benighted, needy brown children of the Empire and the benevolence of mission servants. Nice examples are the late 1930s story books produced by the Church of England Zenana Mission Society, such as *The Sugar-Cane Harvest and Other Stories of India* by Constance M. Bradley. British children were able to imagine what it might be like to be good-natured young Jaya, the outcaste 'Untouchable' boy, and the religious significance of his meeting with the 'Good Samaritan', here a Hindu to Christian convert. Or to appreciate the sharp contrasts of ignorance and knowledge positioning ineffective, local, folk superstition against effective, European medical expertise as found in the story of little Maya and her Hindu grandmother's conviction that the Smallpox Goddess will cure her.

> The doctor mem-sahib sat on a stool and tried to explain to Maya's mother and Raji what vaccination was for. She showed the marks on her own arm and on the nurse's and told them that very few people in England had smallpox after they were vaccinated.
>
> 'The bus driver said that even the King-Emperor and his children believe in this magic', exclaimed Raji. 'Is that true, Doctor?'
>
> (Bradley, 1938, p. 68)

A connection between the assumptions of Empire and Christian missions may seem not only quite apparent in these propaganda fables but indubitably established, judging from Bradley's simplistic penmanship. A construction of dyads is offered in these fables as wholesome fare, positioning what we would now term the 'First World' versus the 'Third'; the benighted versus the educated; magic versus science; squalor versus hygiene; heathen callousness versus Christian kindness. But also, caste exclusion versus faith inclusion; the one 'true' religion versus false gods. Certainly, this kind of reading does not stand the test of time well and where there are easy pickings here for those seeking to draw out and denounce the hegemony of Imperial mission. Yet there is something more going on as well, something quite subversive in its own way: the standard bearer for educated, competent, diligent philanthropy in remote and deprived foreign parts, this splendid, dedicated missionary is a woman and competent, trained physician. It must be said that the oppressive role of these white mission-enamoured memsahibs has been soundly rebuked as imperial cheerleaders (Forbes, 1994; Healey, 2013). Yet what a thrilling example to any young girl reader of the day, taking her far beyond the pretty organisation of the doll house, designed for early preparation of another later. Women too could emulate Livingstone as medical missionaries.

Regular church attendance marked the beginning of the girls' week, where a double shift to Sunday church was ordained, along with solid and realised expectations that the Chalkley daughters would soon step into their Sunday Teacher shoes. There was nothing unusual about attending Sunday School, very many children did. Anglican and Nonconformist Sunday schools opened in 1785 under the Sunday School Society, following the example by Robert Raikes who established the first in Gloucester five years before. Prochaska (2006) duly calculates that by 1915, there were 3,350 Schools operating with 275,000 children enrolled, with far more opening independently of the Society. Sunday Schools not only imparted religious knowledge and values through stories but also provided additional education to the young. Indeed, sometimes it had been the only education offered to children broken in early to waged work (Fraser, 2009).

Post-war Britain has seen a marked decline in church attendance, seriously eroding the social transmission of Christian paths for younger generations, leading to a yet further decline through loss of acculturation. Typically, the Archbishop of Atheism himself, Richard Dawkins (2006), views this demise as a very good thing and condemn religious education as a form of brainwashing child abuse. Others, like Bragg, a former Sunday School boy and child chorister, take issue with Dawkin's damning Manichean judgements of the evils of religion versus the good of atheism:

> But what if that 'indoctrination' is a form of teaching that helps children lead a happier and fuller life?
>
> (Bragg, 2011, p. 203)

Muriel believed that her upbringing, grounded in Christian Methodism, was not only an unquestionable good, but the best of all goodness, grounding her in a faith enabling her to extend loving service to others. She never for one moment viewed her schooling in faith as anything else than literally God sent. It was different for me. As I have written elsewhere, I was raised by troubled parents, poor things, who becoming militant atheists, like Dawkins, scoffing with panicky anger at any infantile interest in Christianity (Ashencaen Crabtree, 2021). For me, at five, such dismissal was experienced as an epistemological and episcopal injury. I have often come across similar levels of angry contempt towards religion and indeed people of faith, but normally from those that I have generally found to be rather unhappy folk, ill-at-ease with themselves and others; religious indifference or disinterest is another matter altogether. I affirm that something precious was denied to me when I was young by this concerted, misguided but probably well-meaning attempt to amputate an unvalidated sense of a numinous moral order in me. I think that had it been fostered or at least tolerated it would helped to anchor a sense of trusting and hopeful security in me, a sense of being eternally watched over and loved, which would have bolstered my endurance and courage to deal with too often an incomprehensible and punitive world. Muriel fortunately knew that beneficence. The Chalkley sisters were enveloped with the sense of a godly, cosmic order held by a loving and capable family, set within a community of corporate and corporal predictability, where if you were obedient, kind, diligent and good little harm was likely to befall you, but if it did God's ineffable comfort remained.

A holy death

Muriel and her elder sister, Betty (Bertha Elizabeth), were six years apart in age and therefore for that alone it is unsurprising that Muriel could not remember too much about their shared childhood. She could recall two memories, although one may have been overlaid by what Bertha told her, but the other was distinct in her mind. The first, being given a mishap of a piggyback by Betty, who fell on her face and banged her nose hard on the floor, because, heroically, she refused to save herself from the fall but held on tight to the plump legs of her little sister. The second, a clearer memory, was told to me thus

MURIEL:[5]   Dorothy and Audrey – they were amusing themselves and I was on my own. Betty took me to cubby hole under the stairs and she drew pictures with me and amused me. I was four. It was her kindness to amuse me because it was a rainy day. I think she would have been a lovely girl.

Betty died in January 1928 in her twelfth year and the quorum of sisters shrank to three. Many families lost a child to death; indeed, the reprobate William and Eliza had lost their eldest daughter, Elizabeth Ethel, aged eight in 1897. Such child losses were by then, if no longer very commonplace sorrows, certainly in a world, pre-antibiotics, not unusual. Betty's death, however, was, as is the loss of any child, tragic, but in her case, particularly horrific. At the same time, how Betty died is also subject to uncertainties, confusions and possibly some obfuscations, remaining unresolved to this day. There are at least two versions of Betty's death of which I am aware held by different relatives, neither of whom witnessed what occurred and each of whom was entirely unaware of the other version. It is not unlikely that within the mythologising families create there are several other versions that circulated; but which is the true version remains unestablished.

There are certain details shared across the two versions: a child on her way home from school; schoolmates at the station; a terrible train accident, the role of a fatal hockey stick; a deathbed hymn. Apart from that the two versions oppose each other, throwing up explanations, understandings and contradictions charged with attitudes, beliefs and ideologies. The two versions of the story I heard at different intervals, the first version was that of Muriel who inferred that she received it from her parents, although whether that was one or the other, separately or together, I do not know. Muriel related this version on other occasions too, never varying in its essence or general details. The second version I heard only once and that years later from a younger member of the family descended from Dorothy, who herself was only two years younger than Betty to whom she was close. Neither Muriel nor Dorothy nor their parents nor any other relative of theirs, so far as it known, witnessed what really happened that day.

Version 1. Muriel's account.

Betty was tragically killed on the railways when Muriel was four years-old.[6] Mother was cooking tea ready for Betty when she got home from Chester grammar school, for Betty was a clever girl who had won the scholarship and this was her first term at the school. To get home Betty had to travel from Chester to the Port Sunlight station by train.

There was a group of girls in the train compartment, Betty's friends. For whatever reason they decided to find an empty carriage at a junction (implying there were others, strangers perhaps, in the carriage they occupied). There was an empty train at the junction they alighted at, which was being linked to the one that they were in and this was in the process of backing up for the link-up. Upon finding the carriage the girls chose, Betty, being a helpful girl, held the train door open for the others to get in first. The train suddenly jerked as it started up. Betty still holding the carriage door and unseen by the driver tripped over her hockey stick, and fell on the lines as the train started. The train ran over her lower legs, one was completely amputated by the wheels and the foot on the other leg was virtually severed and hanging off. Betty did not lose consciousness when the railway workers 'threw her' on a railway trolley and rushed her to Chester Infirmary.

Bertha at home was cooking potato cakes for high tea, quite unaware what had happened, there being no telephone in ordinary homes in those days. It was Frank who knew first, having taken a phone call at the Lever Brothers, where someone phoned him from the pub to tell him what had happened. Muriel was told she had to go and stay with her aunt.

Betty lived for three days in the hospital with her parents sitting beside her bed. She was aware of what had happened and said to her mother, 'I left a leg on the line, didn't I?' She died of shock, but just before she died, she sang 'Jesus loves me, this I know'. Then she simply turned her head and looked at one parent and then the other on either side of the bed, closed her eyes and just went.

MURIEL:[7]   She was a very popular girl, a leader in the Girl Guides, and the Guides carried her coffin at the funeral. There was a photograph of them carrying Betty. She was a clever girl, a caring girl, was Betty'.

Version 2. A family member's account.

Betty was going home from school. She was on the platform waiting for the train to approach and the lads (schoolboys) were chasing her around her hockey stick, messing about. She tripped over the hockey stick and fell on the tracks in front of the train, severing both legs. In the hospital the child was in terrible agony. It was Frank who made her sing 'Jesus wants me for a sunbeam' when she was dying. Bertha was appalled by this act and never forgave him.

In considering these two versions, what are we to make of such discrepancies? While there may be such a thing as an objective truth, we have no hope of recovering that now but can only retreat into a post-structural uncovering of the underlying, dominating meanings in these discourses, supported by the established facts: a dreadful railway accident, a fatal fall, a mutilated and dying child. Our minds can furnish the rest: the gory horror, the screaming children, white-faced passengers, horrified railway workers, the shouts and blowing whistles, the clatter of trolleys, the urgent dash of nurses and doctors, morphia and cold instruments. The hammer blow of the terrible news on a work telephone – 'Chalkley Repairs!'; weeping, overwhelmed, wild-eyed parents; confused, frightened siblings parcelled off to shocked relatives.

Betty in Muriel's version is fatally maimed through performing an act appropriate to a generous, polite and virtuous girl: she holds the carriage door open for her friends to pass to safety first, before taking her seat at what was a precarious juncture in their journey. In the second version, Betty is being a silly, heedless schoolgirl cavorting with the boys, oblivious to caution as the train approaches. The train itself is either stationary and then setting off; or is otherwise approaching the station and about to stop. In one version, Betty seems to be pulled onto the tracks by the train departing and in another, she falls on the tracks as the train comes in. In one scenario, we can imagine railway workers busily linking the train carriages together at the platform and vaguely perhaps aware of the children nearby. Or there are no railway guards on the platform and only an unobservant driver.

The development of each narrative also tallies with the positionalities of the narrator and how they, in turn, position poor Betty. Dorothy, from whom this unnamed family member claimed version 2, was, as Muriel described, popular, sporty, vivacious and pretty. She evidently liked boys and they her. She met her child sweetheart, 'Bran' Davidson at the age of fourteen and married him in 1940; when a widow, she happily remarried. Muriel by contrast, never gravitated towards male company, she never married and her relationship with men was kept to the chaste and collegial. The 'Betty' actor conforms to one of these two female dyads in these constructed narratives.

One most interesting detail refers to the hymn that Betty in both versions sang. The hymns differ, 'Jesus Wants Me for a Sunbeam' of version 2 is not the same song as 'Jesus Loves Me, This I Know', although they can both be easily found on the Internet today as saccharine-sweet, twee hymns aimed at transatlantic child audiences. 'Jesus Loves Me' has a deeper and darker history, being written by American hymnologist, Anna Barnett Warner in the mid-nineteenth century. The verses were swiftly appropriated in a novel written by her sister, Susan Warner (1860) for a deathbed scene of a child, 'little Johnny'. The aptness of these verses in such a heart-breaking context is clearly apparent; but while lending more credibility to Muriel's relating of events in version 1, it does not mean it was so.

Jesus loves me – loves me still,
Though I'm very weak and ill;
From his shining throne on high,
Comes to watch me where I lie.
Jesus loves me – he will stay
Close beside me all the way.
Then his little child will take
Up to heaven for his dear sake

We must ask ourselves then, is it *really* possible that Betty, so terribly injured in such a traumatic and agonising accident, could *actually* have voluntarily sung anything to her grieving parents just before she died of shock? Then again, is it possible that Frank, such a devoted, caring father, could really have forced his cruelly injured, dying child to sing hymns – and that against the wishes of his distraught wife? Either seems hopelessly implausible. Alternative ideas present: is it more likely therefore that these tormented parents so wished to hear their beloved eldest child singing her way to heaven that they simply chose to believe that she had done so? If version 2 is correct, could Bertha have continued to live with Frank if she really held such a deep and terrible grudge against him? Maybe, for many wives of the age did live with despised husbands. The opportunities for earning a living as a married woman with children to support but without any employment experience were poor at best during the depredations of the Depression. So, let us stretch our imagination further and permit the possibility, however slight, that in fact Betty did die in such innocent grace, as version 1 tells us. Noble, brave, altruistic, 'good deaths'; are far from unknown in our human history; and God willing we will also die a good death of our choosing. Then too, the imminently dying often no longer feel terrible physical pain in the same way as they did before, as I have witnessed myself, so maybe Betty *was* one of these blessed mortals who could die such a death.

Some of just these possibilities are mutually exclusive: they cannot all be true. It comes down to what we *choose* to believe and what we can *bear* to believe. So, which assumed reality we pick tells us less about one girl's death and far more about ourselves: how we perceive the world and its actors, their outer and inner motivations, as well as our inter-relational positionalities in it.

Methodists were good at death-bed scenes. So too were the later Victorians, with what has been seen in contemporary times as the maudlin and macabre fetishising of death, particularly when coupled to the new technology of photography; despite the whole-scale graphic photo-documentarising of modern lives, however mundane or intimate. The Romantic Movement was similarly obsessed with the untimely deaths of the young, beautiful and talented. The realities of brief lives were much more visible then than now. The example of John Wesley's death reminded all Methodists that this was not only the portal to eternal life for believers, but as offering glorious opportunities to engage wholeheartedly in dying an exemplary Christian death (Hempton, 2005). Nor were innocently pious children excluded from practising a holy Methodist death, serving as examples of Christian trusting faith and fortitude to the inevitable.

Nearly all younger children begin by looking up to the elder siblings, and sometimes that easy superiority is well-deserved. Even in her nineties,

Muriel remembered Betty's death, as it was told to her, as utter tragedy, but of equal weight, illuminated by the transformational wonder of its holiness. Maybe Muriel's understanding of her so admirable sister's parting was flawed by inaccuracies. Perhaps if the facts had been skewed somewhere down the line, it was done so either unconsciously or deliberately to desperately construct a portrait that partially comforted and compensated for the horror. In this way, an enduring familial Methodist iconography was provided that could be held onto to ease the pain of the loss of this most promising and beloved first-born.

Schooled for labour

Of all her three sisters, Muriel was the only one not to receive a good school education; this she held as entirely owing to her own personal deficiencies. The state grammar school behaved graciously and bestowed on Dorothy, Betty's scholarship. Probably Dorothy would have won the scholarship on her own merit anyway, but it was a generous gesture nonetheless, indicating how far Betty's death affected the community. Bertha then prevailed upon the family to uproot themselves and move away from Port Sunlight. Maybe the memories of former happiness were too painful to endure, or perhaps it was neighbourly sympathy that did it. Port Sunlight, after all, was by design a place where one's neighbour was also a co-worker, so self-imposed moments of oblivion through the monotony of work and the mindlessness of domestic chores would have been rare; and always there was the pity to endure. Muriel justified the move to Little Sutton, a pleasant village in the Wirral, six stops down the railways tracks towards the city of Chester, as her mother's bid for a much-needed change of scenery, and where the family tragedy would have been less known of, if at all. Another explanation offered claimed that this enabled the precious second child to catch the bus to school rather than ill-fated train. Who could argue with a mother over such latter reasoning under these circumstances? At any rate, the family moved to a three-bedroomed terraced house, and which, in turn, years later was bought by Dorothy and her young husband, the multi-talented Bran, who was not only a signpost painter and decorator, but could play the ukulele and compose hilarious recited monologues; ran a Methodist Sunday School and the Methodist Youth Orchestra; and won the highest trophy awarded for amateur dramatics: a mantelpiece ornament of a performing seal on wheels balancing a revolving ball on its head. Marvellous stuff!

As soon as she was old enough, Muriel also took the bus to Chester to attend school, this being the Hunter Street Central School. This school originated from an amalgam of mixed schooling provision for working-class children in the local area. Its roots also lay in the old Chester Ragged

Schools of the early 1850s, supplemented by Sunday School education. But its pedigree was equally derived from the 1918 Education Act under Prime Minister, Lloyd George, raising the leaving age to fourteen, abolishing fees for elementary schools and ensuring that central government funds contributed to at least half the cost of local education (Timmins, 2017). By 1894, this school had been elevated to one for girls with an educational provision that was a cut above the lower levels of schooling, although still below the calibre of the grammar school system that Muriel's sisters enjoyed.

Muriel was far from proud of her academic abilities and regarded herself as something of a 'dunce' at school. As she often repeated, English composition she was good at, but 'sums' were her Waterloo. Her failure in this regard, which seems to have been a view shared by her family, helped to establish her hapless trajectory at school.

The family moved yet again this time going up-market to buy a bigger, solid-looking newly built semi-detached house, number 293, Spital Road, in the Wirral town of Bromborough, an easy cycle ride for Frank to Port Sunlight. Unbeknownst to the family, down the same road the Congregationalist neighbours' son had just gone off to study philosophy, politics and economics (PPE) at Jesus College, University of Oxford. Neither Muriel nor, I believe, her older sisters, ever recognised this exceptionally brilliant, cherubic-cheeked young man, nursing great political aspirations, to be the future Labour Party British Prime Minister, Harold Wilson (Thomas-Symonds, 2022).

The Wilson family rented their Victorian conversion flat in Spiral Road off the father's employers, the Brotherton's Chemical Company, but the Chalkley family were higher on the property ladder. The purchase of one's own home has been a strong and realistic aspiration for Britons in the twentieth century; although a failing one for younger generations by the twenty-first, and by the same token it was an unusually ambitious step to take in the 1930s, However, it was also entirely in line with the embourgeoisement of Methodists, whose doctrine of thrift, simplicity, temperance, diligence and honest hard work made for fiscal prudence. Such virtues, which politicians keenly promote as good 'family values', gradually, pushed Methodist families towards achieving not only spiritual but material comfort, demarcating them as naturally finding their level in the respectable and stolid middle-classes (Hempton, 2005).

The move to Bromborough facilitated Frank's journey, but Muriel was now further away from the Hunter Street Central School and, given the choice between staying there and facing a longer bus journey, or going to the inferior, Elementary Council-run school round the corner, she was unwisely permitted to choose the latter, because, as she said, she 'was not clever'. A case of a self-fulfilling prophecy, if ever there was, for attending the Council school did nothing to raise Muriel's opinion of herself. All for her life, Muriel had a decided inferiority complex about her intelligence, always comparing herself with humble awe to the intellectually very able Audrey.

In common with most children who went through the Elementary school system, Muriel left school at fourteen with no formal qualifications to her name; although such basic education offered none anyway, and therefore precluded the opportunity for either exam passes or failures. Muriel was fortunate in some ways as her parents' generation often left school at twelve and it was only in 1918 in England and Wales that the school-leaving age was raised, a privilege enjoyed by Scottish children since the turn of the century (Bochel and Daly 2009).

Although denominational churches had sought to impress their stamp upon the education of children along sectarian lines (Smith, 2010b), neither Muriel nor her sisters received a Nonconformist school education, beyond their Methodist Sunday Schools. Both the grammar and Central schools, each run by the State, were stamped with the Establishment Church of England association. It seemed to do them no harm as it was not school but the enveloping Methodist ecology of home and church where grounding socio-religious values were deeply imbibed, mandating the necessity and the nobility of labour.

An old photograph found in Muriel's muddled collection. Here she is standing in the front garden wearing a little girl's floral summer frock and white ankle socks, looking every bit the undeveloped child that she still was at fourteen. At this age, Muriel was sent out to work to help financially support her family, and the most obvious source for a weekly pay packet was back at Lever Bros. Her first job was in the 'Tin Box Department', standing in a factory line performing a single task, over and over again, involving finishing off the cardboard cylinders that eventually would be filled with the harsh, scouring soap I remember my own houseproud mother using to punish our kitchen sinks and bathtubs to a relentless shine. For Muriel, it was a horrible and boring job.

MURIEL:[8]   The 'Vim' containers used to have a slit in the lid, which you put your knife in. Behind the slit was sticky paper, and my job was to glue on the paper that covered the slit on the lid. My hands would be covered by glue when I came home. It was terribly noisy – and there were big machines filling the tube with the Vim really near us – and you had this clanging noise nearby. I was fourteen and I did that job for a year – monotonous, tiring because you were standing all day, but it was a job and we needed the money.

Memories and narratives are shaped by the underlying power of discourse where, as we have already seen, particular themes and positions come to the fore. Perhaps therefore it is not altogether surprising that in regards to Muriel, the little factory worker, a different, anonymised hand-me-down recollection circulates in the family to set beside her account.

> Frank told his daughter that she there was nothing for it but for her to go to work in the factory. It was felt that Muriel never forgave her father for that and that she always complained that she had to "stand all day and my hands were red raw".

To me, and I fully admit to a partial and partisan view, Muriel never expressed anything other than comic horror when recounting this first job. If she ever had felt resentment for being thrust into the commonplace miseries of women's unskilled labour so abruptly at such a young age, she showed no trace of it; even if Frank had most likely been instrumental in finding her this monotonous work.

Some begrudging therefore might certainly have been natural, particularly as Muriel was clearly aware of the great contrast between the expectations for girls in the thirties compared to those today. She regularly asked after my work and family, taking a shine to Jonathan and our young daughters, the 'baby' being only twelve at the time, as well as delighting in the basket of kittens I playfully brought round for a visit. She knew full well that my girls were receiving an excellent education and would not leave school until reaching woman's estate. She would often quiz me about their futures, asking what their plans were for when they left school, meaning of course, waged work. It was a difficult question to answer satisfactorily, as we spoke across a generational gulf of expectations regarding formal education and milestones, today ticked off by essential exam results and qualifications. The career life prospects for fourteen-year-old girls now might make those of their counterparts in the 1930s seem threadbare by comparison. Muriel treated it all with curiosity and amusement, even though some of my convoluted answers must have left her none the wiser. What she did know is that my daughter's childhood was allowed to unroll into distances far beyond her ken into that utterly remote, fabled domain: a university education.

For many of Muriel's new female workmates in 1936, wages meant the factory floor and the mechanised tempo of their lives would be measured by the routine clocking-in and clocking-out of the day's humdrum labour. Maybe that was sufficient for some and all that could be aspired to for others; there was probably little reason to think it could be otherwise for this gangly girl child.

Notes

1 Commoners had the right to graze their animals on 'common land'. A right still bestowed in limited parts of England like the ancient 'New Forest'.
2 Muriel Chalkley interview with author 29 October 2013.
3 Muriel Chalkley interviewed by author 29 October 2013.
4 British Library 'Sounds'. Audrey Chalkley interviewed by Caroline Ferris, 1994. Methodist Church Oral Archive. C640/044.
5 Muriel Chalkley, interview with Author. Ibid.
6 Muriel made an error, she was in fact six-years-old when Betty died.
7 Muriel Chalkley, interview with Author. Ibid.
8 Author's interview with Muriel Chalkley 2013.

References

Abrams, L. (2012) Story-telling, women's authority and the 'Old Wife's Tale': 'The story of the bottle of medicine'. *History Workshop Journal*, 73, 95–117.

Ashencaen Crabtree, S. (2021) *Women of Faith and the Quest for Spiritual Authenticity: Comparative Perspectives from Malaysia and Britain*. London/New York: Routledge.

Blythe, R. (1969) *Akenfield: Portrait of an English Village*. London: Penguin Books.

Bochel, H. and Daly, G. (2009) *Social Policy*, 3rd ed. London: Routledge.

Bradley, C.M. (1938) *Sugar-Cane Harvest and Other Stories of India*. London: The Zenith Press.

Bragg, M. (2011) *The Book of Books: The Radical Impact of the King James Bible, 1611–2011*. London: Hodden & Stoughton.

Bragg, M. (1999) *The Soldier's Return*. London: Sceptre.

Davidson, L. (2010) A quest for harmony: The role of music in Robert Owen's New Lanark community. *Utopian Studies*, 21(2), 232–251.

Dawkins, R. (2006) *The God Delusion*. London: Bantam.

Forbes, G. (1994) Medical careers and health care for Indian women: Patterns of control. *Women's History Review*, 3(4), 515–530.

Fraser, D. (2009) *The Evolution of the British Welfare State*. Houndsmill, Basingstoke: Palgrave Macmillan.

Gillett, M. (1978) *Wandering in Talbot Village: A Study of Philanthropy in the Nineteenth Century*. Bournemouth: Bournemouth Local Studies Publication.

Hattersley, R. (2014) *John Wesley A Brand from the Burning*. London: Abacus.

Healey, M. (2013) *Indian Sisters: A History of Nursing and the Estate, 1907–2007*. London: Routledge.

Hempton, D. (2005) *Methodism: Empire of the Spirit*. New Haven, CT: Yale

Henson, D.F. (2017) Fragments and fiction: An autoethnography of past and possibility. *Qualitative Inquiry*, 23(3), 221–224.

Hubbard, E., and Shippobottom, M. (2003) *A Guide to Port Sunlight*. Liverpool: Liverpool University Press.

Jeremy, D.J. (1991) The enlightened paternalist in action: William Hesketh Lever at Port Sunlight before 1914. *Business History*, 33(1), 58–81, https://doi.org/10.1080/00076799100000004

Le Corbusier (2007) *Toward an Architecture*. Translated by John Goodman. Los Angeles, CA: Getty Research Institute.

Liverpool Schools. Available at: http://www.liverpool-schools.co.uk/html/history.html [Accessed 18 March 2022].

Maslen, J. (2013) Autobiographies of a generation? Carolyn Steedman, Luisa Passerini and the memory of 1968. *Memory Studies*, 6(1), 23–36.

McEvoy, L. (2010) *Corset and Codes at Spirella in Letchworth. Great British Life*. Available at: https://www.greatbritishlife.co.uk/homes-and-gardens/places-to-live/corsets-and-codes-at-spirella-in-letchworth-7086106 [Accessed 18 March 2022].

McQueen, A. (2011) *The King of Sunlight: How William Lever Cleaned up the World*. London: Corgi.

Miller, A.J. (1996) *Old Bournemouth: The Story of the Bourne Tregonwell Estate*. Bournemouth: Bournemouth Local Studies Publications.

Orwell, G. (1937, 2001) *The Road to Wigan Pier*. London: Penguin.

Parker, J. (2023) *Analysing the History of British Social Welfare: Compassion, Coercion and beyond*. Bristol: Policy Press.

Prochaska, F. (2006) *Christianity and Social Services in Modern Britain: The Disinherited Spirit*. Oxford: Oxford University Press.

Rowan, J.D. (2003) *Imagining corporate culture: the industrial paternalism of William Hesketh Lever at Port Sunlight, 1888–1925*. PhD Dissertation. Louisiana State University.

Smith, A. (2010a) Discourses of morality and truth in social welfare: The surveillance of British widows of the First World War. *Social Semiotics*, 20(5), 519–535. https://doi.org/10.1080/10350330.2010.513187

Smith, J.T. (2010b) Ecumenism, economic necessity and the disappearance of Methodist elementary schools in England in the twentieth century. *History of Education*, 39(5), 631–657.

Thompson, E.P. (1963) *The Making of the English Working Classes*. New York: Vintage Books.

Thomas-Symonds, N. (2022) *Harold Wilson: The Winner*. London: Weidenfeld & Nicolson.

Timmins, N. (2017) The *Five Giants*. London: William Collins.

Vallely, P. (2020) *Philanthropy*. London: Bloomsbury Continuum.

Ward, S.V. (1990) The garden city tradition re-examined. *Planning Perspective*, 5(3), 249–256. https://doi.org/10.1080/02665439008725706

Warner, S. (1860) *Say and Seal*. Philadelphia, PA: J.B. Lippincott & Co.

Woodruff, W. 2002. *The Road to Nabb End*. London: Eland Publishing.

4 War, mercy, hope and charity

Faith and health

Thematically nursing and religious piety are inseparably clasped in the Chalkley story; one cannot be severed from another: the heart from the hand, the compulsion from the action (Galvin and Todres, 2009). This conjoining of motive to motor is certainly not true of nursing today, an altogether much more secularised business. Individuals may hold a faith but this should be kept strictly away from the workplace and removed in the locker-room metamorphoses of private citizen to nurse. If anything, British 'caring services' of nursing and social work can be actively hostile towards religious beliefs in its staff, with Christianity usually receiving the sternest finger-wagging. Wordsworth's (2015) pleading for a transatlantic British Parish nursing model pointed to a recent case of a community nurse suspended by the UK Nurses and Midwifery Council for offering to pray with a patient.

Although religion is banished from State welfare vocations, they bear deep roots planted in the rich soil of a pervasive religious ambience of English society with its ancient traditions of hospitality and care of the needy (Parker, 2023; Payne, 2005; Prochaska, 2006). The formative years of the Chalkley sisters came at a time of social reform seeking to push beyond individual philanthropy towards reliance on state intervention.

The early twentieth century in Britain was an extraordinary period of social transformation commencing with the Liberals' victory in the General Election in 1906, ousting a decade of Conservative Party rule, thereby enabling the early paving towards a future welfare state (Sullivan, 1996). Miniaturised against these vast upheavals of the interim war years, the Chalkley lives merit magnification, positioning their service within the socio-political mechanics of a fast-changing world of cradle-to-grave welfare provision under Beveridge's sweeping social reforms. This would deliver the National Health Service (NHS) in 1948, under the steely negotiations of 'Nye' Bevan, the Welsh coal-miner's son, and Minister for Health in Clement Atlee's Labour government (Parker, 2023)

DOI: 10.4324/9781003359746-4

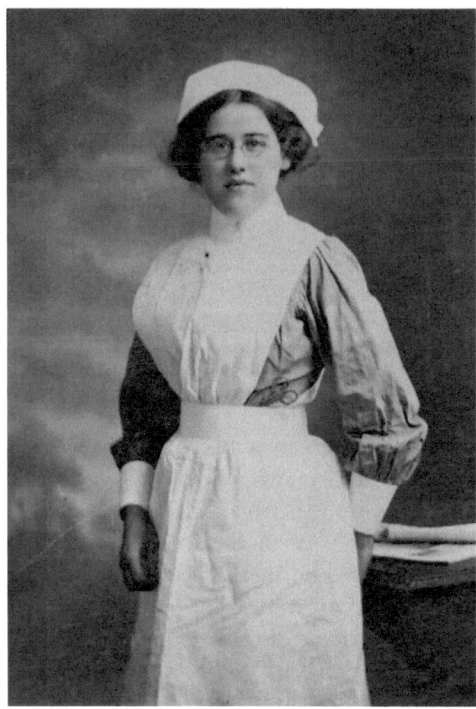

Figure 4.1 Sister Mercy Chalkley. Courtesy of Muriel Chalkley.

Mercy and the war

The youngest of William and Eliza Chalkley's brood, Margaret, was said by family to have been 'humbly' employed; and where we soon lose sight of her in the public records. Mercy, Frank's second younger sister, was quite another matter. A faded, undated photograph shows Mercy, bespectacled and authoritative in a starched nursing uniform, where at the beginning of the First World War, she served in Wrexham Infirmary as a nurse (Figure 4.1).

By 1917, she had moved to another hospital in Garston in South Liverpool, very likely the Sir Alfred Jones Memorial Hospital, which treated the war wounded. By 1918, we find she has moved to a nursing home on elegant Gambier Terrace opposite Liverpool Cathedral. This home may also have nursed seriously incapacitated servicemen. Wilfred Owen's poem 'Disabled' penned in 1917 reminds us of what this could mean:

Some cheered him home, but not as crowds cheer Goal.
Only a solemn man who brought him fruits

Thanked him; and then inquired about his soul.
Now, he will spend a few sick years in Institutes,
And do what things the rules consider wise,
And take whatever pity they may dole.
To-night he noticed how the women's eyes
Passed from him to the strong men that were whole.
How cold and late it is! Why don't they come
And put him into bed? Why don't they come?

For further details of the horror of nursing during the Great War we must turn to Vera Brittain's (1933, 1978) celebrated autobiography and published diaries like that of Sister Edith Appleton's (Cowen, 2012), both being nurses on the Front Line. Suffice to say here, had Mercy been involved in war injury care, as I believe, the impetus for her sharp change of direction is understandable. For by 1919, she was now training for midwifery, gaining her CMB in 1920 where she remained on the Midwives Roll of 1904–1959.

The year 1919 was a pivotal time in the history of British nursing, heralding the Nurses' Registration Act of that year. This had been strenuously lobbied for by a deputation of diverse nursing organisations, including the British Nurses' Association, the Matron's Council, The Registered Nurses' Professional Council, the National Union of Trained Nurses, the Fever Nurses' Association, not forgetting the College of Nursing and the Professional Union of Trained Nurses (The Hospital, 1921). The delay in the implementation of the act was attributed to the difficulty in agreeing on nursing standards between England and Scotland. Eventually, the act would be an important step towards the professionalisation of nursing, establishing State regulation of nurses' working hours and duties; yet standardisation was uneven, with those in the voluntary hospital sector remaining unregulated (Palmer, 2014).

Nonetheless, this was an important beginning for a role hitherto viewed as elementary and integral to the very notion of womanhood, one undertaken in the domestic or neighbourhood sphere. Now nursing as a recognised skilled vocation would set women nurses apart from their sisters through state and cabalistic recognition of their novitiate superiority.

The transition from lay to professional nurse was a pivotal point, emerging from a prolonged patchwork history reflecting the fragmentary, unmonopolised nature of health care in Britain, up to that point. The connection of religious practice and nursing care had been long established across Europe under monastic and convent orders housing the skills of the healer and herbalist. The Reformation under Henry VIII ripped away the ancient mantle of these godly traditions and local healing practices (Payne, 2005). Yet in Protestant, Victorian Britain, the linkage between piety and care was implicit, as was gendered essentialisation of the drudgery of such work, directing women thus employed to the uncounted legions of impoverished, slum-dwelling sick. It was from these ranks that nursing attendants might be found among such communities of deprivation. The late Georgian, early Victorian depictions of nursing were, however, not reassuring images of compassionate, proficient probity. Mrs Poole in *Jane Eyre* is the ignorant and coarse keeper of the mad Mrs Rochester growling in the attic. Mrs Poole's Dickensian counterpart, Sarah Gamp, in *Martin Chuzzlewit* deals in both laying-in and laying-out with equal drunken aplomb (Dickens, 1944, 2004; Healey, 2013; Prochaska, 2006). Ruth, the fallen woman, in Elizabeth Gaskell's (1853) eponymous novel, is a different, more refined creature, redeeming her sinful past by sacrificing her life devotedly nursing an epidemic-struck community, to which till then she has been a stigmatised outsider. Ruth's qualification to nurse is not raised in the novel, for it is her feminine ministration and prayful selflessness that marks her competent. From a heedless Magdalene, Ruth's path to salvation via social acceptability is that of a modest, healing nun.

Appropriately such images were promoted among the London-based Protestant Sisters of Charity, later known as the 1840 'Mrs Fry's Institute for Nursing' together with Ellen Ranyard's 1868 'Bible nurses'. The respectable working classes were the recruiting ground for such nurses and the proposed uniform of dark gown, flannel apron and a tin basin tied around their waists indicated basic, unadorned, female service where carbolic soap hygiene, plain nutritious fare, blankets and patent medicines were their treatments (Prochaska, 2006). The sartorial transformation of dowdy nun-like habits to the twentieth century's smart, militia-type uniforms indicated profound shifts in the religio-social positionality of nursing as a secularised profession (Prochaska, 2006).

The hospital system in England and Wales was a tripartite system that would have been familiar to the Chalkley family. Firstly, there was the privately owned institution for private fee-paying patients; second, there were the voluntary hospitals: those institutions funded by philanthropy and maintained by public subscriptions. Finally, there were public facilities, which had arisen out of the old Poor Law system, and were owned and maintained by municipalities and paid for out of public rates (Gorsky, 2020). Bertha Chalkley believed that because her favourite game was tending a ward of sickly toys, had young Betty lived, she too would have become a nurse. Her three sisters eventually did. Muriel and her surviving sisters would all work with a varied, interspersed but not necessarily interlocking nexus of healthcare up to and following, albeit briefly, the post–Second World War period.

Both Harris (2004) and Porter (1992) argue that the benighted state of health care prior to the monolithic NHS was much exaggerated by its proponents. It is certainly the case that health provision was fragmentary and in need of improvement. The aftermath of the Great War focused attentions on the state of the nation's health with a number of welfare-focused Acts of Parliament arising and the creation of the Ministry of Health in 1919, with notable medical advances made in the interwar period, not least owing to war causalities (Harris, 2004). Timmins (2017) calculates that prior to the Great War, there were 1,334 voluntary hospitals and 1,771 municipal hospitals, but following that the voluntary hospital sector expanded considerably. These voluntary hospitals were hugely varied in capacity and focus, including among their number the large English teaching hospitals holding 500 beds or so, as well as the homely, cottage hospital' that held a mere handful. Old cottage hospitals (often handsome Victorian brick edifices) can still be found all over the country, having been harnessed into NHS service as community clinics for specialist outpatient services.

Municipal hospitals under the local authorities were equally a mixed but inferior bag of health provision containing lunatic asylums, 'fever' and tuberculosis wards (Timmins, 2017), together with various acute, chronic and maternity cases (Porter, 1992). The voluntary hospitals were considered superior to the municipal ones, tainted as the latter were with associations of the old Poor Law welfare care. Consultants and other medical specialists donated their time to the voluntary hospitals *gratis* being subsidised by their private practices, these hospitals tending to operate within urban conurbations. Porter (1992) contends that the voluntary hospitals covered only a minority of health care compared to the municipal institutions upon which the majority of patients relied. Thus, contesting the argument later put forward to justify the establishment of the NHS that both hospitals and general practitioners (GP) were resources unfairly concentrated in affluent locations like Kensington and Bournemouth.

Fees and philanthropy: pre-NHS

Mercy belonged to this changing era of occupational liminality where nursing then was a career wedded to spinsterhood; married nurses would only be more commonly found from the 1940s onwards. Mercy did eventually succumb to the married state. A late marriage was made at the age of forty-two in 1934 to Norman Cardwell. In the same year, she left nursing, with an unimpeachable professional reputation intact, her conduct and work being described on nursing records as 'excellent'. Whether Mercy continued to serve in any particular capacity in the Second World War is uncertain, but as a role model to the growing Chalkley girls her position was assured, where none of the surviving sisters opted for the more traditional housewife route of their own mother.

During these interwar years, Dorothy, now the eldest, set an example by following in Aunt Mercy's footsteps, gaining nursing qualifications and work in both municipal and voluntary hospital settings. Soon married, she stepped into what would become the forerunner of the later occupational health sector by becoming an 'industrial nurse for the gas board', as Muriel and Audrey put it.

Taking German Bismarckian social insurance concepts to heart, Lloyd George had brought the British version to the public, introduced in the Parliamentary Bill of 1911 (Parker, 2023). The new British scheme was aptly coined as the 'ninepence for fourpence' health insurance scheme, in which the insured employee was asked to pay in fourpence, their employer three-pence and the State twopence (Sullivan, 1996). This provided weekly sickness benefit, a disability benefit and a maternity allowance (Harris, 2004). Large employers (like the Gas Board and the Lever Bros.) also provided medical surgeries for their workers, a sensible investment where workers were unlikely to change employment on a whim; although the new social insurance scheme carried limited cover for the insured, and as for their dependents they would need to shift for themselves (Sullivan, 1996).

The role model Mercy offered may have made nursing an obvious choice to her nieces. Although skilled, trained work like nursing was not the readiest means of contributing to a greedy family purse. It was, however, a vocation that was appropriate to the aspirations of grammar school girls of modest but respectable means for whom some kind of waged work was a necessity. Audrey, for instance, was the kind of intellectually gifted girl many grammar schools of the day might encourage to aim high, and indeed she suggests this was so. Unquestionably, she was of university calibre in those days, well before mass education, when only a tiny fraction of the population had an undergraduate degree. However, such illustrious edification likely to secure a prosperous future seems not to have been considered.

AUDREY:[1]   As soon as I was through high school at the age of sixteen, I left; although I was offered opportunity to go on to higher studies. But I felt the family needed my help financially, so I left and got an office job and... learnt to type... at the Stork Margarine works. It was only a ten- or fifteen-minute walk from home.

University was not an ambition that the Chalkley family seriously entertained for their daughters, if thought of at all. Gender may have played an important part in this decision, for some men from deprived working-class backgrounds, like William Woodruff for example, did attain a university education and more, but then he did not come from a Nonconformist background. While the Wesley brothers and their Holy Group were products of the Oxford elite, academic life, the Methodist revolution was not one nurtured in rarefied enclaves generally. Rather the very essence of Methodism in its emphasis on the heart and spirit was one that turned its back on the Enlightenment intellectualism and abstract reasoning. It was not so much *thinking* as *feeling* that fired Methodist passion.

For all of John Wesley's engrossment with and tinkering of theological complexities, emergent Methodism did not appear to offer theologically sophisticated beliefs nor was it an arcane esotericism guarded solely by priesthood. Instead, it offered a counter position of overturned hierarchies and speaking to the heart; to the sensibility and raw experiences of the underprivileged and the ordinary working woman and man, whether they could read and write, or not. Once the split from the Church of England and thereby the state was made, it inevitably meant Methodists like other Nonconformists were excluded from the very Establishment's academic milieu where originally Methodist beliefs had been seeded.

Although Primitive Methodists particularly embraced those from the humblest backgrounds, including women as religious leaders in their own right, the progress towards embourgeoisement, integral to early Methodist values, eventually elevated the social class demographics of its followers (Field, 1997). Nevertheless, with some exceptions, exemplified by E.P. Thompson, a perversely thorny outcrop from a cultivated Methodist family branch (Hempton, 2005), university education, now possible, seems to have lain beyond the aspirations of modern, gifted Methodists like Audrey. Both sisters independently declared that their teenage wages were required to supplement the family income. Although there is no reason to think this to be untrue, daughters leaving school for the workforce, were not commonly associated with the home-owning classes like the Chalkleys.

At any rate, a year was quite enough for Muriel at the Tin Box Department and when another aunt, probably Margaret, mentioned that her friend, the cook of a 'children's' home in a poor part of Liverpool spoke of a vacancy, Muriel, so fond of children, felt this offered a step up and out. The job meant leaving home, like many another domestic 'tweeny' under-servant, which is in fact what she was promptly turned into. The 'home' turned out to be a warehouse for the infants of women in menial employment. Muriel was given charge of twelve unkempt toddlers in an endless round of refereeing infantile thuggery, cleaning, feeding and potty training with few breaks to restore her wits and where her meals were incessantly interrupted by demands; an obese nursery nurse indolently overseeing these struggles from the comfort of her chair. As the youngest assistant Muriel's job was to rise early in the morning to light all the coal fires; exhausted at night, she shared one bed with a light-fingered bully who foisted her own work upon the girl and mocked her mercilessly when Muriel was caught poring over Bible. Not surprisingly, it was all downhill from there.

MURIEL:[2]   I was working far too hard. I didn't last long…I lost weight and was having a breakdown. I loved the children but I remember standing at a window and feeling I wanted to throw myself through it. I was too young and it was too hard.

It was Muriel's friends who galvanised Bertha into maternal action by warning her that Muriel looked terrible: thin and ill. She was returned home in a wretched state and ushered to bed by the doctor, being suspected of having contracted tuberculosis or on the verge of it. Three months of complete rest were prescribed owing to her complete mental and physical prostration.

This was not the first occasion of serious illness Muriel experienced in her childhood and where her parents' grasp of the seriousness of the situation seemed slow off the mark. There was, as we have seen, a serious financial implication involved in seeking medical care, so much so that this punctuated a popular playground skipping song, still in use years after the NHS was established. From memory, I quote one version here:

Miss Polly had a dolly who was sick, sick, sick
Call for the doctor quick, quick, quick
The doctor came
With his high, high hat
And he knocked on the door
With a rat-a-tat-tat.
He looked at the dolly
And he shook his head,
'This little dolly goes straight to bed.
Keep her very warm,
keep her very still,
I'll be back in the morning
with my bill, bill, bill.
Good morning!'

Calling a doctor out seems a luxury today in austerity-worn Britain, with the parlous state of the cherished NHS where services are overstretched, under-resourced and under threat. I am not the only one to shiver at the idea of a Britain stripped of what has been one of its finest achievements. I have experienced health care in countries that relied on personal health insurance, and know what it is like to have to suddenly find money upfront for surgical emergencies or battling with insurance companies to get repaid for sick dependents' care. More recently an adult son of mine, sick with cancer in another country, was praying that his insurance company would not defraud him of his entire life's savings now eaten up by hospital bills.

This is the harsh reality of life without a functioning national health system, free to all citizens at the point of delivery. Young readers like me could glean some vague understanding of the fiscal transactions of health and sickness, pre-NHS, in being introduced to E. Nesbit's (1906) famous Edwardian story, *The Railway Children*. Here Mother is taken ill and Bobbie, the responsible eldest child, approaches Dr Forrest, the kindly but impecunious country doctor, to join his pauper rates medical 'club'. It is, however, the family's benefactor, the rich 'Old Gentleman' who bank-rolls the care Mother really needs. George Eliot's Dr Lydgate may have dreamed of medical philanthropy among the poor, but his tragic misstep leads to serving the monied bourgeoisie and their ailments, real and fancied; the latter the subject of risible hypochondria in Jane Austen's (1815, 1818) novels *Emma* and *Persuasion*.

Yet for those actual families for whom money was tight or indeed, barely enough to keep body and soul together, what then? The answer is obvious: many received no medical care at all and managed their symptoms alone. The best remedy for illness, for those without the money and leisure to nurture a hobby of physical precarity, was likely to be prevention backed by spiritual grace, reflected in the modern connection between cleanliness, morality and godliness, and by the same token, avoiding the contrary: the insanitary, moral baseness and heathenism.

We return to Muriel, aged twelve, who developed sharp pains in her abdomen one day. Her parents comforted her and waited for them to pass. They continued to wait while the pains grew in intensity. They carried on waiting with growing anxiety while the girl experienced physical agony. They waited so long that by the time they finally summoned medical help Muriel's condition was critical and she was rushed to hospital with a perforated appendix and general peritonitis, a condition sufficiently dangerous now and extremely dangerous in the days before antibiotics.

For three days after surgery, Muriel's life was despaired of, while she lay, by distressing coincidence in the same ward that Betty had died in and worse, in the next bed to the one she had occupied and never left alive. Bertha and Frank stayed by Muriel's side for as much of this awful time of suspense as they were permitted. No doubt they bitterly rued their unwise caution now that the youngest child looked as likely to die as the eldest had. Surgery was far from straightforward: the surgeons could not find the ruptured appendix and made several incisions to rummage around searching for it. Finally, Muriel's abdomen was patched together with big stitches and clips around the dangling extrusion of three drainage tubes. She was highly fortunate to survive.

It seems almost incredible that having lost one child at the same age, Frank and Bertha would not have exerted themselves more quickly to summon medical help to their extremely ill child, even if they were unaware of the seriousness of possible appendicitis. Probably they simply did not know what such an acute pain could signify. It is easy to shake one's head over this parental oversight in a time and place when in Britain financial transactions do not stand as barriers to citizens accessing healthcare. Then it was different but it was not uncommon for GPs to waive or reduce their fees in the face of need, if they could afford to. Medical attention was a luxury for common people, a resource that needed to be eked out and rationed. Particularly so if the sick individual was not the main breadwinner, whose loss of income through sickness could potentially destitute the entire family.

> We were married in October 1937 and if we ever wanted to see the doctor the fee was one guinea...we had to be really ill to consider facing up to this. The men did if they were not well enough to go to work, but the women very rarely bothered. My weekly household money was one pound and my husband's total salary was three pounds...
>
> (Timmins, 2017, p. 107)

One doctor's visitation could easily consume over a third of a family's weekly income. Faced with such a financial blow, no wonder people thought twice and thrice before they committed themselves to doctors' fees. Bertha and Frank were lucky that their delay did not cost them more dearly.

We are not sure which hospital Betty and Muriel were admitted to. It was probably the voluntary hospital, the Royal Infirmary in Chester. Muriel said that she was placed in the adult women's ward, so too, therefore, was Betty. The Royal Infirmary had added a children's ward some years prior at the beginning of the Great War and so had the other Chester hospital of note, but neither ward was evidently used in the Chalkley sisters' cases. The latter Chester hospital would eventually be renamed in the late 1940s as the 'City Hospital'; and in fact, it suffered a number of name changes throughout its existence, being briefly renamed St James' Hospital in the 1930s, but starting out originally as the Chester Workhouse infirmary.

The Chester Workhouse infirmary, like other such pauper institutions, was publicly funded and by this period took in a variety of acute contagious and chronic conditions as well as being responsible for psychiatric asylum provision. The pragmatic and ideological construction of the workhouse infirmary would eventually be reconsidered through the 1842 *Sanitary Report* by Poor Law Commissioner and public health social reformer, Edwin Chadwick. This would lift the culpability of the pauper from the stigma of the deplorable agent of contagion, given pauperism was viewed as a social malady. A partial exoneration of the diseased pauper would slowly take place as illness was reframed as arising from conditions of poverty, with the corollary therefore, that public health measures were needed (Dey, 2000).

By 1930, the Chester Corporation had taken over the Workhouse Infirmary as a separate entity from poor relief, and so it is possible that a lower-middle-class family like the Chalkleys might have received medical care at the old, reformed Infirmary. It seems more likely that the girls were admitted to the voluntary sector, given their urgent need and their social background, as these better hospitals offered either general or specialist medical provision for those above baseline poverty. However, the importance of the municipal hospitals in the history of social policy in Britain should not be overlooked,

> As in the field of education, only the armed forces, the felons and the paupers received state medical treatment and it was out of the Poor Law that a rudimentary health service evolved.
>
> (Fraser, 2009, p. 109)

Voluntary hospitals, of which London and Liverpool were well endowed, and unlike the public municipal institutions, had to be more enterprising in maintaining their income streams, particularly as these supported the higher standards of care compared to the municipal institutions. Fundraising was an important source of hospital revenue. Much of the income of voluntary hospital were raised through individual or group subscriptions, as well as through work-place schemes in the form of social insurance against future medical needs for workers. Nevertheless, it was not an uncommon sight or beneath the dignity of the hospital to see nurses from voluntary hospitals holding collection boxes out to the general public in order to inject vital fiscal lifeblood into hospital coffers – a sight that Bevan deplored (Timmins, 2017).

Whichever hospital the sisters were admitted to a year after Betty died, the 1929 Local Government Act changed the way hospitals were owned and run. How far this affected Muriel's hospital care compared to Betty's is much less germane than the issue of the changing status under which patients from less well-off families were admitted. Formerly two large administrative powers governed medical treatment, that of the Poor Law and Public Health departments; the former administration covered the care of paupers, while the latter nominally did not. Under the 1929 Act, a new body the Public Assistance Committee would replace the Poor Law administration (Levene et al., 2006). This was a move that

Florence Nightingale would have approved in early criticising the seeming appropriateness of conjoining an infirmary with a workhouse (Fraser, 2009). Arguably, however, the connection between the workhouse and the associated hospital offered an acknowledgement that serious illness could devastate those groups that politicians today would term, 'hard-working families', by reducing them to utter financial ruin and Parish dependency (Gorsky, 2020). The grating, de facto association would thankfully be abandoned, although shadows from the past would now and again dredge up the grudging and penalising charity of workhouses. For some time to come after the 1929 Act the typical workhouse infirmary patient and provision of services would remain much the same, despite the workhouse label being administratively consigned to the historical rubbish bin.

The stigma of the workhouse had been enormous, to the extent that years after the workhouse had completely disappeared, as had the last generation who had been imprisoned in those grim walls, the shadows remained. Working in geriatric wards and day hospitals as a young social worker, time and again, I had to address the shame and fear that gripped some elderly people in need of social service provision. Too frequently I had to reassure them that any services they received *really* was theirs by citizen entitlement, and unstained by a forbidding past of humiliating, begrudging 'charity'.

Hope, faith and charity

War clouds and the mobilisation of the nation's resources brought new vistas and prospects. Women could find opportunities opening in wartime that had been previously closed to them, and would, in many cases, close again after the servicemen returned home. In the meantime, women could and did experience something like a 'good war' (Nicholson, 2012), although at the beginning, we find Muriel trying to apply herself, like Audrey, to dull clerical work. Having failed to get to grips with Pittman Shorthand at night school, she signed up for a shorthand and typing course with the Greggs School, taking the complicated journey known to many having to daily cross the Mersey: 'bus to Birkenhead (Woodside). Then ferry boat. Then go over the Mersey to Liverpool' followed up with a walk, by no means an exceptional commute. To get to school in Liverpool from the Wirral, Jack, a scholarship school boy, had to first take a bus, then a ferry, then a tram and then run the gauntlet through a rough area lined with resentful hooligans lying in wait for the grammar school kids. Then of course there was the fun of doing it all over again in reverse.

Six months later, Muriel achieved a certificate of completion from the Gregg's School (typing – '80 words a minute'). She treasured this certificate as providing the first evidence of any exam passed to-date. Back at the Lever Bros. Muriel had now climbed a small but important rung from blue-collar overalls to 'white collar and tie' (the young lady's version thereof). She followed in the footsteps of Gladys Mary Baldwin, Harold Wilson's future fiancée, by becoming a Lever Bros typist (Thomas-Symonds, 2022). Now the commencement of war saw the official hurdles into nursing begin to drop. With newlyweds, Bran and Dorothy donning their respective wartime uniforms, the emergency of the war had seen the admittance age for nurse training falling from eighteen to seventeen (Barr, 2007). The reduction in the admission criteria also helped, benefitting even those clever grammar school girls, Dorothy and Audrey, who had matriculated with School certificates at sixteen but had not stayed at school long enough to gain the Higher School certificate, previously required for nurse training. But the nursing entrance exam in mathematics, English and General Knowledge was still too daunting a challenge for academically insecure Muriel until Dorothy announced some welcome news: 'Now's your chance! They've cancelled the exam'. Muriel, aged eighteen, lost no time handing in her notice to Lever Bros. and joining the hospital Dorothy had been based at before transferring to Birkenhead General Hospital to complete her nurse training.

Leasowe Hospital, and unusually given its clientele, was a voluntary rather than municipal Wirral hospital, opened by the Liverpool Children's Society in 1914 to cater for the care of children with tuberculosis of the bones, an extremely, debilitating disease. Operating under the name of the 'Liverpool Open-Air Hospital for Children' until 1948, we know from Muriel's account that in addition to wards for older boys and younger children, were wards for adult women in the 1940s, according to the National Archives. It was here that Muriel would serve as a nursing novitiate.

Following Muriel into nursing came Audrey, who would also serve her apprenticeship in this Leasowe Hospital. Audrey's war began by helping out in the Liverpool Blitz, firefighting and putting out incendiaries that were being relentlessly dropped in Merseyside. Another story interweaves: tiny Jack and his mother stand paralysed with fear on a stricken Mersey ferry now trapped between the Liverpool docks and the Wirral quay, while all around them fall the enemy bombs, lighting the evening sky with deadly explosives.

Liverpool burned and people died. Audrey working in the Stork Margarine offices signed up for first-aid training under the St John's Ambulance service, a logical first step in a lifelong vocation.

AUDREY:[3]   And I thought I don't want to be an office worker all my life, just dealing with papers and so on, so I thought I wanted to go in for nursing or at least I thought let me be a VAD whilst the war's on, you know, a voluntary nurse.

And I spoke about this to my elder sister who was already in nursing. She had done her training and was an industrial nurse, and she said 'oh the war might go on for three or four years and by that time you could have finished your training. You do the same things whether you're a voluntary nurse or a student nurse'. So, she encouraged me to apply for training, which I did.

In the meantime, Muriel, so keen to become a nurse, was not having a particularly good time at Leasowe Hospital, being made to feel but a poor substitute for capable Dorothy who had passed the various institution tests with flying colours. It was a difficult beginning into nursing for her – the work was demanding and deeply demoralising, and now subject to wartime conditions.

The Open-Air Hospital at Leasowe was much in demand, for tuberculosis was still a common malady and responsible for a large proportion of male and female deaths in the late nineteenth century (Harris, 2004). It was also a disease overly romanticised when it affected the precocious and talented (Chopin, Anne and Emily Brontë, Keats, Orwell and D.H. Lawrence), belying its more unpleasant symptoms such as rancorous breath as the lungs putrefied, as grimly noted by Susan Sontag (2009). The truth being that it was not a disease of just the effete intelligentsia, but primarily that of the urban poor (Roberts and Bernard, 2015). As it progresses, tuberculosis can move from the pulmonary and lymph node systems into the bones and joints causing crippling disability. Prior to streptomycin penicillin, there were few effective treatments for it, apart from very long spells of absolute convalescence, involving prolonged bedrest and plenty of fresh air. This is illustrated in extracts from a diary kept by a patient in 1944, describing the strict treatment regime provided in sanatoriums:

The rules are:

1 Absolute and utter rest of mind and body – no bath, no movement except to toilet once a day, no sitting up except propped by pillows and semi-reclining, no deep breath. Lead the life of a log, in fact. Don't try, therefore, to sew, knit, or write, except as occasional relief from reading and sleeping
2 Eat nourishing food and have plenty of fresh air (Hurt, 2004, p. 350).

By 1935, there were 550 such sanatoria in England and Wales, all situated in places where the air was unpolluted (Roberts and Bernard, 2015). Seaside locations were popular and Leasowe between Moreton and Wallasey on the Wirral was one such site. This coastline I knew of through Jack's stories of evacuation from burning Liverpool with his war-weary mum to the Wirral, moving from one set of digs to another, their world held in small cardboard suitcases; the common experience of refugees everywhere. These two events, Jack's early evacuee exodus and Muriel's wartime nursing initiation – not only were contemporaneous but also occurred mere handful of miles from each other. Both cowered under the same bombing raids and shared the same danger.

Muriel's education continued. In nursing wholesome sustenance together with good hygiene were two of the most elementary but important aspects of returning patients to good health before sophisticated pharmacology replaced such measures. A rudimentary line of defence may be but in the face of poverty, a necessary one, so nurses need to be handy cooking.

MURIEL:[4]   milky porridge and milky rice pudding and (beef) mince; very basic but nourishing because they relied on that and the fresh air mainly and rest for curing them'.

In terms of nutrition, there was a certain irony in this hospital's emphasis on a lactose-heavy diet, given that Muriel attributed to the high rates of tuberculosis in the population to the general and avoidable consumption of unpasteurised cow's milk. The simplicity of the diet was more likely owing to unimaginative institutional cooking now under wartime rationing, rather than any particular efficacy to be found in bland, insipid meals. Given the utter monotony and miseries of prolonged hospital care, mealtimes of any kind must have been one of the few routines patients actually looked forward to. This diet being no worse and probably considerably better than those enjoyed at home. The nurses themselves ate a sparse, rationed diet of bread and margarine or dripping supplemented by a spartan meal. On some nights, hunger pangs drove the young nurses to secretly prepare a disgusting and illicit meal of potatoes cooked in liquid paraffin.

At Leasowe, the sea air was fresh and often very cold, as might be expected from an open-air ward in the North of England. The wards themselves were big terrace-type structures with large wooden shutters to keep some of the elements at bay. It must have been simply perishingly cold at times and mothers of the nurses busied themselves knitting mittens for their hard-working daughters. As for the patients themselves, forcibly confined to bed, they were surely liable to die of hypothermia without the nursing staff attending to them constantly with blankets and stone hot-water bottles.

Fresh air fanaticism infected all that British generation, with mine experiencing the tail end of it in the odd belief that regardless of the weather, cold, damp air was inevitably healthier than indoor warmth. Three nasty bouts of COVID-19 in the past two years have made me appreciate fresh air like never before, I must confess; and even my Continental mother developed a strong taste for it upon coming to Britain. This despite the fact that upon giving birth to her firstborn at a London teaching hospital during a freezing, snowy January in the fifties, her tender babe was promptly initiated into English ways by being shoved onto the icy balcony by the nursing staff to bawl her poor little head off.

Nonetheless, with luck for good measure and a strong wind behind one, fresh air evidently could do the trick. Anna Beer's (2016) scholarly account of forgotten women composers makes reference to the significant threat to Elizabeth Maconchy's brilliant musical career in the thirties following a diagnosis of tuberculosis. Refusing to leave England for the picturesque Swiss sanatoriums, newly married Maconchy's self-imposed health regime involved living out-of-doors on the south coast, where she lived, slept and composed. The regime evidently worked for her luckily; unlike her doomed father and younger sister, she eventually made a full recovery.

In these sanatoria, however, the cure for bone tuberculosis demanded more than custard and cold air. The hospital bore its Christian virtues on its ward names of 'Hope', 'Faith' and 'Loyalty' (rather than 'love'). 'Charity' was either dropped off the list somewhere or simply viewed as implicit to a voluntary hospital's institutional fabric.

Sensibly young children were placed on the wards upstairs, being easier to lift in the event of bombing raids. The older children and adult wards were downstairs. Tackling this disease required that such patients: women and children were tied to metal frames with their legs strapped and 'sticking out', lying either face-up or face-down, sometimes for years on end at times. This iron maiden therapy must have been a truly miserable business for the patients, especially for the children who were only permitted to receive parental visits once a month for fear of unsettling them. Such thinking would eventually be reformed by Bowlby's (1969) Attachment theorisation; although for me, a sickly child, too late for most of my forlorn hospital internments. I digress, so back to Leasowe.

Altogether it is hard to imagine a much more miserable cure for any disease short of major surgery without anaesthetics. How much worse it must have been for the patients hearing the Luftwaffe flying overhead, shrapnel spiking the hospital grounds, knowing oneself to be a pinioned 'sitting duck', with absolutely no chance of escape from this infernal metal, medical contraption and a potentially violent death. When the sirens wailed all that could be done for the patients was to close the shutters and shut the usually wide-open front doors, sliding the smaller children, still fixed to their frames, beneath the beds of the older children and to hope and pray for the best. It must have petrifying.

As for the nurses after tending to the patients their safeguards against these dangerous, disrupted nights were to put on their one-piece siren suits and go down to the basement to curl up wherever they could while the raid lasted. Muriel's leering, overly close companion on one such night was the classroom skeleton.

Leasowe hospital was recalled by Muriel as an unhappy place with a high staff turnover. Much preferring the women patients in Loyalty ward, or the girls in Faith ward, she dreaded being sent to the Hope ward, where the bigger boys lay stewing with frustrated boredom and resentment. Unlike Dorothy who appeared to know how to navigate male gaucherie and testosterone-fuelled interest, timid Muriel was frightened of these mischievous boys and felt bullied by them when they ganged up her with unkind pranks to relieve their pent-up male adolescent need for some amusement.

The culture of the hospital seemed a strange combination of care and punishment, deserving of Foucault's judgement. In her old age, Muriel described the hospital to me as a 'terrible place'. One where the child patients tied to their frames would be punished by being placed face down over the open lift shaft and told in no uncertain terms what would happen next if they continued to misbehave. The Matron in true form was a terror to her staff and her will was enforced by the frightening ward sisters, the young nurses devising cunning stratagems to warn each other that these harridans were on the march down the corridors. Hating her time there so much and feeling unfairly treated and put upon, Muriel vowed to leave. Phoning Frank to ask for his permission to hand in her notice, for after all her earnings were a family matter, and receiving a loving assent, she put in her notice and was duly summoned to the Gorgon's lair for the following encounter:[5]

'Stand over there where I can see you', snapped Matron from behind her desk.

'I want to leave', said Muriel stoutly. 'I want to give in my resignation'.

'What! Just when you have been there a year and getting to be of some use to us - and now you want to leave. You signed to say you would say two years'.

But Muriel had no memory of signing anything of the sort. Matron frowned.

'I suppose this is all because of you moving to Hope'.

But seeing Muriel's obstinacy, added mean spiritedly, 'you're not as good as your sister. Knowing your sister as I did, I would never have thought another member of the same family would do such a thing'.

Unfortunately for Muriel she paled in comparison with Dorothy at Leasowe, a popular nurse who managed the intimidating Hope ward boys well.

'I leave a month today then Matron', perfidious Muriel replied with unusual pertness and walked out.

A week later Muriel was summoned back to see Matron who tried a different tack using a charm offensive but rather too late in the day. Muriel wasn't having any of it.

Her next step did not take her so very far away, geographically speaking, unlike Audrey's momentous stride towards remote shores, to which we will now turn.

Notes

1 Interview with Caroline Ferris. 1994. Ibid.
2 Muriel Chalkley, interview with Author. Ibid.
3 Audrey Chalkley, interview with Caroline Ferris. Ibid.
4 Muriel Chalkey interviewed by Fran Biley, 2010.
5 Personal communication with Author, 2015.

References

Austen, J. (1818) *Persuasion*. London: John Murray.

Austen, J. (1815) *Emma*. London: John Murray.

Barr, L. (2007) Nurse training in World War Two. *Journal of Orthopaedic Nursing*, 11, 220–223.

Beer, A. (2016) *Sounds and Sweet Airs: The Forgotten Women of Classical Music*. Oneworld Publications: North America/Great Britain/Australia.

Bowlby, J. (1969). *Attachment and Loss*. Volume 1: Attachment. New York: Basic Books.

Brittain, V. (1933,1978). *Testament of Youth*. London: Virago Press.

Cowen, R. (2012) *A Nurse at the Front: The First World War Diaries of Sister Edith Appleton*. London: Simon & Schuster UK Ltd.

Dey, D. (2000) Pathologizing poverty: The metaphor of contagion from the new poor law to public health, pathologizing poverty. *Journal of Interdisciplinary History of Ideas*, 9(18), 1–27.

Dickens, C (1944, 2004). *Martin Chuzzlewit*. London: Penguin Classics.

Field, C.D. (1997) The social structure of English Methodism: Eighteenth-Twentieth centuries. *British Journal of Sociology*, 28(2), 199–225.

Fraser, D. (2009) *The Evolution of the British Welfare State*. Houndsmill, Basingstoke: Palgrave Macmillan.

Galvin, K. T. and Todres, L. (2009) Embodying nursing openheartedness. *Journal of Holistic Nursing*, 27(2), 141–149.

Gaskell, E. (1853, 1997) *Ruth*. London: Penguin Classics.

Gorsky, M. (2020) Public, private and voluntary hospitals: Economic theory and historical experience in Britain, c. 1800–2010. In Martin Gorsky, Margarita Vilar-Rodriguez and Jerònia Pons-Pons (Eds.), *The Political Economy of the Hospital in History*. Huddersfield: University of Huddersfield.

Harris, B. (2004) *The Origins of the British Welfare State: Social welfare in England and Wales, 1800–1945*. Houndsmill, Basingstoke: Palgrave.

Healey, M. (2013) *Indian Sisters: A History of Nursing and the Estate, 1907–2007*. London: Routledge.

Hempton, D. (2005) *Methodism: Empire of the Spirit*. New Haven, CT: Yale.

Hurt, R. (2004) Tuberculosis sanatorium regimen in the 1940s: A patient's personal diary. *Journal of the Royal Society of Medicine*, 97, 350–353.

Levene, A., Powell, M. and Stewart, J. (2006) The development of municipal general hospitals in English county boroughs in the 1930s. *Medical History*, 50(1), 3–28, https://doi.org/10.1017/s002572730000942x

Nesbit, E. (1906) *The Railway Children*. London: Wells Gardner, Darton & Co.

Nicholson, V. (2012) *Millions Like Us: Women's Lives during the Second World War*. London: Penguin Books.

Palmer, D. (2014) *Who Cared for the Carers?* Manchester: Manchester University Press.

Parker, J. (2023) *Analysing the History of British Social Welfare: Compassion, Coercion and beyond*, Bristol: Policy Press.

Payne, M. (2005) *The Origins of Social Work*. Basingstoke: Palgrave Macmillan.

Porter, A. (2004) *Religion versus Empire? British Protestant Missionaries and Overseas Expansion, 1700–1914*. Manchester: Manchester University Press.

Prochaska, F. (2006) *Christianity and Social Services in Modern Britain: The Disinherited Spirit*. Oxford: Oxford University Press.

Roberts, C.A. and Bernard, M-C. (2015) Tuberculosis: A biosocial study of admissions to a children's sanatorium (1936-1954) in Stannington, Northumberland, England. Tuberculosi., 95 (Supplement 1), S105–S108.

Sontag, S. (2009) *Illness as Metaphor & AIDS and Its Metaphors*. London: Penguin Classics.

Sullivan, M. (1996) *The Development of the British Welfare State*. Prentice Hall: London.

Timmins, N. (2017) The *Five Giants*. London: William Collins.

The Hospital (1921). *Nurses Registration Act, 1919. Agreement in Sight*, July 16. Available at: https://www.ncbi.nlm.nih.gov/pmc/articles/PMC5248270/?page=1 [Accessed 5 April 2022].

Thomas-Symonds, N. (2022) *Harold Wilson: The Winner*. London: Weidenfeld & Nicolson.

Wordsworth, H.A. (2015) *Rediscovering a Ministry of Health*. Eugene, OK: Wipf & Stock.

5 The 'call' to India

Meeting Miss Freethy

The last of the sisters to enter nursing, Audrey was the first to become a missionary nurse, achieving Registered State Nurse in June 1944. Her post-qualifying period before embarking to India as a nurse missionary was brief, for missionaries equipped with crucial, professional skills were greatly in demand. The 1946 Bhore Report revealed that scant hundreds of trained nurses served populations of many millions in India, this intense scarcity was further exposed by in-coming injured serviceman from the Asian theatres of the Second World War (Healey, 2013).

Prior to Audrey's departure, the sisters both worked at Clatterbridge Hospital, initiating some confusion between who was the nursing senior and the junior, resulting in Muriel being given basic tasks at times and Audrey those above her trained station. It was galling for Muriel to be subject to unflattering comparisons with Dorothy in Leasowe, but now it was happening all over again at Clatterbridge, for it was Johnny-come-lately Audrey not Muriel who received a hospital silver medal for student nursing. Professional comparisons, however, would be soon redundant when Audrey heard 'the call'.

Parish churches were centres of community activities, and a church speaker 'talk' attracted respectable gatherings. Christian mission work in remote, foreign parts was always a draw, combining the ethnological with the exotic and the intrepid. It was here that Audrey received that powerful inspiration summoning a life from secular ordinariness to plunge into the depthless channels of peregrinating religious devotion.

AUDREY: ... I'd been there (Clatterbridge) about one year. I went to a missionary meeting nearby and I heard a missionary nurse from South India speaking about the tremendous need in the villages of India; and how far people were from any hospital or doctor ...and a great need for missionary

DOI: 10.4324/9781003359746-5

nurses. It came to me like a knife, you know, a 'call'. This is why I'd been called into nursing from office work.

This was a Damascene moment of piercing clarity, Audrey was struck to the core of her being and never recovered from it. Instead, and with her parents' blessing, unlike the dire disgrace heaped on Carol Graham by her family (Graham, 1980), promptly wrote to the Methodist Mission House offering her services. She was instructed to complete her training in both nursing and midwifery first and having done so, wrote again in 1946. To this letter, she received a positive reply asking where in the Empire she wished to serve. Rather frightened by the boldness of her decision, Audrey proposes India as the 'call' to service had come through the person of an unnamed missionary nurse who was herself either Indian or serving in India, an identity now difficult to establish. Any questionable associations of missionary work and civil unrest in India proved no deterrence, although, for instance, the Amritsar Massacre of 1911 under General Dyer was sparked by colonial outrage at reports of an Anglican English woman missionary being pulled off her bike and severely beaten by nationalist mobs (Pass, 2014).

The timing was propitious and the candidate judged ideal. From this point onwards, Audrey's new life as a missionary was greatly accelerated forward. She was not only promptly invited to interview, but swiftly asked by a Mission House functionary to take up an urgent posting to Madras, owing to serious nursing shortages. All this without any preparatory missionary training, in itself an anomalous start.

A dull-looking archival folder lies in a box file among a multitude of similar boxes stored at SOAS. This is where we must look to find a lively set of correspondence between the Methodist Missionary House[1] at 25, Marylebone, London NW1 and West Park Hospital, Macclesfield, Cheshire. The correspondents are the rather superior, well-educated, 'blue stocking' Miss Mabel Freethy, B.A. of the Women's Work division of the MMS and an earnest young woman by the name of Miss Audrey Chalkley.[2] The matter to hand concerns God's work and the greater good.

On 25 May 1946, Audrey writes to Miss Freethy at Mission House:

Dear Miss Freethy

I understand from Miss Walton that you are very concerned about the urgent need for a nurse in the Madras district, and I am both overjoyed and humbled that she has asked if I am willing to fill this vacancy.

As you will know, I was expecting to begin training at Kingsmead in September, and although I was looking forward to that further preparation for work overseas, yet the more I hear of the great need for missionaries, especially in India in this critical time, the more eager I am to begin the work Christ has for me to do there.

It will be a great pleasure to me, I am sure, to meet you and have a talk about Madras and preparations I shall have to make. I can arrange to come to London at any time after next Sunday, 2nd June, whichever day is most convenient to you.

Hoping to hear from you soon. And to see you in the near future.

Yours sincerely

Audrey M. Chalkley

To which Audrey received a warm and thankful response by mail from Miss Freethy three days later.

Dear Audrey,

Thank you for your letter. You cannot imagine what joy it gives to us at the Mission House to receive a letter showing so fully your desire to serve Christ where-ever He needs you to. I am longing to tell you something of the needs of India, though some of it makes a tragic story. I deeply deplore the fact that this request prevents you going to Kingsmead before you go out to India, but as I see things at present India's need is so desperate that I am led to think it is the right for you to go at the earliest possible moment, but we can talk things over when you come up.

South India's tragedy was one seen first-hand by conscientious Miss Freethy. Apart from extensive reportage expeditions to Asia on behalf of the Methodist Mission, she had been principal of the excellent, Methodist-founded Southland College for girls in Ceylon from 1918 to 1935, over-seeing sweeping improvements and, interestingly, encouraging pupil use of their vernacular mother tongue.

Enterprising new recruits was always sought and so pleased was she by this new petitioner that Audrey was invited to stay at her London house at St John's Wood for closer inspection. By August 1946, plans were speedily afoot for Audrey to sail for India before the year was out. Two months earlier, Miss Freethy issued her new protégé with a raft of administrative information, including life insurance policies (London Life Assurance), next-of-kin forms and a voluntary insurance form for the State Pension. In addition, Audrey received clothing coupons, shopping lists for W.J. Allison and Co., health instructions and a book ordering form, for which she was allocated a generous £10 spending money. In addition, receiving an 'outfit grant' of £37,10 shillings, plus, a £10 bonus; altogether a generous wardrobe budget. Miss Freethy added,

I am giving you the names and addresses of three missionaries home on furlough from the Madras District, who will be able to give you all sorts of information and background knowledge that will be of immense value to you when you actually arrive on the Field. They are:-

Miss Betty Brock, Landour, Pinhoe, nr. Exeter (An industrial worker)
Miss Gladys Holmes, 25 Harcourt Street, Heworth, York (A medical Evangelist)
Miss Audrey Wiggs, 3 Higham Road, Woodford Green, Essex (An evangelistic worker).
Yours affectionately.

These three missionaries, Betty Brock, Gladys Holmes and Audrey Wiggs, reappear across various Methodist Mission records, interviews, correspondence and missionary oral histories. Despite the vast scale of the British Empire, the missionary world could be reassuringly small and intimate. Gladys Holmes, an old Ikkadu Hospital 'hand', would play the wise mentor to the inexperienced Audrey Chalkley. Audrey Wiggs we will meet again in Chapter 6, and not only did she get to know the young woman but also she herself was warmly referred to by the redoubtable missionary doctor, Dr Edith Little[3] in her recorded life story of medical missionary work in South India.

Gladys and Audrey Wiggs were fleetingly important figures for our Audrey, but Betty Brock carried a more immediate role overseeing the Methodist Mission 'Ikkadu Village Industry'. This offered vital employment opportunities to local people, with women and girls trained in the distaff arts of needlework in enterprises more commonly now labelled 'microbusinesses', enabling them to help support themselves and their families. The goods produced were high in quality and, often, quantity, sold locally not to fellow Indians, but to the European contingency, exported to the United States and hawked in the UK by Methodist missionaries on furlough.

After almost eight testing, unrelieved years prior to and throughout the war, poor Miss Brock, finally limped home to receive medical care and a long rest. A series of letters between her, Miss Alice Walton (seemingly her first 'handler') and Miss Freethy in 1945 to 1946, directly refer to Betty's painful neuralgic conditions: a compound fracture of her jaw and nastily compacted dental problems. Betty, decidedly depressed, wrote to Mission House from her parents' home in Exeter on 21 November 1945[4] to express 'very real doubts about whether it would be the right thing for me to return'. Urging them to seek her replacement, she pathetically concluded: 'I was not much good as a missionary'.

This received a prompt response from Miss Walton two days later:

My dear Betty,
I was so very sad to have your letter this morning, for it certainly did come as a surprise to me. I expected that you would arriving home worn out and exhausted, but I had no idea that you were questioning your missionary vocation. I am replying by return, just to say one thing, 'Don't come to any decision just yet and don't talk about it much either!'

Miss Walton clearly believed Betty's misery posed potential disaster for recruitment and fundraising efforts, if it got out, for at the top of this correspondence copy, is typed in paler ink *'Tell Miss Porter not to let her do any deputation work'*.

A later fragment of correspondence dated 30 May 1946 from Miss Freethy to unknown Methodist parties reveals that Miss Brock's return to Ikkadu had become urgent, being,

> an industrial worker is in charge of the Ikkadu Village Industry in which over 120 men and women are employed. This work gives full time employment in an area where the people suffer from desperate poverty and it is essential that the work is maintained.

By 9 December 1946, Miss Freethy congratulates Miss Brock on a clean bill of health and wishing au revoir for her return to Ikkadu, where new recruit, Gladys Spreadbury would help carry her cross.

A year later, Miss Freethy is writing a gossipy letter to Miss Brock dated 19 June 1947, regarding their colleague, Dr Alice Musgrave at Ikkadu Hospital, whose diagnosis of tuberculosis in 1945 had caused alarm.

> I do wonder whether she (Alice Musgrave) will ever be able to put in a full time job as a doctor in India, I am longing to hear that her health is fully restored and that she will be able to carry on without any question.

Like her colleagues, Drs Mary Proudlove and Annie Banks, Dr Musgrave was a birth-right Methodist of a strong Ministerial background (Spencer, 2016). A conjoined Wesleyan and Irish Liverpool heritage produced additionally a brother and sister, missionaries both, working in China and Burma respectively. Dr Musgrave's obituary applauds her long and energetic career in South India, first at Ikkadu and later at Chennai, earning the Order of the British Empire (OBE) in the 1970s for her services to Indian health care (Musgrave, 2011).

Yet caring for others was no protection against personal ill health, rather the reverse. Tuberculosis, particularly for Ikkadu nursing recruits living in unsuitable conditions on-site, was an occupational hazard, one denounced in the Ikkadu Hospital Report of 1940:[5]

> Until they are settled in a decent nurses' home we shall always feel that, to a great extent, the conditions under which they work are responsible for this, and that the fault is ours.

The imminence of *swaraj* (Independence in India) brought among other great changes, the need for overseas missions to become self-sufficient. On notepaper displaying the Ikkadu Village Industry's logo: palms, a hut and winding path, Miss Brock writes to Miss Freethy on 12 July 1947, but the news she shares is not encouraging. Despite, international interest for the Ikkadu goods from England, Hong Kong, Denmark and Sweden, local custom has tailed off.

> It is doubtful whether we shall be able to sell enough things in India when so many Europeans have left. We could weave clothes for Indians but then we should have very little work for the women for they would not want to pay the extra money for hand-stitching. There are so many restrictions that it is all very confusing....Business is still very difficult but many of our customers have not left India yet but I think many more will have left before the end of the month and then after Christmas business may be very slack.

Nonetheless by the 1950s, she has managed to cling on, her name briefly mentioned in the Methodist Report of 1951. How long she remained in Ikkadu is unclear, but by 1983, Audrey Wiggs (by then Lea) describes poor Miss Brock as dying a 'tragic death'.[6] The original Ikkadu Village Industry collapsed but was later revived by an accomplished handloom weaver: 'Mr Jacob' as Audrey Chalkley referred to him, whose story is picked up in Chapter 6. The Ikkadu Village Industry was endangered many times, but Miss Brock would have been happy to know that her legacy lived on. In its precarious incarnations under Mr Jacob, the new Ikkadu Cottage Industry, now 'The Brock Memorial Building', was expanded through the active fund-raising activities of Audrey Wiggs. Mr Jacob expressed ful-some gratitude in an elaborate verse that names all who had helped him and the 'Outcaste' workers of Ikkadu, particularly Audrey Lea.

> It was a miracle this lady with humble hands
> Was able to raise a huge sum of forty thousands.
> She managed to transfer the amount for this noble cause
> The Brock Memorial Building now stands the fruit of her task.[7]
> (Jacob Ratnum, undated, stanza 19)

Returning to our Audrey, the aspiring missionary and novice nurse, Miss Freethy made it clear that the young woman's hand having been put firmly to the mission plough was not to be retracted. But the galloping pace of parting from dear ones was not easy for Audrey, the pulling of heartstrings revealed in paper. On 25 September 1946, she writes,

> Dear Miss Freethy,
>   You asked me to let you know when I was ready to sail, and I am pleased to tell you that all my preparations are now completed, so that I could be ready to sail at very short notice.

I should be glad, however, if you could give me an idea as to how the passages are going, and whether I am now near the top of the list and likely to be offered a passage soon. The real reason for my asking this is that if it seems unlikely that I shall be sailing before, say, the 10th October, I should very much like to go and visit my friends in Ireland to say 'Goodbye' to them, as they are very anxious to see me again, and my friend Kathleen Hay is arranging to go there for a fortnight's holiday on October 2nd. Facilities for travelling to and from Ireland are better now than in the summer months, and no sailing tickets are necessary as from October 1st, so that if I could receive notice of my passage while in Ireland I could come straight back and be home the following morning, as the boats between Liverpool and Belfast sail by night. Our friends live actually in Eire but quite near to the border of N. Ireland.

The address is:-

Mrs A. Armstrong
Cornaught
Carrigallen,
County Leitrim, Eire.

I do hope you can agree to this arrangement, for I have given the matter much prayerful consideration, and I shall be glad to receive your reply at your earliest convenience.

With all good wishes,
Yours very sincerely

However, Miss Freethy was evidently having none of it, and having obtained such a promising candidate in Audrey was determined to ship her off to India at the first opportunity. She wrote back on the following day to firmly deter Audrey from any other adventures.

Dear Audrey,

I wish it were possible for me to say that it would be quite safe for you to go and visit your friends in Ireland but I am perfectly certain it would be extremely unwise for you to do this. I know that travelling between England and Ireland is considerably easier than it was, but the only woman missionary who has sailed recently was one from Ireland and she had an extremely awkward time getting over to Liverpool in time to catch her boat. I know that you would be greatly distressed if you missed a boat through having gone for a holiday.

I really cannot tell you anything at all about passages except that your name is high up on our list. You may be offered a passage at any moment; on the other hand, you may have to wait for several weeks, but we had quite an unexpected offer of eight passages a couple of day ago and this may be repeated. May I remind you again that if you leave

your home even for a few hours, let it be possible for us to get touch with you by telephone or wire without delay,
    Yours with love

A few days later on 4 October, Audrey conceded, giving up the idea of Ireland. Who exactly Kathleen Hay and Mrs Armstrong were is unknown, but for a notably quiet type Audrey enjoyed some strong and long-lasting friendships. However, there is a peculiar emphasis in the term 'prayful consideration' that draws attention. An irresistible suggestion arises that this Irish trip was important to Audrey emotionally, and also perhaps offering some powerful temptations.

What kind of visit to friends might require the power of such earnest prayer? Disembarking from Liverpool at Belfast, Audrey would, if permitted, have travelled down through Northern Ireland into the small village of Carrigallen in the Irish Republic, where her female friends resided. Such a journey would very likely have taken her through Armagh, slanting diagonally down to her destination, or alternatively across to Omagh and then down to Carrigallen. Said quickly to the untutored ear both names sound very similar, and if Muriel was correct, Audrey had an admirer: a young Irishman who was very sweet on her. Audrey was, like Dorothy, not unattractive to men, 'walking out' with a few boyfriends in her time prior to becoming a missionary. According to Muriel, an Irish swain had begged Audrey to marry him, but she resisted the offer in favour of an altogether different life. It is not unreasonable to suppose that the journey upon which Audrey deliberated so hard involved a difficult parting, for the distance to India was immense, even with modern transportation, and expensive. Long-distance romantic liaisons were so difficult to maintain that partings were likely to be permanent.

A man could be a married missionary, for women, it was a spinster's vocation. At Ikkadu, Dr Proudlove's happy occasion received this abrupt response[8] in an unsigned copy of a letter from the MWW dated 8 July 1947:

Dr Bolton has spoken to me and to the other Officers about your proposed marriage. I should be very grateful if you could come and seem me so that we could talk over the many implications of this proposal.

Pass (2011) in her study of Anglican women missionaries in India states that the SPG, unlike the CMS, automatically removed married missionary women from their employment lists. Furthermore, she points to the example of a 'Miss Henderson' a spinster in her forties offered for missionary work by her family as a surplus woman of no other particular use (Forbes, 1994b, p. 157; Pass, 2011). We know how much their parents, or at least Frank, approved of the mission path the sisters took. Perhaps it was deemed particularly suited to them simply because they had not taken the commonly accepted path of marriage.

Whatever the truth of the matter, Audrey appeared to make her peace with Miss Freethy's decision and a few days later in early October she wrote back to humbly comply: 'I must just be patient and wait for my passage'. Adding a little plaintively, 'I expect you can understand me feeling a little restless at times after the busy and absorbing life of the hospital'. This time she requests with more success to be permitted to go and see a 'Pageant of the time of John Wesley' the following week where she will be staying with her friends in Macclesfield, providing both the address and the telephone number in case she needs to be urgently contacted by Mission House. A few days Audrey hears that she is to sail on the 18 October believing she has reason to bless Miss Freethy for arranging her passage with Gladys Holmes, now declared to be quite an 'old friend'. The speed of mission operations, the distance and distinctiveness of the role meant acquaintances were rapidly promoted to close friendships.

On the day of departure, the P&O steamer, the 'Empress of Scotland' left Liverpool bound for Bombay with Audrey on board. The list of passengers records predominantly British male professionals with their memsahibs. We find a Scottish tea planter and 'housewife', a Chemist and his; ditto a Civil Servant; a geologist and a professor with 'housewife' spouses, and so on; some encumbered with children and some without. Of the ten women recorded on many listed passenger pages, only three women are employed: a teacher, disembarking at Port Said; a nursing auperintendent by the name of Mary Costello and Audrey, listed as a 'nurse'.

Farewell to England

The new generation of steamships like the Empress of Scotland had cut down sailing times to a mere fraction of the voyage that once confronted passengers heading out to India, like the wretched 'fishing fleet' of unmarried women seeking colonial husbands, such as Miss Quested in a *Passage to India* (Forster, 1924). Under sail, the voyage had been both a dreadful and hazardous experience lasting months, but by 1830, steam had replaced sail and over time the voyage improved, became associated with leisure and pleasure *en route* to Imperial business (MacMillan, 1998). The social hierarchies remained rigid with Government officials and Army officers taking precedence over planters, common troops and other lower ranks, where Macmillan (1998, p. 23) claims that 'missionaries were shunned by common consent'. If so, Audrey seemed oblivious to it, recalling a very pleasant trip of 'deck games and swimming'. By 1959, Wendy Gray Rogerson (2018) on her virgin trip to Borneo as a new missionary nurse experienced the social life on board ship as marvellous fun.

Audrey's ship, the Empress of Scotland, built in Glasgow in 1930, was a Canadian Pacific liner of speed, commodiousness and beauty. She acquired a quick name change from the earlier appellation of the Empress of Japan, deemed quite unsuitable when Japan became part of the hated Axis power. Her transformation from luxury liner to troop ship was effected very early in the Second World War. Nonetheless, after a post-war brush-up-and-polish back in Glasgow, the Empress of Scotland was back in business for cruises departing from Liverpool.

Despite my initial scepticism, Audrey's recollections of swimming on board in 1947 were entirely correct, for some photographs of the ship can be found online showing delightful first- and tourist-class accommodation, complete with a small but classically elegant swimming pool. Audrey's photos of later voyages show less formality and more fun, snapping high jinks of passengers in swimming costumes balancing astride 'the greasy pole' – nothing improper, merely a slippery metal pipe suspended over the pool.

The luxuriousness of the Empress was testified to as the vessel which brought Princess Elizabeth and the Duke of Edinburgh home from their Canadian tour in 1951, according to the Liverpool Ships website. It must have been a somewhat unusual social and leisure experience for a lower-middle-class woman like Audrey, whose natural sophistication would not, as a rule, have stretched to a cruise ship of this glamorous calibre.

Soon after arriving in India on 6 November 1946, Audrey is once again writing to Miss Freethy from Mylapore, Madras, to tell her of her exciting journey and arrival. She and Glady Holmes shared an airy cabin coming over, with four other adults and four children, but this was no hardship as they enjoyed their own individual portholes as well as the cabin's shared bathroom. A ship's cabin holding ten people today might be thought to represent something less than comfort, mentally downgrading the luxuriousness of ship a notch or two. But Audrey stoutly reports that she spent her time learning Tamil with Gladys and two Church of England medical missionaries. She was, moreover, 'very pleased, too, to find that at meals we had the company of Mr Spear, Mr and Mrs Hooper, and Lady Wadsworth, so there was plenty of interesting and enlightening conversation for me to absorb'. Mr Spear may have been a relative of Mary Spear, a Methodist missionary friend of Edith Little's stationed in Dharapuram. The Hoopers may have been part of the famous Anglican Kenyan missionary family (Cassons, 1998), but on those speculations, Audrey throws no further light. Instead, she breathlessly reports meeting a host of well-wishers.

At Nugari we were greeted by Margaret Valentine, Mr & Mrs Binke, and several of the Indians, and I had my first flower garland! It was a very exciting, although we only stopped for a few minutes. At Trivellore we only had time to wave at Miss Pronsdon.

We arrived in Madras about 7 p.m. on Monday, 4th, and were welcomed by Mr Payler, Mr & Mrs Foulger, Joan Smith, Evelyn Green, Pearl Kidd and Helen Witter. I soon found myself at Dovetown Lodge. And Joan and Evelyn have made me very much at home. I went out to Guindy yesterday with Mrs Foulger and met Margaret Horwood, Mr & Mrs Luckcock and Mr and Mrs Pettet.

A more nuanced reflection was offered by Audrey in the Sounds recording:

I sailed from Liverpool and said goodbye to my parents, I can see them now waving on the side as the ship steamed out. Well, for me it was quite an adventure. And I arrived at Bombay. I remember the thrill of going through the gateway of India, and we went to the home of a missionary for the night and then he put us on the train for Madras the next day. It was a thirty-six-hour journey from Bombay to Madras, with Gladys Holmes. She was excited about going back of course, and she expected me to be excited too, but I wasn't, I was quiet. I suppose I was taking it all in. Only… it was an adventure (but) there was some fear and apprehension, I suppose. And I arrived in Madras Central Station on November 4th and this was my introduction to Madras. I was welcomed at the railway station by a large number of Methodist missionaries. I think altogether we numbered over forty in the Madras district.

The first impressions of India in all its colourful, scented, dusty, animal-laden and people-crowded diversity could be quite overwhelming to foreign visitors unused to such a sensory tsunami. MacMillan (1998, p. 33) describes contrasting attitudes among British women on their first encounter to the vast subcontinent, 'India was too big, too untidy, too crowded - in fact, too much India' with its cavalcade of bullock carts and scandalously semi-nude and rudely greedy Madras boatmen. Some colonials fell in love with India and some wanted to run away from it. Audrey observed and pondered and did neither.

Newly arrived, and with unfamiliar chirpiness, Audrey continued recounting to Miss Freethy, relating that she spied a fellow tyro.

I have only peeped at Zoe Weylandt so far, as she is sitting her Tamil exam. Mr Foulger tells me that Zoe is going to Ikkadu at first, as of course, she will be more use than I would there, and here in Madras I shall be able to concentrate mostly on Tamil, and help a little (and incidentally learn a great deal) at the Kalyani Hospital. I am to have no administrative responsibilities at the hospital, so am hoping for plenty of time for study. That is the arrangement at the moment, and I am quite happy about it and eager to begin.

Miss Freethy remained in close and often affectionate contact with all her women missionaries. A cache of letters held at SOAS concerning Zoe Weylandt reveals that she arrived in India before Audrey, picking up the baton from Gladys Holmes, soon to be relocated to another village twenty-five miles away to begin again the good work she had started in Ikkadu two decades before.

In terms of local language acquisition, Porter (2004) notes that for *zenana* workers in India, this was not deemed vital. Commensurately, Kent (1999, p. 130) comments on how hampered foreign female missionaries were by the immense cultural gaps that were virtually unbridgeable without a shared language. This handicap was one Miss Freethy fully aware of and determined to overcome, reinforcing the importance of acquiring the 'vernacular'. Writing to Zoe Weylandt in 1946,[9] she stated,

It is extremely important that a nurse should have a good knowledge of the vernacular or it will be extremely difficult for her to tackle her job. You will not only have to talk in Tamil to your patients, but we hope that before long you will be helping to train nurses, using Tamil as the medium of instruction.

Accordingly, prior to sailing out, Zoe was to study Tamil under the tutelage of Reverend Basil Matthews, the Tamil tutor at SOAS, with Miss Freethy suggesting that she should even seek temporary accommodation with a Tamil speaker. In due course, Miss Freethy wrote to Zoe on 30 April 1947 to congratulate her on her 'splendid success' in the Tamil examination.

Owing to the rush to get Audrey to India, she missed out again on a formal period of preparation; this time in respect of university language tuition, but dedicated herself to cramming Tamil in Madras, while helping out at the local hospital.

By 22 November 1946, a few weeks after Audrey's arrival in Madras, Miss Freethy is writing[10] approvingly to Dr Musgrave.

Audrey Chalkley seemed to me to be particularly keen on missionary work, well-balanced and mature and with her head screwed on straight.

Adding with regret,

She has gone out without any time at Kingsmead, which is a pity, but I hope the District will keep in mind our request to send her home at the end of three years for further training.

Kingsmead

Kingsmead became a training college for British Methodists under the Selly Oak Foundation; however, it commenced life in 1905 through the Friends' Foreign Mission Overseas Association, joining Woodbrooke, a Quaker college established by George Cadbury in 1903 at Selly Oak in Birmingham (Pass, 2011). With a strongly ecumenical ethos, the Foundation was not solely Nonconformist but offered a home to Church of England training institutions, like the College of the Ascension, established by the Anglican SPG (Cadbury, 1937).

During the Great War, Kingsmead drew in Methodist women missionaries for training and gradually the Methodist influence prevailed over the college. Pass (2011) notes the more rigorous missionary training imposed by the SPG on women candidates over that of men, presumably resting on entrenched patriarchal assumptions of the natural order of male competence and female ineptness. Whether this influenced Methodist thinking is less clear. Kingsmead was not a short course, some like Muriel Chalkley and earlier, Dr Edith Little, stayed two terms there, others like Christine Macqueen, a 1950s India-bound missionary teacher, stayed longer.

Recalling Kingsmead in the late 1960s onwards, Mosley (2004) recalls it as an international community of diverse residents, representing twenty-six nationalities, including the African nations, South India, Hong Kong and North Europe, and not all were Christians. A group photograph taken of Muriel's cohort at Kingsmead shows while a number of Asian and African faces among the white Caucasian faces. In fact, although a Methodist lay preacher, fully versed in Scriptures, she related[11] that she found her time at Kingsmead a terrible bore and burden, struggling with essays on the Ancient Hebrews and other theological esoterica; dismissing this tuition as entirely impractical.

Kingsmead was admittedly geared towards the more scholarly, discursive outlook, offering lectures on the Old and New Testaments; encouraging interfaith dialogue, political and economic knowledge, socio-religio-cultural awareness and sensitivity. It conceded eventually, supplementing the high-brow with the low- through essential skills training like car maintenance. It was a shame, faced with a stubborn combustion engine Muriel would have been good with a toolbox.

Psychological and spiritual robustness in the mission field was vital and Kingsmead sought to prepare candidates for it:

> Though I cannot point to a place where it was explicitly spelt out, it seemed to me that the period of Kingsmead was to help people going to serve overseas to be *spiritually tough*, to be *sensitive* and to be *receptive*.
>
> (Mosley, 2004, p. 2)

In Audrey's case, religious rigour combined with socio-cultural sensitivity and receptivity had yet to be proven. No wonder that the earlier rush to ship her out had been such a cause of vexation to Miss Freethy. It was an additional loss for Audrey who would probably have relished the scholarly experience. But the over-riding necessity of the day was for competent, qualified nurses over and above that of merely educated missionaries. Spencer (2016, p. 48) duly quotes Miss Freethy in a letter to Dr Mary Proudlove in South India, agonising over the scores of unfilled missionary vacancies that the war had caused in terms of recruitment, retention, and the disruption to international mobility.

> I sometimes wonder whether even devoted Christian people have as yet as great a sense of responsibility to the world as they have to their own land.

The missionary attrition rates wrought by matrimony added to unpropitious wartime conditions, deterring young women from mission work; and of those that applied, some fell by the wayside (Spencer, 2016). Perhaps it was not only the hazards of missing her ship that lay at the back of Miss Freethy's mind in effectively ordering Audrey to abort her Irish trip. However, a further letter from Miss Freethy to Dr Musgrave, dated 12 June 1947 was highly commendatory of the new recruits:

> Madras has scored during the last twelve months in getting Audrey Chalkley and Gladys Spreadbury so we are not sending another new recruit this year.

By May 1947, Audrey had passed her first-year exam in Tamil and a few months after was the Nursing Superintendent at Ikkadu Hospital. No wonder, she felt daunted to be promoted to this position for Audrey had become a qualified State Registered Nurse (SRN) only eighteen months before. Now her responsibilities included assisting three doctors, supervising eight nurses, tutoring a bevy of student nurses and managing all the hospital domestic staff.

Women in medicine

In 1916, writing for private circulation for the Methodist worthies, F.P. Wigfield considered the future direction of the Wesleyan Methodist Missionary Society. Noting the tremendous need for medical missionaries to work in the 'non-Christian world', he concluded that the training of local people in modern medicine was the obvious policy to address the demand.

This was not an innovative idea for the medical training of Indians chimed with the established views of the colonial authorities and the underpinning rationale for the Countess of Dufferin Fund (Forbes, 1994a). The health of high-caste Indian women and girls, particularly, was not just a cause célèbre, but a well-acknowledged issue (Forbes, 1994b). By the 1880s, a Bombay business made a generous offer to build a hospital for local women run by women doctors. This proposal was counterproductively rejected by the colonial Bombay government, demanding that women doctors should be supervised by 'male superior staff' (MacMillan, 1998, p. 209). Even missionary committees could deprioritise women's medical authority over a preoccupation with their gender, as Jane Birkett, a qualified doctor in Rajasthan, discovered in 1904 when told she was ineligible to sit on the mission committee, owing to her sex (Hardiman, 2008).

The Bombay authorities were out-of-step with the socio-politico-cultural sentiment in India and among British missions, where Women's Work (for women by women) was deemed not merely a gesture towards the fairer sex but an essential component of the imperial drive towards a nation that was healthy, productive, educated and ideally, compliant to the colonial rule of law and order. Women's health in India demanded a veritable army of women doctors and where they went, so too should skilled nursing help. This was aided by the towering figure of Florence Nightingale in the Empire, especially so in India where her work with the Royal Sanitary Commission on the Health of the Army in India outlined a strong need for nursing care; in addition to her strenuous campaign to concentrate Imperial minds on improving health and sanitation there (Healey, 2013).

The histories of British women physicians more generally speak of serious discrimination towards aspiring women physicians, hungry for a vocation, where India was the most obvious destination for many. It offered the greatest opportunities for, particularly, single, European women hungry to give themselves to highly skilled, professional work, which medicine, that esoteric and jealous priesthood, represented. This is subject to revisionist critiques accusatory of intersectional oppressive practices wielded by European women medics over Indian counterparts (Healey, 2013). Nevertheless, an important subtheme points to the conspicuous success women doctors could achieve in the greatest of the Crown colonies.

A plaque at Ikkadu Hospital reveals the name of its medical superintendents from the hospital's founder, the Reverend William Goudie in 1889, onwards. Here, engraved, are mainly Anglo-Saxon names. Rather quaintly, when women, their marital status is indicated. Thus, Dr is followed in brackets by anomalous unmarried female status. In 1899, the Superintendent for one decade was Dr (Miss) Palmer. Eventually, we arrive at 1916–1939 where three doctors are listed, including Dr Proudlove, whose omitted 'Miss' proves the rule; until we reach 1939–1942, finding Dr (Miss) Alice Musgrave, followed in 1946–1949 by Dr (Miss) Smith. Thereafter, we find Dr Musgrave has returned to the same superintendent role between 1955 and 1958, albeit still obstinately, a 'Miss'. We then come across Dr (Miss) Mary Koshy, an Indian doctor, unusually unmarried, with whom Audrey worked; and the final woman incumbent, carefully noted to be a 'Mrs'.

One such history serves as a motif, Edith Little went to South India as a very young doctor with a brand-new medical certificate upon which the ink had barely dried. Although she worked at Kalyani Hospital in Chennai, at Ikkadu Hospital as well as Mysore and Hyderabad, Edith and Audrey were not contemporaneous, for Dr Little's post-war was not that of Audrey's, but the aftermath of the Great War. She embarked for India in obedience to the will of her late father who had himself served in the Madras region for thirty years. This was the well-respected Reverend Henry Little, a Methodist convert and missionary of unimpeachable character, albeit 'autocratic' ways, as the SOAS archives puts matters, whose good works with his first wife included the care of seventy-one Indian children left orphaned by famine and the founding of a school bent towards their Christian education and apprenticeship skills.

According to Edith, her father died not only virtually bankrupt but deeply disappointed to have produced two superfluous daughters instead of sons to continue his mission legacy in India. A burdensome legacy then but one Edith shouldered, securing a medical education at the voluntary Royal Free Hospital, supported by two small grants. One came from the 'excessively holy' Medical Missionary Association, as Edith put it, which still functions. The other, supporting the training of women, came via the auspices of Margaret Bondfield. She was heavily involved in several groups from which funding may have come, including the National Federation of Women Workers, the Women's Labour League and the Women's Co-operative Guild. Of Bondfield herself, this eminent and remarkable Englishwoman, now largely forgotten, was the tenth child of a West Country lace-worker, a Christian socialist, a magistrate and women's emancipation activist, founding the first trade union for women. A political career was the natural outlet for Bondfield's talents, becoming the first ever woman Parliamentary Minister under a Labour government, and eventually the Minister for Labour in the 1929 government (Oakley, 2019; Sparks, 2021). Young Edith's petition for money to pursue a medical education could have received no better feminist patronage.

The automatic sexism of the day together with sympathy for returning Servicemen ensured that plum opportunities for medical practice were taken by men. Edith's preparatory training for her future work in India was 'wonderful', but only on the missionary front. With little medical training, she was sent on a cargo boat to India ending up eventually at Ikkadu Hospital under Dr Edith Tucker for whom she deputised. The medical responsibilities set against her levels of her ignorance terrified Edith, swotting in bed at night by the light of a lantern, and by day relying heavily on a 'very, very good Indian' woman doctor. Although junior in knowledge seemingly Edith outranked this unnamed other, thus illustrative of both a racialised pecking order and the whitewashing of intersectional colonial history.

It took years of campaigning for British women to be permitted to qualify as physicians. Edith Pechey and Sophia Jex-Blake in the vanguard at the University of Edinburgh, decamped to Switzerland to receive their awards (Forbes, 1994b). Pechey sought better career prospects in India, becoming the chief medical officer of the Carna Hospital for Women and Children in Bombay (Forbes, 1994b), following Dr Fanny Butler, already in situ, running a *zenana* hospital in Bhagalpur. Sophia Jex-Blake instead stayed in England to flout the medical establishment by founding the London School of Medicine for Women (Roberts, 1993). Lest she be forgotten yet again, let us remember Elizabeth Blackwell, born in 1821, Bristol educated and medically qualified in America. A friend of Florence Nightingale, Blackwell was the first woman to have her name placed on the British Medical Register in 1859. Her incredible determination in the face of enormous prejudice and opposition finally broke the barbican erected against women medics (Nimura, 2022; Wright, 1995).

Quite unexpectedly I happened to stumble across Elizabeth Blackwell's grave on a family holiday in Scotland while in the middle of writing this chapter. She lies in rest beneath a prominent Celtic cross in the peaceful, if vertically challenging, Scottish churchyard at St Kilmun overlooking Holy Loch in Argyll and Bute; her grave annually tended by the women doctors of Glasgow (Wright, 1995).

Higher castes were an influential sector of society that the Raj benefited from cultivating. *Purdah*, deplored as benighted (and indeed the forthright Dr Underhill has much to say on that subject and none of it good), provided an unparalleled opportunity for British women working in medicine to voyage to the 'land of secular career opportunities' (Forbes, 1994b, p. 518). As Porter (2004) observes, mission and medicine enabled women's mobilisation to combine respected work, foreign travel and adventure.

In the Indian mission stations, away from the *zenana*, high caste and government-funded hospital institutions, women doctors, however hard pressed, overworked and under-resourced were engaging in work second-to-none in being conspicuously vital and necessary. They were duly held in high esteem (Compton Brouwer, 1990), and where the missionary records across the churches operating in India mentions the names of women physicians and medical superintendents time and again. It was under these figures of authority that Audrey now raised up to nursing superintendent, was now chief handmaiden in this most unusual 'woman's' world.

Notes

1 The British Methodist Church relocated from this splendid central London address in January 2023 to less impressive, smaller quarters. Readers must draw their own conclusions regarding the implications of that.
2 Audrey Chalkley Correspondence. WM Missionary letters. Madras Diocese 1946–1948. Special Collections, SOAS. MM Box 1305.
3 British Library 'Sounds' Dr Edith Little interviewed by Betty Hares, 1992. British Library (BL) Methodist Church Oral Archive. C640/010.
4 Betty Brock Correspondence. WW Madres Missionaries Letters 1939–1945. Special Collections, SOAS, MM Box 1305.
5 Ikkadu Hospital Report, 1940. Special Collection, SOAS. MMSL INS-T91.
6 Copy of a letter to Mr Barnes from G. Audrey Lea. Dates 7 October 1983. Audrey Chalkley's personal effects.
7 Bearing the inked stamp of Ikkadu Cottage Industry Brock Memorial Building a 22-stanza poem entitled *A Profile* written by Jacob Ratnum (no date). Audrey Chalkley's personal effects.
8 Mary Proudlove correspondence. WW Missionary letters. Madras Diocese 1946–1948. Special Collections, SOAS. MM Box 1305.
9 Zoe Weylander Correspondence. WW Missionary letters. Madras Diocese 1946–1948. Special Collections, SOAS. MM Box 1305.
10 Alice Musgrave Correspondence. Special Collections. MM Box 1305.
11 Muriel Chalkley, interview with Caroline Ferris. Ibid.

References

Cadbury, E. (1937) The Selly Oak Colleges. *International Review of Mission*, 26(1), 119–121.

Cassons, J. (1998) 'To plant a garden city in the slums of Paganism....': Handley Hooper, the Kikuyu and the future of Africa. *Journal of Religion in Africa*, XXVIII, 387–410.

Compton Brouwer, R. (1990) *New Women for God: Canadian Presbyterian Women and India Missions, 1876–14*. Toronto: University of Toronto Press.

Forbes, G. (1994a) Managing midwifery in India. In Dagmar Engels and Shula Marks (Eds.), *Contesting Colonial Hegemony: State and Society in Africa and India*. London: British Academic Press, pp. 152–172.

Forbes, G. (1994b) Medical careers and health care for Indian women: Patterns of control. *Women's History Review*, 3(4), 515–530.

Forster, E.M. (1924, 2005) *A Passage to India*. London: Penguin Classics.

Graham, C. (1980) *Between Two Worlds*. Madras: Selly Oak College.

Gray Rogerson, W. with Fox, B. (2018) *Midwife of Borneo*. London: SPCK.

Hardiman, D. (2008) *Missionaries and Their Medicine: A Christian Modernity for Tribal India*. Manchester: Manchester University Press.

Healey, M. (2013) *Indian Sisters: A History of Nursing and the Estate, 1907–2007*. London: Routledge.

Kent, E. F. (1999) Tamil Bible women and the zenana mission of colonial South India. *History of Religions*, 39(2), 117–149.

Liverpool ships (No date) Liverpool based British Ocean Liners of the post world war 2 period from 1946 www.liverpoolships.org. Available at: http://www.liverpoolships.org/empress_of_scotland_canadian_pacific.html [Accessed 3 January 2023].

MacMillan, M. (1998) *Women of the Raj*. German Democratic Republic: Thames and Hudson.

Mosley, A. (2004) *Kingsmead, 1969–1977: Preparing for Mission Overseas*. Methodist Missionary History Project. Available at: http://www.methodistheritage.org.uk/missionaryhistory-historyproject-listbyauthor.htm [Accessed 7 July 2022].

Musgrave, D. (2011) Alice Musgrave obituary. *Guardian*, Tues 13 December, Available at: https://www.theguardian.com/theguardian/2011/dec/13/alice-musgrave-obituary [Accessed 14 July 2022].

Nimura, J.P. (2022) *The Doctors Blackwell*. New York: W.W. Norton & Co.

Oakley, A. (2019) *Women, Peace and Welfare: A Suppressed History of Social Reform, 1880–1920*. Bristol: Policy Press.

Pass, A. (2014) Swaraj, the Raj, and the British woman missionary in India, c. 1917–1950. *Transformations*, 31(3), 175–188.

Pass, A. (2011) *British women missionaries in India c. 1917–1950*. PhD Dissertation. University of Oxford.

Porter, A. (2004) *Religion versus Empire? British Protestant Missionaries and Overseas Expansion, 1700–1914*. Manchester: Manchester University Press.

Roberts, S. (1993) *Sophia Jex-Blake: A Woman Pioneer in Nineteenth-Century Medical Reform*. London: Routledge.

Sparks, K. (2021) 'Prisons and the Public', by Margaret Bondfield, JP. *The Howard Journal*, 66(SI), 38–46. https://doi.org/10.1111/hojo.12439

Spencer, B.B. (2016) *'Ours is a Great Work': British Women Medical Missionaries in Twentieth-Century Colonial India*. PhD Dissertation. Georgia State University, 2016.

Wright, M. (1995) *Elizabeth Blackwell of Bristol*. Bristol: Bristol Branch of Historical Association Local History Pamphlets.

6 Medical mission in India and the confluence of worlds

The Ikkadu medical mission

The first Protestant missionaries to Tamil Nadu were Germans recruited by Frederick IV of Denmark, translating the Bible into Tamil as early as 1796 (Blair, 2008). By the mid-1920s, Beach and Fahs (1925) reported in their Missionary Atlas that thirteen foreign religious institutions were at work in the wider Madras region, including eight American and Canadian societies. The British societies included the CMS, the LMS, the Salvation Army, the SPG and finally, the WMMS. Given the crowded field of Protestant evangelists, a natural conclusion might be that gathering heathen souls was either highly promising or discouragingly competitive. This did not deter cooperation across missions. In a published report in 1946, Miss Freethy commented on the support given to Methodist medical missions in South India by other churches, which Methodist missionary Ruth Anstey[1] affirmed as occurring within education too.

The sanctified enshrinement of enlightened individuals in an unfolding tapestry of hagiography forms venerated Methodist tradition. At Ikkadu in Tamil Nadu, this commenced with nineteenth-century missionary, Reverend William Burgess, founder of the Methodist Mission in Hyderabad and Secunderabad. Ikkadu was a village community of Hindu caste families separated from the 'Untouchable' Outcaste quarters. According to Audrey[2] the name meant 'fly forest', offering unsavoury connotations of disease. Undeterred, Burgess embarked on his third project to create a new Methodist Mission. A photograph of him reveals an intense, if unimpressive, figure of English manhood. The fires, however, burned hot in his slight frame, for Burgess served across South India, leaving missions in his wake, and overcame the tragedy of losing wife and son in a shipwreck in 1892, en route from London

DOI: 10.4324/9781003359746-6

to India with the task of delivering a church bell. His courageous fortitude became an ornament to the Methodist tradition.

AUDREY: On entering the outcast village Burgess was confronted with a tall, scowling devil priest who was carrying a spade. When Burgess began to speak to him of Christ the devil priest said angrily 'I'll smash your head'. Burgess continued to speak to him quietly about Christ and the devil priest became silent, wondering. The fearlessness of this white man amazed him. After further visits by Burgess the devil priest became the first convert of the Ikkadu village and soon others followed until there were three hundred baptized Christians there. Then the caste Hindus began to sit up and take notice but not sympathetically.

It was not heathenism that daunted evangelists, interpreting this as an amoral, latent state of ignorance awaiting revelation. Rather it was heathenism and idolatry combined with active hostility towards Christianity that suggested anti-Christ practices; implying, moral and spiritual dangers to add to mere physical ones.

AUDREY: William Goudie took over Burgess' work and when he first walked through the village of Ikkadu he was stoned and cursed. But like Burgess, Goudie too was unafraid and even built a bungalow and settled down to live in Ikkadu. He used to be up in the very early morning and out tramping to the many villages around, and would often come walking home, carrying on his big shoulders an unwanted and uncared for child. Soon an orphanage was started and Goudie realised the great needs of the people in the area. He saw the poverty, the unemployment, disease and illiteracy.

According to Mohanraj's (2018) respectfully affectionate account, Goudie had great sympathy for the Outcaste people, becoming one of their strongest advocates. By 1902, he had overseen the building of the Wesley Church in Ikkadu (Mohanraj, 2018), previously a mud hut on an insalubrious site. Goudie set out on a thoroughly comprehensive overhaul of Ikkadu, harnessing all the steam-driven, God-fearing, zealously energetic love-of one's-fellow-man of that formidable generation of Bible-bearing, gung-ho Victorians, absolutely determined to improve the lives of the heathens whether they desired it or not.

Goudie seems to have thought of everything: A children's home established, it was then transformed into separate Girls' Home and Boys' Home to which was attached their own farm; home-grown industries were started up to help local women; a dispensary was opened up, run by Goudie and Miss Palmer, an Anglo-Indian nurse, later qualified doctor and hospital supervisor. Fundraising enabled its conversion to a small hospital, of which Goudie claimed,

> It was built by the love of Christian people, and stands as a monument of that love to all who may either receive or observe the ministry of kindness for which it was erected.
>
> (Findlay and Holdsworth, 1924, p. 236)

By 1904, the fruit of labour was a Mission House, the hospital, the 'Burnham Children's Home', the 'Southern Cross Home', the 'Lace Hall', and a chapel, comely and strong. By the time Audrey joined the Ikkadu Hospital in 1947, it catered for 100 in-patients, building on the legacies of both Goudie and the remarkable Miss Palmer (Figures 6.1 and 6.2).

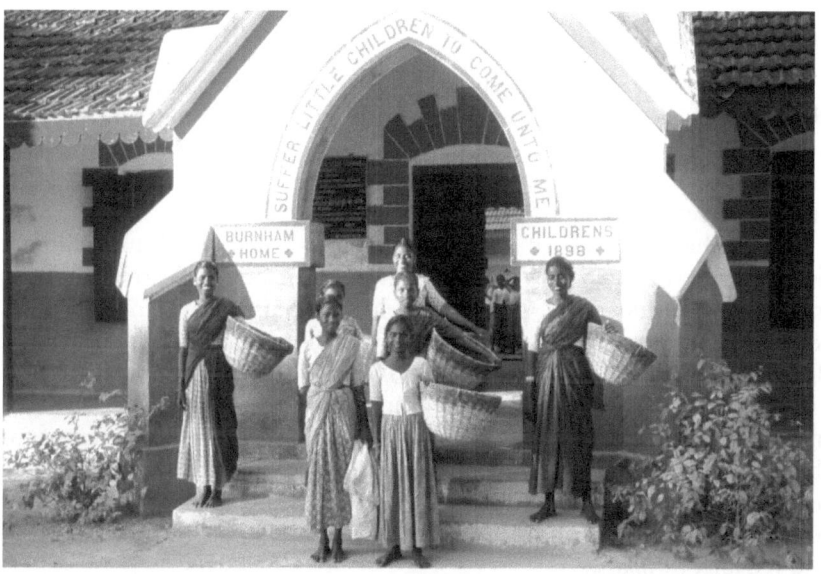

Figure 6.1 Burnham Home, Photograph Audrey Chalkley. Courtesy of Muriel Chalkley.

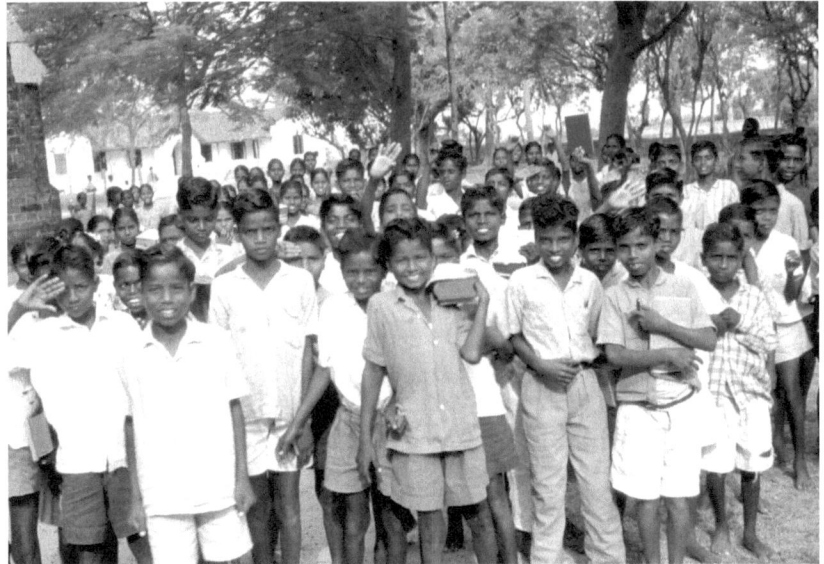

Figure 6.2 Ikkadu Boys' Home. Photograph by Audrey Chalkley. Courtesy of Muriel Chalkley.

Stigma by proxy

Mabel Freethy was no metropolitan pen-pusher idly spinning the desk globe to plot the whereabouts of her various missionaries but an exemplar of her fin-de-siècle Ladies Auxiliary forebear, Caroline Meta Wiseman, both eager to expand the scope and influence of women's Methodist leadership overseas.

Conflict had just finished across both theatres of action. Virtually immediately arms were laid down Miss Freethy undertook a 'Secretarial' fact-finding tour of India and Ceylon with her colleague, Reverend Hickman Johnson, authoring two reports of how mission had fared during the disastrous years of the Second World War (Freethy, 1946; Johnson and Freethy, 1946). The report offered grim findings: 'Indian colleagues have made a splendid contribution, but these have been far too few in number' – the huge shortage of trained staff seemed impossible to fill, but 'friends' had helped and Methodist missionaries were being diverted from China to India. 'the need for ministry of healing' is 'urgent' and diseases, diverse and terrible, rampage.

Shortages of food, in some places lack of water, in others good rains have resulted in widespread epidemics; cholera, dysentery, plague, smallpox are among the diseases that are mentioned in nearly every medical report.

(Freethy, 1946, p. 2).

There was not only a critical need for hands-on healing but for public health education too. Starvation was a spectre the poorest lived with. Families were found surviving on one meagre meal a day; when the monsoon failed, there was no work and no pay. The period of 1945–1946 was a very testing time in India, illustrating that Miss Freethy had so wished to impart to Audrey in her fond letter in May 1946.

There were silver linings notwithstanding: in Ikkadu Hospital, an 'Indian laboratory technician is rendering valuable service', having conducted 13,528 laboratory tests, of which 8,475 were microscopic examinations; playing an important role in the 120 blood transfusions that had been carried out in the hospital since January 1941 (Freethy, 1946, p. 3).

Additionally, a number of qualified midwives stood to readiness, an important means of supporting national future independence (Johnson and Freethy, 1946). Yet the problems of recruiting local people to medical roles, particularly nursing, related to caste issues and gender propriety – it was simply not deemed a respectable occupation for caste Hindu (Vosler, 2010) or Muslim women (Spencer, 2016).

On the debit side, heroic efforts by mission hospitals were pitifully insufficient to stem the tide of human affliction (Healey, 2013). While the zenana hospitals and government health facilities tended to work with those in urban areas and those from caste groups, the mission hospitals in rural areas treated the poorest and lowliest communities. At the bottom of the social heap were the Outcaste groups, the 'depressed classes'.

Attempting to care for patients across caste groups was riven with difficulties. Working with those in greatest need, normally Outcaste communities, meant foreign missionary medical staff also became stigmatised by association.

EDITH LITTLE: No one would go near them or touch them. If you touched them, you couldn't touch other people.

Furthermore, referrals of seriously ill Outcaste patients to specialist or better-equipped hospital facilities were also blocked on the grounds of ritual pollution. The Ikkadu Hospital report stating that demands for private rooms far outstripped availability, implicating caste:

In one case a child, very ill with typhoid, was taken home because there was no means of providing her with a private ward. We were very sorry to hear a few days later that she had died.[3]

Demarcations by caste at Ikkadu Hospital were wisely subverted by relabelling via repurposing:

> Formerly the wards were more of less rigidly separated by caste, as evidenced by the names, Brahmin's ward, Caste ward etc. Now all of this has been altered. The Brahmin ward is the maternity septic ward. The caste ward is the surgical ward. The non-caste ward is chiefly medical, and on its back verandah we have the typhoid patients. The children's ward and end ward are now one big children's ward, which is really a very happy ward.

The problems of providing medical and nursing care were legion. The perpetual problem of funding shortfalls and the balancing of books is a case in point. With an undeveloped clerical-administrative arm available, hospital superintendents were personally responsible for the financial viability of their hospitals, managing toppling medical caseloads, essential administration, accountancy and expanding resources.

AUDREY: We didn't have any office staff …So the medical superintendent used to do the accounts, and I can remember Alice (Musgrave) especially poring over the hospital accounts late at night while I would get the admissions and discharges book up to date and mark nurses' test papers

Charity when predicated on bureaucracy, demanded efficient and trustworthy administrative book-keeping, which became one of the main, if unexpected tasks, falling to the lot of many female missionaries. The work was relentless: a continual round of shortages of staff and funds in the face of ongoing crises.

AUDREY: A cholera epidemic found Dr Joan (Smith) and I working together trying to save lives. The only help we could get from the District Medical Officer was a supply of cholera vaccine, which we soon used up, and a small thatched shed put in a field, to which cholera sufferers were brought. We visited people at their home to persuade them to have the injection, but some hid themselves. Then they would fall sick and die within a few hours. I recall the sad death of a mother who left ten children, all of whom survived because they had the injection.

Frustrations towards local superstition and ignorance could run high among missionary medical staff. In 1928, Dr Proudlove expressed utter exasperation over an Indian patient who, having contracted smallpox immediately after giving birth, refused to be quarantined in a room inauspiciously close to the morgue; thereafter discharging herself and new-born back to her village to spread the disease around at leisure (Spencer, 2016). The basic concept of hygiene appeared meaningless to many local patients. The incomprehensible practices of 'Western' medicine, its regimes and routines, presented chasms of misunderstandings between staff and their obstinate, ill patients. Christian 'love', the driver of mission work, could not always dissipate the ambivalence aroused in missionaries for the communities they served (Spencer, 2016, p. 4).

Under the fresh efforts of a new generation of missionary doctors and nurses at Ikkadu, nineteen years later, matters had not noticeably improved. The gods of chaos and order continually battled for supremacy in offering skilled medical care under gruelling rudimentary conditions. The daily efforts of staff must have been nothing short of heroic.

AUDREY: Besides care of the patients, there was a constant struggle to try to keep the hospital reasonably clean, neat and quiet. We battled against flies, bed-bugs and other insects, wild dogs and cats, rats, monkeys and crows.

Firewood, cooking utensils and bedding etc. were brought in by a group of relatives who all wanted to stay with the patient, sleeping under and between beds. We always seemed to having to calm distressed relatives and angry, shouting servants and even nurses. It now seems incredible that so many surgical operations and deliveries took place with success, when I think of the poor facilities and lack of hygiene. Often there was no running water, no light except a storm lantern or torch, and only primus stoves, charcoal or wood for heating water and for sterilising. I was often amazed to see our Indian staff 'making do' without complaining, under great difficulties. I learned a lot from them.

As they had decades before, sick people were brought to the hospital, when they came at all, by bullock cart from remote villages (Figure 6.3).

If local curative resorts failed, patients were often seriously ill before setting out on the long journey. For the medical staff, a correct diagnosis involved a frantic detective hunt deciphering unfamiliar Tamil neighbourhood dialects to question 'well-meaning relatives and village practitioners' about symptoms spotted and remedies tried. Who could be saved or sorrowfully lost to death was ever in the balance. Some patients were blinded by traditional remedies applied to their eyes in the villages, claimed Audrey.[4] Others given such strong purgatives to loosen the sickness that

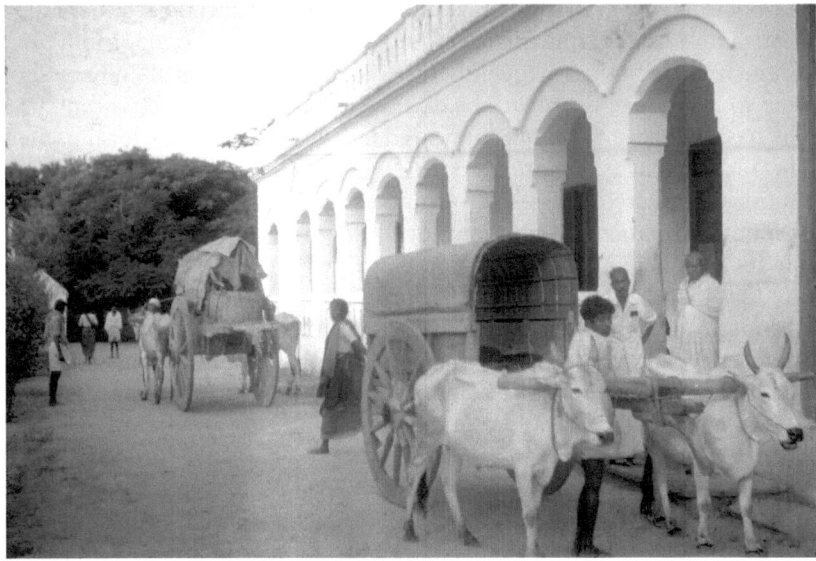

Figure 6.3 Bullock Cart to Ikkadu Hospital. Photograph by Audrey Chalkley. Courtesy of Muriel Chalkley.

their stomachs became dangerously distended. Local remedies could cause very serious deteriorations in health conditions and not infrequently death.

AUDREY: How grateful they were and how we would thank God for answered prayer when a patient recovered who had been brought in almost dead. Some were brought too late and there were sad unnecessary deaths. But there was also miracles of healing which sometimes resulted in conversion from Hinduism.

Audrey and her colleagues dealt with leprosy, smallpox, tuberculosis, malaria, sepsis, cholera, typhoid outbreaks, even the Plague, which from the nineteenth century into the twenty-first, periodically infected Tamil Nadu and beyond (Singhai et al., 2021) Chronic anaemia, trauma injuries, skin diseases, filariasis and other parasitical invasions, miscellaneous diseases, infections and childbirth were all seen. Even the 'baby show' at the annual Ikkadu 'Hospital (fundraising) Day was a parade of infantile debilities.

AUDREY: And out of about forty babies I remember …We chose the two healthiest for first and second prizes. And nearly every one of them had scabies, ringworm, discharging eyes… (hook and round) worms and many had nutritional deficiencies. Every baby was given some prize however, to encourage the mothers.

Although a trained midwife, Audrey comments less about her involvement here, although the hospital offered antenatal care. Maybe it was less memorable to her compared to the hiatus of other emergencies concerning diseases by then rarely, if ever, seen in Europe.

Childbirth: purity and defilement

Audrey Chalkley's (1987a,b) authored Indian textbooks obviously cover midwifery, but this did not map easily onto the socio-cultural vernacular of India or the picture of traditional village home births. Childbirth was not a time when cultural ritual was suspended but deeply embedded within it. Birth was as governed by the strict demands of caste, as all other aspects of Hindu life, preoccupied by and premised on concepts of the clean and the unclean, the sacred and the profane. This, to the extent that such considerations compartmentalised aspects of birth into that representing ritual pollution and the uncontaminated. These Manichean dichotomies were described and denounced by Lilian Underhill,[5] the Indian-born, physician and polemicist, daughter of the valiant Lilian Starr, the missionary nurse and bemedalled 'Heroine of Peshawar'.

> Caste and custom are the deciding factors, and to understand this I would ask you for a moment to unlearn all your knowledge, and specially what you mean by clean and unclean, sceptic and aseptic. Instead hold the popular Indian belief that dirt, germs and filth do not define, but that food cooked by a person of a lower caste than yourself – and, among the orthodox Hindus, even the shadow of that person crossing your food – does, that to touch a dead body or a woman in labour is absolute defilement by religious law.
>
> This idea, that a woman is ceremonially 'unclean' at the time of her confinement, however high caste she may be, decides all that is done. The worst and not the best…are good enough at such a time; old waste rags are collected, ready for the event, and there is no real preparation in the way of new clothes, for that is unlucky. Instead of the best room, some outhouse, a corner of the courtyard, or the flat roof … is used. I remember attending a case in a big rich house, and yet the tiny dark room in which the woman lay was no larger than a cupboard…. There were no windows, and we worked by the light of tiny wicks in saucers of oil. If there are windows they will be shut and barred to prevent the evil spirits and those that bring tetanus from entering.
>
> (Underhill, undated, p. 2)

All bodily effluent of the birthing Hindu mother are pollutants that cannot be touched by any caste person. The house must be ritually cleansed before others may enter. The disposer of unclean items is an Outcaste woman, the *dai*. She will specialise in this aspect of the birth, because only she is of such lowly status that she has no caste to pollute and is too lowly for contamination to effect. Outcastes specialised in all essential jobs in Indian society that were too vile for caste people to do: butchery, leather tanning, the gathering and disposal of human and animal excrement; so too was birth their specialism – or rather post-birth, as Sarah Pinto explains,

> A firm distinction between work that comes before (and during) delivery and that which comes afterwards; between respectively work that can be done by anyone and that which is the purview of 'untouchable' specialists.
>
> (Pinto, 2008, p. 41)

It is curious from a Western perspective to view birthing attendance as that which anyone can do. But in her contemporary ethnographic study of birth and village life, Pinto (2008) comments that birthing women often did not remember who had helped with the delivery. Those actors performing at the high point in the drama of birth in other cultures were less memorable to these mothers than those involved in the ritualistically postpartum business:

> The latter, spread over three to six days' time, includes a matrix of bodily work and cleaning: cutting the umbilical cord, rubbing the baby with ground-up dirt, bathing the infant, massaging infant and mother, removing placenta and trash from the house (or burying or burning the placenta inside the house) ....
>
> (Pinto, 2008, p. 41)

A hereditary role with expertise ritually demarcated to the postpartum period cannot translate into the concept of a conventional midwife. Perhaps, as both Audrey (1987) and Pinto (2008) observe, the concept of a 'traditional birth attendant' is more accurate; although in the latter's recent study some woman birthed alone, only afterwards summoned the *dai*.

Whenever Audrey delivered babies as a European midwife (the before, during and after-birth), then she too became both polluted and a pollutant of others. The reputation of the *dai* has been dire in many colonial reports, probably coloured by the culturally translated stigma of caste, compounded by engrained, British class prejudice (Forbes, 1994a). Nevertheless, the purported suffering of Indian women in childbirth stirred the Empress of India, Queen Victoria, to compassion and action (Lang, 2005).

Katherine Mayo, the peregrinating and demonised American journalist, also referred to the *dai* with undiluted horror. Mayo's travelogue study in India of the 1920s, clearly sympathetic to the British Raj, covered a host of topics, with some official statistical data and direct observation to support her claims. Largely focusing on the plight of women and girls in Hindu society, Mayo passed judgement on child marriage, femicide, *purdah*, childbirth and the ritual ostracisation of widows. Her publication, *Mother India* (Mayo, 1929), resulted in a furore of outrage, from Hindus in the main, and was strongly condemned as partisan, Hindu-phobic and ill informed (Mukherjee, 2017). Even today post-colonial writers are swift to distance themselves by dismissing the work as 'notorious' (Pass, 2011, p. 173). Mayo claimed to have witnessed births herself, offering hair-raising account of the practices of the Untouchable *dhai*, described as dirty, aged, palsied and partially sighted:

> Such labour may last, three, four, five or even six days…She (*dhai*) kneads the patients with her fist; stands her against the wall and butts her in the head; props her up-right on the bare ground, seizes her hands and shoves against her thighs with gruesome bare feet…. Or, she lays the woman flat and walks up and down her body, like one treading grapes.
>
> (Mayo, 1927, pp. 92–93)

If there is any truth in these accounts it might explain why an Indian commentator wrote in 1866 that 'the risk of dying in childbirth was so high that Indian mothers would eat a specially prepared death meal before going into labour, in the presence of her family and friends (Lang, 2005, p. 365). However, there was another major culprit in childbirth mortality rates in India, excising Dr Underhill (1935), namely child marriage and therefore pregnancy in immature female bodies.

A point of some unresolved confusion relates to Underhill and Mayo describing the worst examples of birthing problems and midwifery malpractice, rather than the post-puerperal role we otherwise understand the *dai* to occupy. Reputational rescue of the *dai* is launched by Lang (2005) and Pinto (2008), among others; not unreasonably so, as logic persuades that many births must have progressed safely. Cutting through a polarised, partisan debate, Audrey the mediator, brings an authoritative voice to the topic (Figure 6.4)

> Untrained Dais are often a cause of maternal and newborn deaths, but with training many of them are of great value in the MCH (Maternal and Child Health) services.
>
> (Chalkley, 1987, p. 9)

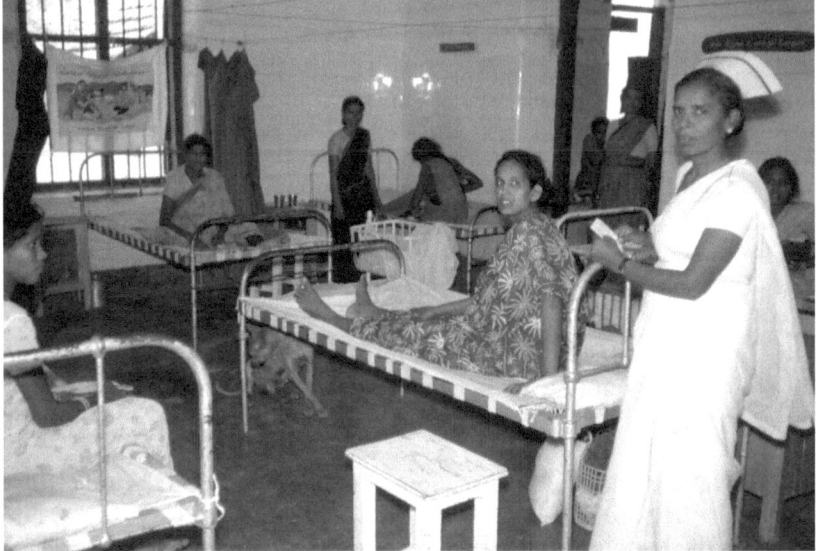

Figure 6.4 Ikkadu Hospital Midwifery Ward. Photograph by Audrey Chalkley. Courtesy of Muriel Chalkley.

Outcaste communities

Of the Indian communities that Miss Freethy saw, few were poorer than Ikkadu, yet this was also a location of evangelising energy. Missionary proselyting is the target of postcolonial critiques where these activities and underlying rationale are attacked as usurping, interfering, alienating and disinheriting of indigenous people from their natural or original allegiances to native religions (Burton and Burton, 2007). Missionary work is accused of disrupted traditional healing traditions, indigenous aetiologies and explanatory frameworks (Barimah and van Teijlingen, 2008), replacing these with confusingly unfamiliar biomedical schemas and practices (Good, 1987). This 'take-no-prisoners' approach was one that Fran adopted on this issue. Indophile and mental health nurse by training he was keen to explore the healing pretentions of the allopathic medical tradition and its harm to developing countries in interview with our sisters. The unwanted chaff may intermingle with the good wheat, even so, Audrey's narrated experiences told a different story to the one Fran held (Figure 6.5).

AUDREY: But how grateful they (patient) were and how we would
              thank God for answered prayer when a patient recov-
              ered, having been brought in almost dead. We had many

cases like and they followed our feet in grateful thanks and sometimes they would ask us 'why do you this? Why have you come?' And that was an opportunity to share with them…that the reason we've come is in the name of Jesus to help them as He helped people when He was on earth. And some of them used to say to us 'why has nobody come to our village to tell us about these things?' And in the Hospital itself we had prayers every morning and we also had a service on a Sunday to which all the patients were invited and relatives as far as possible they would come and hear about Jesus. And so many conversions would occur on people's stay in hospital.

Although Christianity purportedly set foot in India through St Thomas, its influence was regionally contained and culturally constrained. Opposition to Christian missionary work was not inhibited solely by Hindu worship, or later, Indian nationalism, but also suppressed by British vested interest, particularly the British East India Trading Company (Frykenberg, 2005). Even afterwards, Queen Victoria promised no interference in the religious life of India (Neill, 1964, 1979). The question of caste was one viewed as integral to Hinduism and therefore, from the state's point of view, demanded a laissez-faire approach. This was an antithetical position

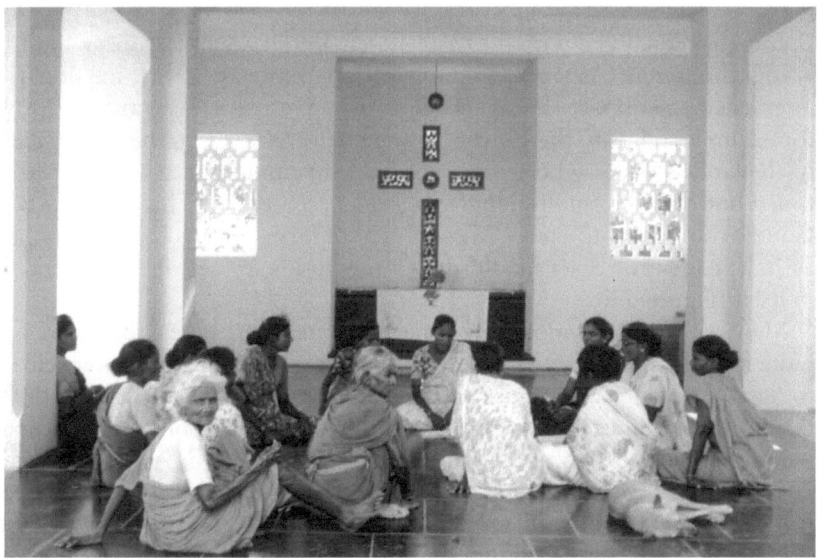

Figure 6.5 Chapel Worship at Ikkadu Hospital. Photograph by Audrey Chalkley. Courtesy of Muriel Chalkley.

so far as missionaries were concerned. Nonconformist missions especially, regarded the caste system as a social and spiritual evil (Forrester, 1980); an ossified rigidification of a social structure condemning a whole, vast sector of society to unredeemable and bestial degradation of effective enslavement (Mohan, 2016).

The concept of caste, although differing across North and South India (Gupta, 2017), captured the British imagination in its awful inexorableness. Neither piety, pity nor prize could ever wipe out the daily implications of exacting and remorseless conditions of differences it imposed upon Hindu social relations and virtually every condition of life. Charlotte Brontë summoned up caste for her gothic tale of socially proscribed intimacy across stern class boundaries. Jane Eyre, both the child and the woman, is observant of the taboo of 'caste' transgression: 'I was not heroic enough to purchase liberty at the price of caste' (Chapter 3, p. 57) and later, 'He is not of your order: keep to your caste' (Chapter 17, p. 192).

Yet in comparing Hindu caste with English class barriers, however daring the fictional transgression of class by Jane and Rochester, the analogy was weak.

> But in India the bounds of caste are of steel; and as soon may a black puppy-dog be changed into a white one as a barber become a Brahman.
> (Phillips, 1912, p. 4)

Becoming acquainted with the caste system in the age of European anthropological interest (Ashencaen Crabtree, 2012; Rawat, 2016), missionaries intervened to support the underdog in decisive ways. Viswanath (2009), for example, refers to the concept of the 'man-mortgage' of hereditary debt to the landed castes who owned not only the land upon which Outcastes toiled but also the small plots for subsidence survival. This explains why Goudie took pains to create Mission school farms for his Outcaste pupils, as independent of caste landlords – a revolutionary act of empowerment in itself (Figure 6.6).

Many rules were imposed by force on Outcaste peoples, they were forbidden to touch caste people; the main roads and thoroughfares were closed to them; forbidden also to use sandals, or wear loincloths of any length for men, or cover upper bodies. Any attempt to cover their breasts by women would be fined through the extortionate *Mulakaram* 'breast tax' (Gupta, 2017, p. 21). Reduced to scavengers and beggars they were excluded from education or any advancement in their reviled and subjugated state (Graham, 1980). Intersectional oppressions weighed the most heavily on Outcaste women, subjugated as they were by patriarchal Hindu society, by caste and via sexual violence (Sharma and Geetha, 2021); psychological

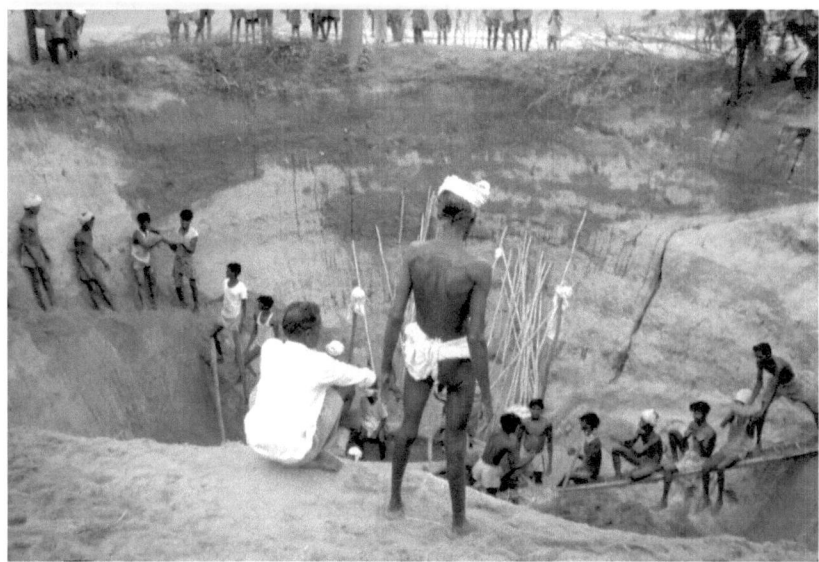

Figure 6.6 Dalit Labourers. Photograph by Audrey Chalkley. Courtesy of Muriel
Chalkley.

and bodily insults, which continue to this day, as a mere cursory search of
the international news will testify to (Bajoria, 2021; Biswas, 2020).

Returning to conversions, evangelists were not to be deterred. The *zenana*
missions had achieved little of that during their time (MacMillan, 1998).
Missionaries had found the well-to-do Hindu and Muslim burghers largely
unmoved by Christian messages, offering little in the way of hope to the
yearning Christian heart (Vosler, 2010). If they made small progress in the
great urban conurbations of India, and even less among the privileged, it was
in the Southern rural areas, among the least privileged, where European missionaries found the flock that most needed their loving care. Thus, from the
1850s onwards it was becoming clearer who might listen to the Good News
of the Gospel. These were the Outcaste communities, the Untouchables, the
Pariahs, later to be dignified with the name 'Dalits'. By 1855, caste slavery
had been abolished in India (Mohan, 2016), but the condition of the Dalits
remained deeply oppressed within Indian society. Even within the Christian
Church, the indigenous and Syrian caste Christians found it difficult to shed
a history of engrained prejudice for their Outcaste brothers and sisters in
Christ, leading to a rise of new Dalit churches (Mohan, 2016). Moreover, a
good number of Indian priests existed with the mooted hope of eventually
heralding in indigenous bishops (Porter, 2004), a hope finally realised in
1912 (Billington Harper, 2000).

By the early twentieth century, thousands of conversions to Christianity were being claimed. In 1903, a remarkable Indian Anglican priest from a low-caste community, the Nadars, began his mission in Telugu as Assistant Bishop to the progressive Bishop of Madras, Henry Whitehead. This individual was Vedanayagam Samuel Azariah whose self-appointed mission was to bring grace to the people of Donerkal of Telugu. Carol Graham, who served with huge admiration directly under the future Bishop Azariah, describes the Herculean task Dornekal presented to the evangelist.

> The village people among whom they work lay were certainly backward beyond belief. The jungle reached the railway on either side and there were no roads. Even literacy, much less education, was practically unknown. Ignorance, drunkenness and dire poverty from within, oppression and corruption from without, combined to keep the outcastes in a state that was almost sub-human.
>
> (Graham, 1946, p. 84)

Azariah set to with a determined mind to improve the Outcaste people to models of respectable peasant society: sexually and morally continent, clean and sober in their habits and dress. Graham (1946) attributes the mass conversions Azariah achieved to a communal mindset (no doubt reinforced by the deep insularity of geographically and socially static communities) together with a fired but hitherto unfulfilled desire for self-improvement (Figure 6.7).

The Methodists also reaped mass conversions among the Dalit communities. Reverend J.J. Ellis, for instance, unexpectedly recouped a great harvest of converted souls in the Anglican stronghold of Trichinopoly in 1913. The archival trove of Missionary Methodist interviews in the 1990s includes a number of recitations of missionary achievements in the field. It is here we find modern morality tales of the conversion of the Indian downtrodden to the path of Christ, combining the allegorical with the prosaic. One such story is narrated by Dr Little who worked with Reverend Ellis, for whom she had the highest respect.

> An Outcaste man walks to a far-off temple to thank the gods for the birth of a son. He bears a heavy trunk as a gift to the temple. Greatly fatigued he arrives at the foot of the long temple staircase preparing himself for obeisance of gratitude. Instead, the priest is too indolent to deal with his request and sends him away on the pretext that the god is sleeping. Very disappointed the new father leaves downhearted, but on the road meets a missionary. Upon hearing this woeful tale tells him that the one truth Christian God, unlike the false Hindu god he visited, never sleeps on the job.

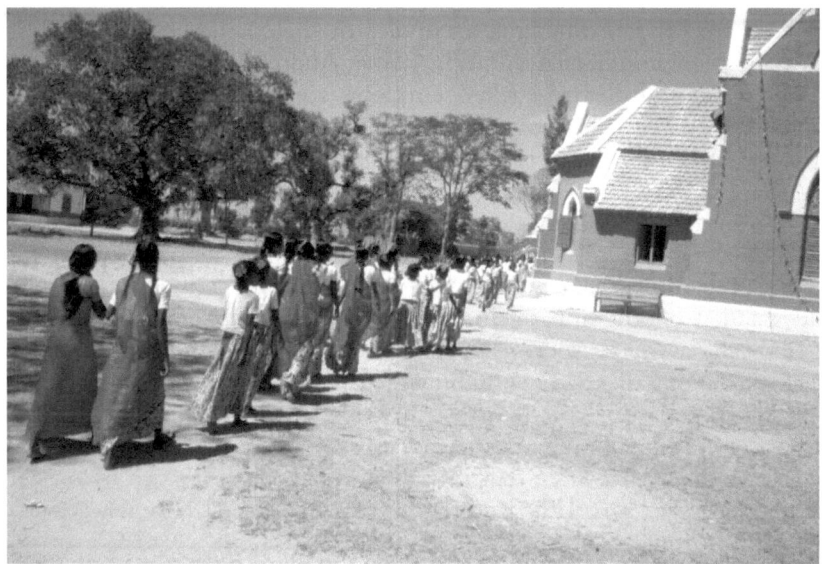

Figure 6.7 The Wesleyan Church, Ikkadu. Photograph by Audrey Chalkley. Courtesy of Muriel Chalkley.

Wonders abounded: curiosity about the strange, foreign religion grew among two itinerant Indian weavers, Alagan and Kuppan. Requesting a Methodist missionary for their village, they received two: Reverend J.J. Ellis and his companion in Christ, Paul Rangaramanujam. The Hindu landlords hearing of this became enraged and frightened off the villagers except stalwart Alagan who demanded baptism because Swami Christ shed His precious blood for a mere Outcaste like him (Manickam, 1977). Slowly thereafter baptisms began to grow and the message about Christianity was passed from mouth to mouth, village to village. The slow trickle of converts turned into a current and then an unstoppable, surging tide.

Paul Rangaramanujam had been a Brahmin convert in his youth. Christian conversions of the despised Outcaste could be inflammatory enough in Hindu society, resulting in serious intimidation, but the conversion of members of the most revered caste of all was treated as an absolute outrage. Rangaramanujam and his boyhood companion, John Krishnaswami, were students under the care of Ellis, then vice-principal of the mission college they attended. Inspired, the boys ran away from their homes on Christmas Day to seek Church baptism. Recaptured pressure was applied to force the youths to renounce their allegiance to the false foreign faith. They prevailed, despite all persuasions, and eventually each was ordained a Methodist Minister.

These are yet more tangible examples of the Methodist hoarding of the apocryphal and hagiographical. Among Audrey's personal effects was an interesting cardboard-backed envelope containing some preciously guarded documents, including a snipped newspaper obituary and some letters written to a Miss Eva Barnes in England from a certain Methodist minister, the Reverend Theophilus Subrahmanyam.

The obituary described Rev. Subrahmanyan, who died in 1933, as 'a much-loved Indian Minister and Saint', a man of modesty, humility, quiet and gentle bearing. At home in both South India and England, we find a faded photograph set in Swanswick Missionary Summer School in Derbyshire, where Audrey has crossed out the date of 1926 (question mark) in favour of 1921. Subrahmanyan is caught smiling and at ease with his relaxed, dog-collared fraternity, his hands in the pockets of his summer tweeds. Subrahmanyan was so respected and admired by his British Methodist brethren that his living legacy was captured by one of the photographed seven, the Reverend C.H. Monahan (1922), who served in Madras for many years.

Subrahmanyam was born into a prominent Brahmin family and given the name Lakshmī-Krishna Subrahamanya Aiyar together with a strictly orthodox upbringing. Eventually enrolled in the Wesleyan Mission High School by his widowed mother, Subrahmanyam began the long, slow and painful journey towards abandoning his Brahmanic upbringing and embracing Methodism. In this transition, we find some familiar imagery: the sheltered, privileged background, the shock of challenging new realities, the intense inner battle between two competing beliefs and ontologies. We find the drama of Biblical revelations through a devastatingly vivid vision, as Subrahmanyan described to his amanuensis. On the left stood Brahmins, fair-skinned, clean and proud, and on the right were the poor, ill-clad Pariahs with dark complexions.

> Then… a glorious fiery hand descended upon me and, plucking me from amongst those proud Brāhmans, placed me amongst the pisācas, those untouchables, dirty outcastes, whom the Brāhmans despise. The hand rose up high and again descended on my head with a marvellous pressure which I feel to this day. It was as though a fiery current was passing through me from head to foot. With the pressure of the hand, a voice said: 'Follow thou Me'. Immediately there was thick darkness in the room, and a fairy sleep overtook me and I slept.
>
> (Monahan, 2021, p. 58)

To describe Subrahmanyam's agonising departure from the Brahmin fold as by no means easy is a feeble understatement. His was a veritable martyrdom. Drugged and held hostage by his relatives, he was tortured: beaten and branded with hot pokers for two days to try to force him to renounce Christianity. He life was seriously imperilled had his sister not managed to smuggle him out to be hidden, during his manhunt, under the protection of an Indian Christian train guard on an outward-bound train. No one better knew how dangerous the social consequences were regarding baptism of Hindus. On 8 May 1924,[6] Subrahmanyam wrote to his dear friend Eva Banks, about an attack on Dalit villagers he had been working with:

> But suddenly the caste people very stealthily carried them away to a distant village and kept them there. Further such as were unwilling to accede to the words of the caste folk were beaten badly and were threatened with setting of fire to their huts.

Regular correspondence with Eva Barnes kept her abreast of developments. On the 20 August 1929 Subrahmanyam informed Eva of the new orphanage, the 'Isaac Home', and how well her sponsored pupil protege, Jacob Ratnam of Poonamalle Orphanage, fared. Astounded Subrahmanyam writes,

> This is the first time in my Christian life (about 39 years), I have come across a gentleman, an Indian Christian, offering to help me in the work. And I praise the Lord for it. I hope this is be the beginning of a train of devoted souls coming to my help in this great work.

The dependence of Indian Christians on continuing Western financial support was a genuine concern for missions, given the dearth of local fund-raising. How serious a situation this was can be estimated by Subrahmanyam's surprise at any local financial contribution at all. For there is more remarkable news to impart to Eva:

> You will be delighted to hear that a brahmin gentleman, a lawyer, offered to give a small subscription of Rs 2/- a month towards the support of a child; a pariah child to be helped by a brahmin! Just imagine the work of the spirit of the Lord.

Providentially, as Subrahmanyam would undoubtedly attribute it, a Brahmin orphaned infant was placed in his orphanage. Much later in 1983, Audrey Lea née Wiggs[7] writes to a 'Mr. Barnes' in Kent, England, some close male relative to the now late Eva Barnes. Her information concerns this Brahmin infant, now 'a distinguished headmaster and a wonderful Christian', to whose son she is the godmother.

At this point, all the Subrahmanyam's correspondence to Eva Barnes that Audrey possessed closes, although the 'saintly' Reverend is mentioned again in this trove of cherished documents. One being a long paeon of gratitude to Reverend Subrahmanyam and for significant donations made by Eva Barnes and Audrey Lea, written by the adult, Ratnum Jacob, a father of seven, whose Christian life labours revived the Ikkadu Cottage Industry, despite all the odds, after Betty Brock's original venture was closed down by the Methodist Mission. Bizarrely, this closure was said to be owing to 'communist infiltration', according to Audrey Lea's letter to Mr Barnes.

Audrey Lea returned home permanently to Britain in the early 1940s, where she met Eva Brooks. By doing so, she missed witnessing at first one of the most remarkable sagas of Christian endeavours in Indian history: the establishment of the united Church of South India (CSI) in 1947.

The internecine differences across the Protestant denominations in Britain, and competition across overseas mission churches, were unfavourable to the growth of Christianity in India or China. Such differences impeded Christian development in socio-cultural contexts that paradoxically had known of Christianity for centuries, venerably so, in the case of India, but remaining largely aloof to its appeal and inhospitable to its expansion. Ecumenism was the theme of the seminal Edinburgh World Missionary Conference in 1910 – a matter of genuine interest to Indian, African and Chinese delegates, but the Conference did not go so far as to outline policies towards realising it (Pass, 2011). That year also saw church union between Presbyterians and Congregationalists in South India (Pass, 2011), but this too did not go far enough. Close to the action, Carol Graham (1946) later stated that Bishop Azariah believed it vital to have Union in non-Christian countries but this had to be achieved with, at the minimum, equanimity from the Church of England.

> He realized, none better, that no union would be possible or worth having in India unless it radically altered the relations of similar Churches at home. 'No happy home is possible for young couple if their parents are not on speaking terms!'
>
> (Graham, 1946, p. 110)

After decades of tentatively exploring how union could possibly work, Azariah pleaded the case at Lambeth Palace, the eyrie of the Archbishop of Canterbury. The scheme, proposed in 1929, drew sufficient support to move towards fruition immediately post-War (Graham, 1946).

The CSI was a monumental milestone in Protestant history, bringing together thousands of Anglicans, Methodists, Presbyterians, Congregationalists, the Church of Scotland and others. Sectarian differences were abandoned in favour of common allegiances. It was heady stuff; too much so for some. Audrey arrived in India the year that the Church of Scotland, 'India old hand' missionary, Lesslie Newbigin, was made the CSI's Bishop of Madurai and Ramnad, one of fourteen such bishoprics. His strong support of the 'South India Scheme' (the future CSI) as forming an excellent example for Anglicans to follow, fired such highly charged exchanges with Archbishop Fisher, Newbigin was virtually ejected from Lambeth Palace on one memorable occasion (Laing, 2009).

Anglican churches in Britain and their missions looked askance at this new development eroding the distinctiveness of the Established Church, where Holy Communion was feared degraded by its delivery at the hands of the episcopally non-ordained, as Methodism permitted (Pass, 2011). The Anglican Mothers' Union and the SPG were particularly opposed to the new status subsuming Anglicanism into ecumenicalism in India, duly threatening withdrawal of their support and resources (Graham, 1980; Pass, 2011). The bitterness felt by many in the Church of England poisoned a happy concord, where on a return visit home Carol Graham found proponents, such as she, shunned, with notices pinned to Churches banning Holy Communion to heretics who had joined the CSI. It was a profound blow.

> It is hard to understand in view of all that has happened since then but the experience of coming from something that seemed so utterly satisfying and God-given to find oneself largely estranged from what had been such a wonderful heritage was very bitter and left a wound which took a long time to heal.
>
> (Graham, 1980, p. 51)

Some High Anglican missionaries refused to stay in India after the CSI was established, says Ruth Ansty,[8] who observed shrewdly that those who worked the hardest to connect and adapt to Unity, with acceptance of new religious forms and practices, were those who made by far the most spiritual progress.

RUTH ANSTY: To me it seemed entirely right, natural and desirable thing to happen. I didn't have any theological problems. As Christians we should be together, especially in country like India where Christians are only a minority.

As for Audrey Chalkely,[9] she remembered the inauguration of the CSI as a glorious occasion:

AUDREY: The following month, on 27th September 1947, I was privileged to see the birth of the Church of South India and to take part in that thrilling service, with communion celebration by clergy of all the uniting churches. Soon we discovered the fruits of union as we worked together with those of other traditions.

Methodists, like Audrey Chalkely and Ruth Ansty, and Anglicans like Carol Graham, put aside redundant sectarian identities, continuing their work in India under the CSI's guiding Ministry, the ecclesiastical body to which they were now answerable. They did so joyfully and without hesitation. In so doing, they offered a modest but powerful challenge to the petty demarcations of difference seeding distrust and disunity, threatening to poison the wellsprings of human compassion and human dignity.

1947 – Independence, unity and discord

Year 1947 is naturally far more remembered and celebrated as the year that India claimed independence (*swaraj*) from Britain than the founding of the CSI, understandably so. Missionaries had been discouraged from dabbling in politics (Porter, 2004), but the implications of *swaraj* was not lost on them. Methodist mission overseas held uncertainties in this new post-war world, but that they would retain a foothold in India was a firm conviction. On their tour of India and Ceylon Rev. Johnson and Miss Freethy explored what *swaraj* would mean for Methodist ministry in India, being reassured by the answers they received.

> Wherever they go asking knowledgeable Indian ministers and laymen about the implications for swaraj on the Christian church they meet with the unanimity 'Whatever it may mean, we are ready for it' 'Nothing can happen that can destroy the Church, even if missionaries were driven out and funds cut off, we should, of course suffer gravely but we should survive'.
>
> (Johnson and Freethy, 1945, p. 17)

The revered figure of Mahatma Gandhi, a colossus in modern Indian history, is forever associated with the mass protests against British colonialism from India through the 'Quit India' campaigns of 1942 (Pass, 2011). His call for resistance rose from personal and political humiliations experienced under colonialism, and corollary conditions of racism and marginalisation. If some, like Carol Graham (1980), chose to live simply, other colonials lived in opulence and most could afford a lifestyle in India that would have been beyond their means back home. Yet colonials were not a homogenous community and if India represented a time, place and opportunity for energetic women missionaries, these co-existed alongside the Raj's idler memsahibs, as exemplified by Lois Carden's[10] diaries. Lois, a lady of leisure married to Dickie, recorded a life in Calcutta from the mid-1930s up to 1947, consisting effervescently of clubs, dinner, drinkies, parties and shopping.

If Lois was a typical example of over-indulged colonial womanhood, to which ordinary Indians might reasonably object, there were worse insults to bear. Mary Spear described how she and Audrey Wiggs, voyaged to

India together as raw recruits.[11] While the colonial Madam and her family travelled first class, their young Indian *ayah* (nursemaid) was kennelled in a stiflingly hot hut at the back of the ship. The disgusted young missionaries invited the timid girl to use their cabin whenever she needed it, because apart from the 'insupportable heat' she was also completely unprotected against sexual exploitation by the 'lascar' sailors (surely not them alone). For which pains the two received 'a "raspberry" from the Purser because she was only a servant etc. etc. But it didn't stop us'.

Nonetheless, even without wholesale, united hostility towards British Rule, the drawing to the end of the British Empire was nigh. British colonials, scenting the smell of change in the air, turned their thoughts to the English Home Counties. All that was really needed was an agreement on how and when Independence should happen with many headaches to be sorted out first. Britain was exhausted and bankrupt after a hugely expensive war; heavily indebted to the United States for war loans, and India was costly and troublesome. Its independence therefore was far from unwelcome to the Labour Party, which in the general elections had just ousted the grizzled and defiant son of Empire, Winston Churchill. Imperialism was no longer how Britain could afford to define itself and, if less fervently than Gandhi, Clement Attlee,[12] the new Labour Prime Minister, also wanted out of India (Attlee, 1946). The former Supreme Allied Commander for South-East Asia, Lord Louis Mountbatten, was despatched to India to be its last and briefly tenured Viceroy, bearing Attlee's orders to bring down the final curtain on the British Raj.

Gandhi's campaigns and general protests against the British had proven remarkably successful, but it was pushing at a door that was creaking open. Nonetheless, India was far from united about the question of Independence, given its vast size, the great socio-cultural, religious and ethnic difference of its people, the variety and locus of constellations of vested power in different regions and princely states – and what might be gained or lost through *swaraj*. Nothing was clear or simple, the complexities immense, the politics hotly contested (Pangrahi, 2004; Pearce, 2014).

Gandhi's vision of a united India was based on the realisation of a complete pan-Hinduism, a conceptualisation of *Ram Rajya* (Lord Rama's perfect rule), claims Guru (2016): nothing less than a *Hind swaraj*. There was, however, the question of Muslims and other minorities in India, already feeling alarmed by a vacuum of power caused by *swaraj*, and what this might mean in terms of religious freedoms and political control of Congress by a Hindu majority (Ambedkar, 1940).

For Gandhi, a powerful and influential man like Bishop Azariah of the CSI, who regarded his Christian faith as the way, saw the flaws of the British Empire but also credited it with bringing religious salvation to India; a man of faith who persuaded others to be reborn in Christ, such an individual could only be viewed as the enemy, argues Billington

Harper (2000). Azariah was Gandhi's contemporary and counterpoise: both moved in illustrious circles but reached out to the common people; one came from a high caste and one from the lowest, one a Hindu, the other a Christian, one educated abroad and the other at the local school, one travelled by modern conveyance and the other by bullock cart, one donned the loin cloth, the other, the cassock, Both regarded themselves as unshakeable patriots with a deep love for India and its people (Billington Harper, 2000). Today, the legacy of Azariah is long eclipsed, while Gandhi's has been elevated to virtual sanctification.

Gerard Baader, writing in the 1930s, also viewed Gandhi as 'India's greatest saint' (Baader, 1937, p. 6), a powerful proponent for a united India and self-appointed saviour of the 'Untouchables'. This group, millions in number, Gandhi sought to incorporate into an idealised vision of *Hind Swaraj,* but there was a contradiction at work for racism and social exclusion were hardly vices of Colonial Rule, but underpinned the caste edifice of Hinduism.

To extemporise, Gandhi rejected the stigmatising labels of 'Untouchable' and 'Pariah', in favour of the term *Harijan* (Children of God). This was an improvement in nice ambiguities, but it was still exclusionary, for if 'known to God', the *Harijan* would remain effectively unrecognised by everyone else. The name 'Dalit', however, has shown an evolutionary fitness that has easily outstripped the rather coy Gandhian term; and for good reasons, as the former Madras-based, Methodist missionary school teacher, Christine Macqueen was quick to point out.[13]

> Dalit means 'oppressed'. If you tell people they are oppressed they will get up and fight. If you call them 'Children of God' they will just sit on the lower rung.

Writing prior to the famous Quit India campaigns, Baader (1937) saluted the contemporaneous oppositional position of Dr B.R. Ambedkar, a postgraduate of the progressive London School of Economics, and a brilliant, eloquent, rising star in Indian politics. Remarkably (considering the overwhelming barriers to social mobility), Ambedkar came from the downtrodden Dalit community himself and spoke powerfully for their political enfranchisement and liberation from Hindu oppression, whilst pointing out the dangers for all minorities in India in the internecine and unequal battle to fill the power vacuum of the departing Raj.

> Are the Hindus to be the ruling race and the Muslims and other minorities to be subject races under Swaraj? On that, Muslims and other minorities have taken a definite stand. They are not prepared to accept the position of subject races.
>
> (Ambedkar, 1940, p. 40)

With analytic precision, Ambedkar pointed out that India was constructed on the intractable binary oppositions of *Puruskrut Bharat* (ideal, pure India) and its counterpoint, *Bahiskrut Bharat* (real and polluting), embodied by the Dalits. Only an India based on the qualities of enlightened inclusivity and equality (the *Prabuddha Bharat*) could escape polarities hindering unity (Guru, 2016).

For Gandhi, a re-commitment to the idealised Hindu village offered symbolic opposition to Western, capitalist modernity; the path to emancipation from colonialism, sartorially signified by the peasant loin cloth. Hinduism, for Gandhi, needed to be purged of the taint of caste. For Ambedkar, a modernist, impeccably dressed in English suits, starched collars and ties, caste was integral to Hinduism and therefore an enemy to the Dalit people (Guru, 2016). This was so apparent to him that Ambedkar renounced Hinduism in favour of another indigenised religion, Buddhism (Hans, 2016). Yet neither Buddhism nor Islam had altered the social conditions of the Dalits over centuries, whereas contemporary Christianity had righteously taken the side of the Dalit underdog, promising elevation from degradation spiritually, ideologically and practically. Through them also came the benefits of the modern world: education, health, and access to public, civil life (Mohan, 2016).

The seen but unseen (or entirely overlooked) enforced degradation of the Dalits was a ubiquitous feature of Indian life and their ritualised role essential to the inflexible structure of Hindu society. In his striking novel, *The Untouchable*, Muluk Raj Anand delineated the hideous reality of Outcaste life and the wholesale wastage of human potential.

> He seemed a true child of the outcaste colony, where there are no drains, no light, no water; of the marshlands where people live among the latrines of the townsmen, and in the stink of their own dung, scattered about here, there and everywhere.
>
> (Anand, 1935, pp. 71–72)

The Outcaste anti-hero of the story, Bahkha, is a relentlessly humiliated, thwarted soul and a symbol of negative capability. His physical superiority over the weedy physiques but overweening social superiority of the caste townsmen is emphasised, reminiscently so. Consider the divisive Court room scene in Forster's *A Passage to India*, where the ignored, Outcaste *punkah wallah* is casually elevated to a tragic, Grecian nobility in prose of wistful, pained melancholy.

> Almost naked, and splendidly formed, he (*punkah wallah*) sat on a raised platform near the back...He had the strength and beauty that sometimes come to flower in Indians of low birth. When that strange race nears the dust and is condemned as untouchable, then nature

remembers the physical perfection that she accomplished elsewhere, and threw out a god – not many, but one here and there, to prove to society how little its categories impress her. This man would have been notable anywhere; among the thin-hammed, flat-chested mediocrities of Chandrapore he stood out as divine; yet he was of the city, its garbage had nourished him, he would end on its rubbish-heaps.

(Forster, 1924, 2005, p. 205)

In Anand's novel, it is not the evangelism of the deranged and thereby dis-credited, colonial Salvation Army officer that offers Burkha psychic liberation, but encountering Gandhi and his famous quest to uplift the 'Harijan', the 'Children of God'.

Tellingly Mohan (2016) comments that the height of Dalit activist mobilisation waned post-Independence. Now the momentous day of Independence arrived – greeted with huge public rejoicing, together with minority group trepidation, plus a mixture of chagrin and resignation by some disappointed, dispossessed colonials, although unshared sentiments for many missionaries (Macmillan, 1998). Altogether it was without question an extraordinary occasion. Methodist missionaries there at that time remembered the day as one of celebration, especially since religious freedom was affirmed for newly Independent India.

AUDREY CHALKELY: I was there on August 15th in Ikkadu, 1947, when India got her independence and I remember going to the village open space and seeing the children all gathered for the flag-hoisting. What a joy it was when the British flag came down and the Indian flag went up and everybody rejoiced and sang the Indian national anthem and the children were all given sweets

Her comrade-in-Christ, Ruth Ansty, in Trichinopoly threw herself into the celebrations with gusto.

RUTH ANSTY:[14] The 'QUIT INDIA' signs in the bazaar were soon no longer necessary. On 15th August 1947, India celebrated Independence, and in 'Trichy', as elsewhere, there was great rejoicing. As Captain of the school Guide Company, I was thrilled to march in the Independence Day Parade on Trichy maidan, to sing with thousands of others Indian's New National

Anthem, and to watch Trichy schoolchildren
dance and give obeisance to 'Mother India'.

The following day on 16 August, Louis and Edwina Mountbatten drove
in state from Viceregal Lodge as first Governor-General of Independent
India through massed crowds held back by troops and police lining the
streets. The crowd surged forwards breaking through the cordon to sur-
round the carriage. A dramatic photograph of the time shows the couple
surrounded by hordes of people spilling over themselves to reach into their
carriage. Nothing, actually, could have stopped the Mountbattens from
being hurled out had the masses so wanted, but in fact what was bran-
dished at the amazingly composed couple are multiple hands to shake and
a standing ovation.

'Surely nothing', Graham (1980, p. 42) reflected later 'became the
British Raj more than the manner of their departure and nothing showed
the greatness of Jawaharlal Nehru better than his willingness to give all the
glory to the Englishman who had done so much to make this day possible'.

If India exulted in 1947, the horrors of 1948 would leave indelible stains
in a fateful year witnessing the results of Partition and the assassination
of Gandhi. Mountbatten's in-depth negotiations concerning the future
of Independent India with Jawaharlal Nehru, whom he found a genial
companion, and Mohammed Jinnah, whom he found quite the reverse,
shaped the agreed outcome. In the approach to these critical discussions
and throughout, the distrust felt towards a Hindu majority control of Congress to the detriment of minority groups led to protracted and convoluted
proposals, revisions and rejections. All of which ultimately and probably
inexorably led to the Partitioning of India, with the unforeseen but infa-
mous outcome of chaotic mass migration by millions of people at the forging of two new countries. Britain and Mountbatten have received much
opprobrium for the Partition of 1948 and the way it was achieved (Brass,
2003; Butalia, 2000). But many observers of the time, like Carol Graham
(1980), saw no other alternative to Partition in a country which, for the
British administration, had become entirely ungovernable.

Whether a different matrix of divisions based on variables other than
religion and elementary geography or some extra months of delay would
have made a real difference in saving so many from butchery at the hands
of organised mobs and neighbours is entirely uncertain. The impact of
Partition and the accounts of those caught up in the maelstrom are still
emerging today (Puri, 2019). Indian women were the main victims of mass
abduction, rape, enforced pregnancy and torture, not forgetting of course,
murder on a vast scale, brutal and bloody, where even male relatives willingly slaughtered their own daughters, sisters and wives to prevent them
being violated by the enemy (Butalia, 2000).

At least they were not entirely abandoned:

> The Christian community rallied, doctors, nurses, social workers and others went up from South India together or alone, to rescue abducted women and girls, and carry on in hospitals from which staff had fled.
>
> (Graham, 1980, p. 42)

The Methodist Mission dutifully chronicled these events in their annual reports incorrigibly focused on finding any ray of light within even the darkest night:

> ten million people on the move between India and Pakistan, driven by fear and the tragic memories of brutality suffered and inflicted; the assassination of Mahatma Gandhi, the beloved peace-maker; the withdrawal of British forces; the death of Mr. Jinnah; trouble in Kashmir; trouble in Hyderabad... the story of 1948 in India provides enough explosive material to start a score of revolutions and tax the resources of any Government, hoary in experience.
>
> (MMS, 1948)

Their optimism and faith remained justified for it was also reported that *swaraj* had at last persuaded Indian Methodists to draw out their wallets. Moreover, the same report carried the eager words of an Indian Methodist minister, of whom, a cynic might diagnose as succumbing to the Methodist disease of incurable optimism.

> Gandhiji's death has meant a great victory for the Cross of Christ in Tumkur as everywhere in the country... where I had the privilege of addressing a huge gathering of nearly 8,000 people near the market-place. I presented the death of Gandhiji in the light of the Cross of Jesus Christ. The people listened with rapt attention and during the following week there was an earnest demand for Gospels and New Testaments. Since then the people are getting more eager to listen to the Gospel.
>
> (MMS, 1948, p. 9)

Helping to lead the way undaunted by the terrible year of 1948 and vouch-safed by the good covenants of 1947, the Lord's work in India would go on.

Notes

1 British Library 'Sounds'. Ruth Ansty interviewed by Caroline Ferris, 1994. Methodist Church Oral Archive. C640/043.
2 Audrey Chalkley interview with Caroline Ferris. Ibid.

3 Ikkadu Hospital Report, 1940. Ibid.
4 Such indigenous treatments were practised on Brahmin-turned-Methodist Reverend Theophilus Subrahmanyan in his boyhood, nearly causing blindness (Monahan, 1922).
5 Typescript notes of a talk given by Dr Underhill to the Croyden Branch of the Midwives Institute, 13 September 1932. Cadbury Library, University of Birmingham, CMS/ACC1027 F4/1.
6 Audrey Chalkley's personal effects. Torn extract of correspondence to Eva Brooks (no address visible) from Rev. T Subrahmanyam, Wesleyan Mission, Poonamallee South India. Date written in Audrey's hand 8 May 1924.
7 Audrey Chalkley's personal effects. Letter to Mr Barnes from Audrey Lea.
8 Ruth Ansty, Interview with Caroline Ferris. Ibid.
9 '1786–1986 Celebrate Together' Methodist Church Overseas Division. SOAS, MMS 120.
10 Diaries and miscellaneous papers of Lois Carden. University of Birmingham Cadbury Research Library, Special Collections GB 150 MS119.
11 Methodist Church Oral Archives. Ibid.
12 Clement Attlee's address to the House of Commons, 15 March, 1946.
13 British Library 'Sounds'. Christine Macqueen interviewed by Caroline Ferris, 1993. Methodist Church Oral Archives. C649/054.
14 '1786–1986 Celebrate Together' Methodist Mission history project. SOAS MMS, box 120.

References

Ambedkar, B.R. (Dr.) (1940) *Pakistan or the Partition of India*. Bombay: Thackers Bajoria, J. 2021.

Anand, M.R. (1935, 2014) *Untouchable*. London: Penguin Classics.

Ashencaen Crabtree, S. (2012) *A Rainforest Asylum: The Enduring Legacy of Colonial Psychiatric Care in Malaysia*. London: Whiting & Birch.

Attlee, C. (1946) *Address given by Clement Attlee to the House of Commons (15 March 1946.)* Parliamentary Debates. Houses of Commons-Official Report. First session of the Thirty-Eighth Parliament of the United Kingdom of Great Britain and Northern Ireland. Dir. of publ. Hansard. 1946, No 420; fifth series. London: His Majesty's Stationery Office.

Baader, G. (1937) The Depressed classes of India: Their struggle for emancipation. *Studies: An Irish Quarterly Review*, 26(105), 399–417.

Bajoria, J. (2021) Indian girl's alleged rape and murder sparks protests. *Human Rights Watch*. Available at: https://www.hrw.org/reports/1999/india/India994-11.htm [Accessed 6 August 2022].

Barimah, K.B. and van Teijlingen, E.R. (2008) The use of traditional medicine by Ghanaians in Canada. *BMC Complementary and Alternative Medicine*, 16(8), 30. https://doi.org/10.1186/1472-6882-8-30.

Beach, H.P. and Fahs, C.H. (1925) *World Missionary Atlas*. New York: Institute of Social & Religious Research.

Billington Harper, S. (2000) *In the Shadow of the Mahatma: Bishop V.S. Azariah and the Travails of Christianity in British India*. London/New York: Routledge.

Biswas, S. (2020) Hathras case: Dalit women are among the most oppressed in the world. *BBC*, 6 October. Available at: https://www.bbc.co.uk/news/world-asia-india-54418513 [Accessed 7 January 2023].

Blair, C.F. (2008) *Christian Mission in India: Contributions to Some Missions to Social Change*. PhD Dissertation. Unpublished. Simon Fraser University.

Brass, P.R. (2003) The partition of India and retributive genocide in the Punjab, 1946–7: Means, methods and purposes. *Journal of Genocide Research*, 5(1), 71–101.

Burton, J. and Burton, O.A. (2007) Some reflections on anthropology's missionary positions. *Journal of the Royal Anthropological Institute*, 13, 209–217.

Butalia, U. (2000) *The Other Side of Silence: Voices from Partition*. London: Penguin.

Cadbury, E. (1937) The Selly Oak Colleges. *International Review of Mission*, 26(1), 119–121.

Cassons, J. (1998) 'To plant a garden city in the slums of Paganism....': Handley Hooper, the Kikuyu and the future of Africa. *Journal of Religion in Africa*, XXVIII, 387–410.

Chalkley, A.M. (1974a, 1987) *A Textbook for the Health Worker (ANM)*. Volume 1. New Delhi: Wiley Eastern Limited.

Chalkley, A.M. (1974b, 1986) *A Textbook for the Health Worker (ANM)*. Volume 2. Madras: The Christian Literature Society.

Findlay, G.G. and Holdsworth, W.W. (1924) *The History of the Wesleyan Methodist Missionary Society*, Vol V. London: The Epworth Press, p. 159.

Forbes, G. (1994a) Managing midwifery in India. In Dagmar Engels and Shula Marks (Eds.), *Contesting Colonial Hegemony: State and Society in Africa and India*. London: British Academic Press, pp. 152–172.

Forrester, D.B. (1980) *Caste and Christianity*. London: Curzon Press.

Forster, E.M. (1924, 2005) *A Passage to India*. London: Penguin Classics.

Freethy, M. (1946) *Impressions of Our Tour through India and Ceylon 1945–46*. London: Methodist Missionary Society Women's Work.

Frykenberg, R.E. (2005) Christian missions in the Raj. In Norman Etherington (Ed.), *Missions and Empire*. Oxford: Oxford University Press, pp. 107–131.

Good, C. M. (1987) *Ethnomedical Systems in Africa: Patterns of Traditional Medicine in Rural and Urban Kenya*. New York/London: The Guildford Press.

Good, C.M. (1991) Pioneer medical missions in colonial Africa. *Social Science & Medicine*, 32(1), 1–10.

Graham, C. (1980) *Between Two Worlds*. Madras: Selly Oak College.

Graham, C. (1946) *Azariah of Dornakal*. London: SCM.

Gray Rogerson, W. with Fox, B. (2018) *Midwife of Borneo*. London: SPCK.

Gupta, V. (2017) Breast Tax: Social oppression of Dalit women. *Contemporary Social Sciences*, 26(3), 17–26.

Guru, G. (2016) The Indian nation and its egalitarian concept. In: Ramnarayan S. Rawat and S. Satyanarayana (Eds.), *Dalit Studies*. Durham/London: Duke University Press, pp. 31–52.

Hans, R.K. (2016) Making sense of Dalit history. Writing Dalit History. In Ramnarayan S. Rawat and S. Satyanarayana (Eds.), *Dalit Studies*. Durham/London: Duke University Press, pp. 131–151.

Hardiman, D. (2008) *Missionaries and Their Medicine: A Christian Modernity for Tribal India*. Manchester: Manchester University Press.

Healey, M. (2013) *Indian Sisters: A History of Nursing and the Estate, 1907–2007*. London: Routledge.

Hickman Johnson, G.E. and Freethy, M. (1946) *Report of a Secretarial Visit to India and Ceylon/ With comments on the General Synod Held in Myosore, February 21–27, 1956*. London: Methodist Missionary Society.

Kent, E.F. (1999) Tamil Bible women and the zenana mission of colonial South India. *History of Religions*, 39(2), 117–149.

Laing, M. (2009) The international impact of the Church of South India: Bishop Newbigin versus the Anglican Fathers. *International Bulletin of Missionary Research*, 33(1), 18–24. https://doi.org/10.1177/239693930903300107

Lang, S. (2005) Drop the demon dai: Maternal morality and the State in colonial Madras, 1840–1875. *Social History of Medicine*, 18(3), 357–377.

MacMillan, M. (1998) *Women of the Raj*. German Democratic Republic: Thames and Hudson.

Manickam, S. (1977) *The Social Setting of Christian Conversion in South India*. Wiesbaden: Franz Steiner Verlag.

Mayo, K. (1927) *Mother India*. Newcastle-under-Lyme: Howard Baker Limited.

MMS (1948) *Signs of Victory. The Report of 1948, the 163rd Year of the Methodists Mission*. London: Methodist Mission.

Mohan, P.S. (2016) Social space, civil society, and dalit agency in twentieth-century Kerala. In Ramnarayan S. Rawat and K. Satyanarayana (Eds.), *Dalit Studies*. Durham, NC/London: Duke University Press, pp. 74–103.

Mohanraj, D. (2018) *William Goudie – a veritable apostle to Ikkadu*. Boston University. Available at: https://www.bu.edu/missiology/goudie-william-1857-1922/ [Accessed 21 July 2022].

Monahan, C.H. (1922) *Theophilus Subrahmanyan: The Story of a Pilgrimage*. London: Wesleyan Methodist Missionary Society.

Mosley, A. (2004) *Kingsmead, 1969–1977: Preparing for mission overseas*. Methodist Missionary History Project. Available at: http://www.methodistheritage.org.uk/missionaryhistory-historyproject-listbyauthor.htm [Accessed 7 July 2022].

Mukherjee, S. (2017) Katherine Mayo's *Mother India* (1927) and its critique by the diaspora. *Proceedings of the Indian History Congress*, 78, 820–827. https://www.jstor.org/stable/26906156

Neill, S. (1964, 1979) *A History of Christian Missions*. Harmondsworth, Middx: Penguin.

Oakley, A. (2019) *Women, Peace and Welfare: A Suppressed History of Social Reform, 1880–1920*. Bristol: Policy Press.

Pangrahi, D.N. (2004) *India's Partition: The Story of Imperialism in Retreat*. London: Routledge.

Pass, A. (2011) British women missionaries in India c. 1917–1950. PhD Dissertation. University of Oxford.

Pearce, R. (2014) *Profiles in Power, Attlee*. Abingdon: Routledge.

Phillips, G.E. (2012) *The Outcastes' Hope*. London: Church Missionary Society.

Pinto, S. (2008) *Where There Is No Midwife: Birth and Loss in Rural India*. New York: Berghahn Books.

Porter, A. (2004) *Religion versus Empire? British Protestant Missionaries and Overseas Expansion, 1700–1914*. Manchester: Manchester University Press.

Puri, K. (2019) *Partition Voices: Untold British Stories*. London: Bloomsbury Publishing.

Rawat, R.S. (2016) Colonial archive versus colonial sociology: Writing dalit history. In Ramnarayan S. Rawat and S. Satyanarayana (Eds.), *Dalit Studies*. Durham, NC/London: Duke University Press, pp. 53–73.

Rev. Hickman Johnson, G.E. and Freethy, M. (1956) *Report of A Secretarial Visit to India and Ceylon, by October 1945 February 1946. With comments on the General Synod held in Myosore, February 21-27, 1956*. London: Methodist Missionary Society.

Sharma, B. and Geetha, K.A. (2021) Casteing gender: Intersectional oppression of Dalit Women. *Journal of International Women's Studies*, 22(10), 1–7.

Singhai, M., Shah, Y., Gupta, N., Bala, M, Kulsange, S., Kataria, J., and Singh, S.K. (2021) Chronicle down memory lane: India's sixty years of plague experience. *Indian Journal of Medical Microbiology*, 39, 279–285.

Sparks, K. (2021) 'Prisons and the Public', by Margaret Bondfield, JP. *The Howard Journal*, 66(SI), 38-46. https://doi.org/10.1111/hojo.12439

Spencer, B.B. (2016) *'Ours is a Great Work': British Women Medical Missionaries in Twentieth-Century Colonial India*. PhD Dissertation. Georgia State University.

Underhill, L. (1932). *Customs of Midwifery in India by Mrs L. Underhill*. Published paper presented to the Croydon Branch of the Midwives Institute, 13 September, 1932. London: Midwives Institute, pp. 1–5.

Underhill, L.A. (1935) *Extremes Meet: Some Acts about India's Women*. London: Highway Press.

Viswanath, R. (2009) Spiritual slavery, material malaise: 'Untouchables' and religious neutrality in colonial South India. *Historical Research*, 83(219), 124–145. https://doi.org/10.1111/j.1468-2281.

Vosler, B. (2010) Making his way to the heart of India: British missionaries, Indian nationalism, and religious belonging in post-World War I India. *British Scholar*, III(1), 61–78.

7   The road to Maua

Moulding the new nurse

Escaping from the oppressive atmosphere at the tuberculosis hospital at Leasowe, Muriel sped to Clatterbridge General Hospital for three years of SRN training. Audrey, in comparison, provided only the briefest references to her truncated nursing activities in Britain prior to leaving for India. One senses that Audrey's real life began in India, so her experiences in Britain are little remarked on. Muriel's narratives are far more detailed in this respect. Her nursing career prior to becoming a missionary was longer, more fulfilling and certainly more descriptively vivid. Furthermore, Muriel's mission years were more interspersed by nursing periods back in Britain, each location being full of activity and change. The basic differences between these sisters thereby emerge strongly set side-by-side: one seems reticent to the point of disappearing entirely from view at times. The other is vibrantly and unmistakably present. One is self-effacing, reserved and remote, the other a dynamo of eccentric energy and tragi-comedic turns: a picaresque heroine and foil to Fortune's caprice.

Tracking Muriel's movements requires some complicated plotting of place and position, not aided by her very faded, part-typed, part hand-scrawled, half-page employment record bearing the scantiest employment details, written before the trend for bloated *curriculum vitae/resume*. Furthermore, Muriel's recollections of her time at one hospital often seemed to merge with those of the many others she had known. The emphasis she placed also differed according to the interviewer, offering not so much a triangulation of data, but revealing multifaceted and tonal complexities of an energetic and restless life.

Fran, fascinated by the minutiae of British nursing, focused on this aspect of Muriel's life. From her, we learn of the everyday realities of nursing work in post-war Britain, the routines of practice and proprieties

DOI: 10.4324/9781003359746-7

governing nurses' lives. Training then was expected to be undertaken in the nurses' spare time, sieving out unsuitable candidates. This pseudo-military command-and-control culture fostered both camaraderie and bullying. It was important to quickly learn who were the better-tempered senior staff and who likely to rebuff younger charges with a violently hurled object.

It was very hard work climbing up from the lowest ranks to the respectable status of trained nurse. Muriel showed aptitude: where some of her peers failed, she passed, and was told she was a born nurse – and midwife too. Astonished by her capabilities, Muriel learned quickly, witnessing many new treatments. She saw the early use of Fleming's discovery, Penicillin, that had become a vital part of the Allies pharmaceutical armaments during the late 1943 (Hopwood, 2007; Lesch, 2006). For the public, no longer was death from casual infection to be feared in the same way. She also witnessed medical cruelty too: an agonising rib-resection for a lung abscess performed (unusually) by a woman surgeon under local anaesthetic only; Muriel and her fellow nurses holding down the screaming, writhing patient. This harrowing episode became indelibly inscribed on her memory.

Muriel surprisingly evinced no real interest in midwifery at that time. Instead, she found deep satisfaction in her nursing duties. She liked the simple routine tasks: taking temperatures, sterilising equipment, dressing wounds, plumping pillows. Nor did she object to emptying bedpans or the strong-arm lifting of patients; despite causing her chronic back problems.

In 1944, at Clatterbridge General Hospital, midwifery training had just become available. Muriel and four other nurses were selected to be the first batch of student midwives. Her new goal, under peer persuasion, was to obtain further qualifications (Part 1) in midwifery. It was Audrey, herself involved in midwifery training, who persuaded Muriel to undertake Part 2 at Macclesfield, and so obediently she put herself forward for it in 1945. This involved three months under supervision at Macclesfield and three months in district community midwifery.

The image of the district midwife, smartly and energetically cycling to her next labouring patient, at all hours of the day and night, has become nostalgically familiar to the millions of devoted British viewers tuning into the highly successful BBC series 'Call the Midwife', inspired by Jennifer Worth's (2002) autobiography of the same name. Worth worked as a community midwife in the 1950s Docklands of East London under the auspices of the religious Order of St Raymond Nonnatus (he of the unnatural birth – *non-natus*) whose nuns, qualified in nursing and midwifery, diligently plied their healing skills among the impoverished, working-class masses spilling from this squalid, overfilled, underfed London neighbourhood.

The messy realities depicted in this adored series are merely a televised reflection of those faced by all community midwives across the country then.

MURIEL:[1]   An urgent call came from a boy on a bicycle that this girl was in strong labour and they wanted a midwife quickly so the midwife said to me 'you go on ahead and I'll join you when I finish here'. I followed this boy on our bicycles. Someone was on the street waving their arms saying 'come quickly, the baby's coming!' We rushed up the stairs. Nothing was prepared, I didn't even have my nursing bag. This young, single girl was on the bed – she was having her first baby, only a young girl. She was pushing and I could see the baby's head. I just said, 'if you've got a bowl of water?' They're supposed to have a box of things there but anyway they hadn't got much. All I could think was what am I going to tie the cord with? So, they brought me a bowl of water and soap and I washed my hands and told this girl to push gently and rest in-between. She was very good, the girl and I said to her mum 'have you got any tape?" So, they said, 'Oh I don't know'...they go to have look... came back and said, 'we haven't got any but so-and-so has gone to Woolworths for some'....And they brought it back just in time for me to soak it in pure Dettol. I remember doing that and I delivered this first baby without a tear, beautifully. She was ever such a good girl! She did everything I said. She was a very good patient. Calm. I got the placenta out and it was all over before the midwife came. My first delivery on my own and before I was qualified. I felt quite proud of myself. The midwife said that I'd 'done very well'. So that made me more keen on midwifery.

Worth (2002) attributes the increased professionalisation of midwifery to social policy changes enacted in 1902 through the First Midwives Act (seventeen years prior to nurse registration), for which groups like the Nonnatus nuns had actively pressed. These legal changes instigated the Central Midwives Board (Leap and Hunter, 1993), tasked with establishing a practising midwife's role where unregistered bona fide midwife practitioners of one year's standing could apply for registration. After three years, the registration roll was closed (Dingwall et al., 1988). Of the thousands of women applying across the country, many were deemed to be unsuitable owing to holding no qualifications, being illiterate, elderly, unhygienic in their person, dress or home circumstances; or failing to be of good personal conduct. The lack of registration was ostensibly designed to oust amateur birthing practitioners in a reframing towards specialist, feminised work, now fast becoming strictly monitored by professional bodies, and thus out-of-bounds to the layperson. The targeted incorrigible that professional midwifery was designed to exclude was the neighbourhood, working-class, delivery helpmate and the local 'handywoman'. Morally occupying the same demonised status as the traditional birth attendant, the Indian *dai*, the English 'handywoman' was condemned and parodied using similarly pejorative terms. Oft cited, Dicken's grotesque, laying-in/laying-out' Sariey Gamp, a 'sloppy, dirty, drunkard and hired attendant of the poor', became a byword among the professionals for lay incompetence and ignorance (Leap and Hunter, 1993, p. 6). Worth (2002, p. 5) in turn describes the 'insanitary' work of handywomen as implicated in a 'frightening mortality rate' and that their casual services were socially 'uncontrolled'. Although often viewed as a valued and respected member of her community, the Third Midwives Act of 1926 even went so far as to describe the handywoman as 'the foe' (Hunter, 2012, p. 9).

Although most births took place at home, midwife registration provided the legislative ability to weed out the unwanted handywoman role. This process was facilitated throughout the 1930s by the greater uptake of antenatal services and hospitalised births that were increasingly encouraged. Women did not necessarily resist the move towards hospitalised births, particularly as midwives were not permitted to administer stronger analgesics than gas-and-air, unlike the chloroform, qualified obstetrician administered in hospitals (Leap and Hunter, 1993). Dingwall et al. (1988) argue that these childbirth analgesia distinctions were a deliberate ploy marking out professional turf boundaries, akin to those permitted to use the stethoscope or pulse watch. Such symbolically demarcated territory served as a reminder of the qualified (masculinised), higher-status doctor and the lower-status, subaltern (feminised) nursing role.

The Second World War gave a purposive morale boost to the inevitably high national birth rate, where contraceptives were difficult and expensive to obtain, and abortion illegal. 'Pronatalist' propaganda abounded, licit propagation was recast as a patriotic act, a '"one in the eye" for Hitler', blow against the Nazis (Davis, 2014, p. 260). The birth rate subsequently rose to a peak by 1946 (Hunter, 2012).

It was during this period that the Chalkley sisters were moving into midwifery themselves: part of the skilled, female workforce administering to the wartime baby boom. Some young married women resented this call to reproduction for the sake of Britain, with others driven to desperation and backstreet abortions to get rid of unwanted pregnancies. Nonetheless, the welfare of pregnant women and their infants was firmly on the government agenda through the endeavours of Lord Woolton, a former social worker and witness of the effects of privation among the Liverpudlian poor. Now expectant wartime mothers would receive proper vitamin supplements and larger protein rations (Davis, 2014).

Questions arose concerning where pregnant women could deliver their babies safely. Leachman observes that wartime severely constrained the choice of maternity provisions in city areas, where resources were transferred to areas away from enemy bombing raids, leaving city maternity provision scant (Leachman, 2020). Rurally located maternity homes were set up in existing, remote hospitals or converted country houses, necessitating the evacuation of pregnant women, as well as city children, with the district midwife in tow (Leap and Hunter, 1993).

Such precautions, however inconvenient, were not premature. In May 1941, the year that Muriel was transferring from Leasowe to Clatterbridge, the Mill Road Hospital in Liverpool was catastrophically bombed with great loss of life of patients, medical and auxiliary staff. A ward of injured soldiers received no causalities, but in the maternity ward next door, many women and their newborns were killed (Hogan, 2014). One wonders if perhaps this event, a shocking contemporary massacre of the innocents, added a fresh impetus to Audrey to leave Stork Margarine and become a nurse, as she did at some point in her twenty-third year after August 1941.

From the late 1950s onwards, the services of religious communities of nuns dedicated to serving local people, such as St Raymond Nonnatus and the Community of St John the Divine (the latter serving the Poplar community of East London, the chosen site of the BBC series), would become gradually redundant under the sweeping new broom of the confident, young NHS, forging ahead with hospital birth promotion. This realised a prophecy put forward by the Royal College of Obstetricians and Gynaecologists in 1944 recommending that hospital maternity facilities should be expanded to accommodate 70% of birth; by the 1950s, a 100% increase was anticipated (Hunter 2012).

Whether births took place in hospitals or at home, the position and practices of midwives changed for good. Booked directly by patients, the midwife had been an autonomous professional who made referrals to GPs, *if* she deemed it required. Now the midwife was placed further down the chain of control, being the one to whom a GP made referrals – it was a clear fall in status and independence (Hunter, 2012).

The professional perceptions of a promiscuously prolific army of unqualified, local handywomen requiring curbing, was not matched by numbers of approved birth attendants. In fact, there was a scarcity of registered, qualified midwives. One assertion voiced in the 1960 *British Medical Journal* was that midwifery scarcities existed only in hospital settings owing to the removal of birth from the home context, leaving community-based midwives sitting on idle hands. This statement was roundly challenged in a well-informed letter by E.D. Irvine to the journal arguing that in the Devon city of Exeter, in 1958, there remained a shortage of domiciliary midwives as well as their hospital counterparts; for although there were 483,971 hospitals births, a further 273,032 of births took place at home.

The health of the nation: old and new regimes

The immediate post-war period forging the new hierarchies of health care enabled all to be equally nursed. The old voluntary and municipal hospitals changed both their names and status in Beverage's 'National Health Service' (NHS) of 1948. This had been wrought from a wrangle of earlier negotiations between 'Nye' Bevan, the minister for health in Clement Attlee's Labour government, and the British Medical authorities, opposed to any loss of professional autonomy and income (Timmins, 2017). Yet, it would take time for practices to change.

By December 1945, Muriel, a registered SRN, had transferred to West Park Hospital in Macclesfield, which confusingly, if correctly, she also called 'Macclesfield Municipal'. This hospital was formerly the Macclesfield Poor Law Union Workhouse and Infirmary, a municipal hospital catering for sectors of society unable to attend the superior 'voluntary' hospitals (Timmins, 2017). The infirmary, a necessary, humanitarian attachment to the workhouse, for the care of sick and infirm inmates, eventually evolved to admit non-paupers; although the stigma of the institutions would remain in memory, if not in name, for some time to come.

Higginbotham (2023) has compiled a considerable amount of historical information online about the workhouse system, commenting that until the 1870s the workhouse infirmary was both inadequate in facilities and in expertise. This is discernible from records: in 1886, a St Pancras Coroner's Court[2] records the death of a 'very heavy woman' inmate, who died after being lifted by 'two very aged women, one the help and the other an aged and infirm patient'. The patient fell back on the bed screaming having sustained a fractured arm and dislocated shoulder. The coroner noted a delay of two hours before the medical officer was called. The subsequent death was recorded as acute rheumatism aggravated by a fractured arm. The inadvisability of employing elderly nurses formally noted.

An outcome of the Poor Law Amendment Act, 1834 was the rise of workhouse admissions of the infirm and incapacitated. No longer was 'outdoor relief' provided to sustain the impoverished and sick in their own homes, but where now the principle of 'lesser eligibility' ensured that the workhouse would be viewed as the very last resort of those unable to support themselves (Parker, 2023). By 1861, the workhouse infirmary system was caring for 50,000 sick people, as opposed to 11,000 in the voluntary hospitals (Dingwall et al., 1988). The enclosed citadels of the nineteenth-century asylum system, containing miscellaneous human debris of the Industrial Revolution, would, of necessity, require that patients were cared for by others (Ashencaen Crabtree, 2012). Likewise for the workhouse. Under the directions of the (now) qualified medical officer or the Matron (conveniently often married to the workhouse 'Master') inmate pauper nurses could expect to be paid in gin for the more disagreeable of their caring duties (Dingwall et al., 1988).

Appeals for improvement in the workhouse infirmary were eventually demanded. A paper delivered[3] to a medical conference in Wales in 1892 argued for properly trained workhouse nurses, quoting from a Local Government Board of 1864 recommending (in vain) that examples of better practice should be taken from the voluntary hospitals to inform work-house infirmary practices.

By April 1930, the Poor Law workhouses and their infirmaries passed to the local municipal authorities, along with their 'guardians': the workhouse staff (Parker, 2023). Fifteen years forward the revamped Macclesfield Poor Law Union Workhouse and Infirmary, now entirely renamed, became the third hospital to employ young Muriel Chalkley.

In Muriel's day, the values of lofty piety and lowly humility governing the institutional ethos remained intact. Nurses were expected to kneel and pray for their patients, a familiar public performance to Muriel, given her family background. Furthermore, the passive disengagement and helplessness of the economically dependent, particularly elderly patients, was still assumed in nursing practice. Such values were reflected in the social geography of Macclesfield Municipal, where geriatric care took place in the sacramental waiting room to death.

MURIEL:[4]   [the] old people were all kept in bed in those days. The old men I remember were in the chapel…This had been an old workhouse they'd made into a hospital and the chapel was a ward for old men. And I can remember these old men who were just kept in bed all day and when I think of it now, I can remember it. And they used to be incontinent and we'd used to change dirty sheets and it was terrible really, the nursing.

Macclesfield Municipal née Workhouse Infirmary was a small hospital that 'punched above its weight'. It had grown in expertise and capacity from humble beginnings. By Muriel's day, it now provided general medicine, orthopaedics, surgery and gynaecology. A 'male ward' was matched by a corresponding 'female ward', to which Muriel was promoted to run, for now she was a qualified and proud 'Sister in blue'.

The Matron seeing the writing on the wall regarding the future of small, municipal institutions under a transforming national health scheme, asked Muriel to widen its community value by developing a midwifery ward carved out of an adjacent wide corridor. It was good preparation for the missionary future, for Muriel now ran the women's ward, and antenatal clinics together with the labour ward, undertaking shifts with one other nurse colleague to manage birthing patients, day and night.

One anachronistic oddity was there were no resident doctors for the women's ward, instead each woman was attended to by their own GP. Although they carried superior status to the midwives and were not averse to showing it, these medical practitioners did not always know better.

MURIEL:[5]   I remember one patient and it was a breech presentation. Her own doctor came and said it was a normal head (presentation). I said it was breech and she was pushing and he went to wash his hands and he got a junior medical student and while this was happening and I delivered the breech. I was right. Of course it was a breech! And when he came back washing his hands he said to the medical student, 'was it a breech?' and he said 'yes', and he was amazed. The woman said she pushed hard because she wanted *me* to deliver the baby.

The GP visiting arrangement was not atypical of many other small hospitals and good maternity homes, where the matron, the midwives and the auxiliary nursing staff ran the day-to-day business of institutional childbirth. Women were admitted, often for rest or to await the birth of their babies, and some of these homes could be very comfortable indeed. When he was fifteen, Jack, a brilliant, 'ragged scholar', if ever there were, ran away from Liverpudlian, Dickensian misery of sharing one bed with two belligerent, moronically 'gormless' older step-brothers in the home of his rough but not unkindly docker, ex-boxer step-father, to set himself up in country house modelled on a stately home operating as an upmarket maternity home. Here he had his own quilted and chintz-curtained quarters offset by tutoring the privileged but dim scion of the 'Major and Matron', an ill-matched married couple, who owned and ran the Home (reminiscences of workhouse marital, managerial arrangements). There Jack dined with the mothers-to-be off sumptuous breakfasts of devilled kidneys, bacon, black pudding and eggs or Raj-style kedgeree, all served on silver platters; with two further large meals and teatime to look forward to. This was undreamed of bounty and comfort, until sadly the NHS sounded the death knell of such homes.

Back in the women's ward, under a less luxurious regime, Muriel found herself one night in charge of five women in labour, with three advancing rapidly towards the dénouement of delivery and only auxiliary nurses to help. This was multi-tasking with a vengeance. One woman, a less urgent case, calling for Muriel's attention was promptly sedated while she rushed off to see to the others, each in separate labour rooms, with Muriel popping in and out to deal with each. The first was given gas-and-air and encouraged not to push, while the second imminent mother-to-be was dropping her infant. Having slowed the delivery of one woman down, Muriel encouraged the other to birth her baby quickly into Muriel's impatient hands, with no time to cut the umbilical cord. Rushing back to the first mother, Muriel, with a swift changing of surgical gloves, delivered the next baby. Having extracted the placenta, she raced back next door to the second mother to extract hers. Then she galloped off to the third patient; after which she raced to help a fourth. Just towards the end of her shift, a labouring woman, moments from birth, arrived by taxi and had to be delivered on the hospital trolley. This was a legendary challenge by anyone's standards and duly deserved high praise, which in a cool, understated and very English way she got. She continued to do so, between 1940 and 1955, Muriel peregrinated from post to post across her North-west stamping ground, mopping up professional experiences and qualifications across the changing landscape of post-war health care.

The crisis

Muriel experienced the power of two overwhelming spiritual crises in her youth roughly a decade apart. These years divided the robust, maturing woman from the simple, unfinished girl. Each event thrusting her into a new consciousness, imbued an already generous spirit to radiantly recast service, and ultimately radically shaped the direction and meaning of a life already set in accelerated motion.

Muriel's time at Clatterbridge was a success: she was engaged in skilled work and her studies towards SRN qualification progressed commendably. She had friends at work and was able to visit her family regularly, yet, she was troubled in spirit, deeply so. On one particular Sunday, she awoke strangely miserable, overcome with dark shadows portending a meaningless existence. Cycling home on her Sunday afternoon off, her wretchedness was overtaken by a sudden suicidal madness.

MURIEL:[6] I was cycling home and I had to go down a hill, round a corner and up another hill. And I cycled in the middle of the road with my eyes closed, hoping to be knocked down. Just wanted to die. I just wanted to end it all. I can't tell you why, this is just how I felt. But of course, when I opened my eyes I was at home, wasn't I?

The traffic on the road then was light, but even so it was a crazily dangerous act to cycle blind miles up-hill, down, and around corners. Miraculously, and to her despair, she arrived home at the family front door completely unscathed by any collisions. Muriel's misery continued all that day. Refusing to go to Church with her family, she ill-temperedly chased them out with cries of 'Oh, go the lot of you!' Fortunately, her salvation was to hand, as I have recorded elsewhere:

> I knelt down, 'Oh God, if you are real come to me now!' And it was absolutely amazing. When I knelt down, I wanted the door to open, a hole to appear and for me to end my life. I don't know why. Well, there was a complete transformation – waves and waves of love came pouring over me. It was absolutely amazing. God just filled me with my love and I knew He was real. I wanted to sing every hymn in the book. Amazing. Complete transformation from utter misery to ecstasy. I wanted to tell everyone there. I went to the top of the road to look for them coming from Church – I knew now that God was real. I've never forgotten it. I was twenty-two then and now I am ninety-two.
>
> (Ashencaen Crabtree, 2021, p. 156)

To her family's great rejoicing, their heaven-directed petitions were swiftly and decisively answered. Muriel met them on the road with the pronouncement: 'I am saved, aren't I?' It was indeed apparent to her happy onlookers that it was so.

What is one to make of this epiphany? As Hempton (2005) states, testimonies of conversion form a significant narrative pillar with hundreds of similar Methodist attestations, both written and oral, from the eighteenth century onwards. Given this established tradition and placed beside it, Muriel's experiences were not exceptional. Her 'experience' – a wan word in the light of an occurrence of such devastating and revelatory beneficence – was not peculiar to Methodist soteriological beliefs, but was perhaps increasingly anachronistic. Green (1992) argues that whilst few did not doubt that genuine Christian commitment arose from a powerfully personal experience of conversion, these emotive, dramatic encounters with God became less expected than more rational and systematic decision-making spiritual exercises.

Nonetheless, if vivid religious rebirths were perhaps declining in the post-Edwardian period, many such accounts formed a significant corpus of Methodist history and emotive sensibility. In considering Methodist conversion testimonies as a genre, Hempton suggests that certain themes can be detected:

> Most occurred during teenage years; most betray such some sense of deep psychological distress; most contain within them an explicit or implicit

fear of death; many seem to take place in communities experiencing rapid social change or an unusual degree of social dislocation; and most converts had some preexisting religious knowledge.

(Hempton, 2005, p. 63)

Such features do appear to connect with and illuminate Muriel's revelations. Her crisis takes place at around the age of twenty-one. The war, providing her with the opportunity to enter this much-desired but previously closed world of nursing, was continuing in Europe. Unbeknownst to contemporaries, it was now in its middle phases, a dreary and wearing period of ongoing hardship for Britons; a time of endurance straining at the cheerful 'make do and mend' mentality the population was encouraged to evince. The hierarchical regime of nursing was always hard on its novitiates and tougher still under wartime conditions. At home, the beloved and promising first-born Chalkley child is long dead, the equally loved but less promising youngest child has survived, and strives to 'make good' and be a credit to her family and her upbringing.

Durkheim's concept of anomie may offer a partial solution to the conundrum but despite, material, social and existential threats abounding the manifestations of anomie were not wide-scale. The war for Britons did not seem to undermine confidence in the moral or hierarchical structures they knew, but rather reinforced the fundamental values of the country and created new tropes of triumph. Churchill, the lion-hearted, British bulldog, fiercely defiant against the superior forces of the enemy; King George IV and the Royal Family showing backbone during the bombing of the London Blitz. If death could strike suddenly from the air, the underground train shelters offered some safety and a sing-song. If black-marketeering went on, government rationing offered an example of what genuine social fairness could mean. If some trade unions went on strike during wartime, elsewhere women gallantly stepped up in their utility trousers and service uniforms to help run the country. If this is merely simplistic red, white and blue propaganda myth-making (as it is) and an imperfect picture of wartime Britain, then reveal a better one that contains as much truth. As importantly, it was the story that many Britons told themselves during those tediously dangerous days and lived their lives accordingly.

We must return to Muriel's state of grace both prior to and post this dramatic conversion. Raised with her sisters in the bosom of Methodism, these were children of the most ardent of lay preachers. Frank was devoid of inhibitions about unquenchable public preaching, happily collapsing to his knees to pray for shared salvation; an unusual sight one might think in the restrained North of England, traditionally uncomfortable with unseemly expressed emotion or excessive excitement. The girls were naturally expected to be pious participants in Fellowship, fundraising for Missions, leading Sunday Schools; and becoming lay preachers themselves, as Audrey and Muriel did. Yet, Muriel confessed[7] that she was not moved then by Methodist spiritual barn-storming. Her crises arose from despair at a spiritual disconnect between service in God's name and authentically being with Him in spirit. A personal relationship with God was unfelt, until, like Saint Thomas, in her desperation, she demands proof of God's existence – and receives that in abundance. Like Saint Theresa, overcome by the overwhelming visitation of divine rapture, thereafter transmogrified into a new self: the Christian believer's rebirth, from which there should be no return to doubt. Saved, she is imbued with earthly 'prevenient grace' (Wilson, 2011), with precious certainty of God's will to serve. In short, life once again became worth living for Muriel, elevated into newly God-given meaning and purpose, although His intentions had yet to be discerned. In the meantime, to celebrate her full and inner conversion, Frank, typically, presented his daughter with a book entitled *Prayer and the Bible*, bidding her to both pray and read a passage of the Bible each day. It was in Africa, however, that Muriel would eventually discover both the meaning and the messenger of God's love.

The call

By 1953, Muriel, armed with her SRN Part 1 certificate, beat nursing competition, better equipped with Part 2, to the position of Midwife Teacher at Derby City Hospital. This was a much-needed fillip for her, having earlier failed the practical element of the Midwife Teaching Diploma, introduced by the 1936 Midwife Act (Hunter, 2012), under the incomprehensibly fierce examination of an elderly, curmudgeonly male consultant. Her second attempt under a sensible woman consultant gained her the coveted new qualification. Now in charge of three labour wards, an antenatal clinic and a bevy of student midwives, these were extremely happy and fulfilling days for Muriel. With her student and friend, pretty, curly-headed Pat Tuffrey,[8] Muriel started a Nursing Christian Fellowship for like-minded nurses. She took up tennis, playing doubles with the doctors, to win a silver tennis trophy. The countryside was beautiful and she even found herself the object of romantic admiration.

Altogether the job at Derby was absolutely 'ideal'. But wisely or otherwise, Muriel had struck a secret bargain with God to serve wherever He sent her, if only she could pass her midwifery tutor exam. Now this vow began to trouble her Christian conscience. At first, the nudges to hear the 'Call' and take up the missionary baton were light, but increasingly they became uncomfortable. On furlough from India Audrey was invited to undertake deputation talks about her missionary work at local Methodist churches. Inevitably someone would ask discomfited Muriel, 'what about you? Shouldn't you be there?' Meaning the mission field. These reproaches followed her back to Derby: through the post came unwanted newspaper cuttings forwarded by encouraging Methodists about the need for missionary nurses in Africa. To cap it all, a colleague from her Nursing Christian Fellowship reproached her, saying, 'if I were you, I'd be abroad as a missionary. I think you should do that'.

However, a missionary's life was not what Muriel wanted at all. She had never visualised herself like this, despite her religious awakening. Nor had she ever travelled 100 miles beyond the North-west circuit of the Wirral. Obedient to her father's example and the laudable Methodist tradition of women's spiritual authority, she had become a lay preacher and a good one at that, having an ardent spirit and a rousing voice. Yet, like Jane Eyre fearfully resisting the implacable will of St John Rivers to take up the missionary's staff and follow, her heart was 'mute'. Muriel simply did not recognise herself as having a missionary vocation at all. The path she wished to follow was here in Derby. The pressure grew in intensity, singling her out for a fate she did not want or seek.

MURIEL:[9]   One day I went with some of the others to a Christian meeting and the speaker was talking about there are two roads in life, there is the broad, easy road and there is sometimes a narrow, difficult road. But as a Christian we have to choose the road God chooses for us. He looked straight at me and said 'for all I know there might be someone here tonight who ought to out on the mission field' and he pointed his finger straight at me it seemed. I thought, it's no good, I've got to offer.

It was a bitter pill to swallow and she hesitated. Offering oneself to missionary work meant being sent anywhere in the world for an indefinite period, in effect for as long as one was capable of serving. Maybe it brought to mind Luke 22:42 where Christ contemplates in agony the thorny way of sacrifice before Him.

Saying, Father, if thou be willing, remove this cup from me: nevertheless not my will, but thine, be done.

A Methodist rally was held nearby and like a moth, Muriel was drawn to it. A missionary doctor was speaking to the audience appealing for nurses, particularly those qualified to teach. With a heavy heart Muriel picked up a leaflet upon which was emblazoned 'WANTED URGENTLY NURSES TRAINED TO TEACH', this legend heavily encircled in a halo of ink.

MURIEL: I thought that seals it. I can't refuse it any longer. God helped me get this [diploma, I must use it wherever he wants. I knelt down and prayed this: 'Use me Lord. Use even me, just as you will, when and where'.

And the Lord did. Muriel went home to tell her parents she would offer herself to Mission House. Frank was glad, Bertha much less so at the prospect of losing yet another daughter to long years overseas.

Throughout the mission selection process in 1954, Muriel half-hoped they would decline her offer, whereupon she could honourably return to Derby duty done. No such luck, for first she was thoroughly vetted by an experienced Methodist mission family, then sent to be judged by the recruitment committee. Conscious of Audrey's esteemed reputation, Muriel was defiantly determined to show herself to the committee, led by Miss Walton, in a Cromwellian light: 'warts and all'. Asked what hobbies she had, she replied 'tennis'. Questioned about sewing retorted, 'Oh no, Audrey does that'. Knitting then? 'Oh no! Mother does that'.

Unsurprisingly, the committee looked askance at this unimpressive performance but grudgingly packed her off to Kingsmead for six months with

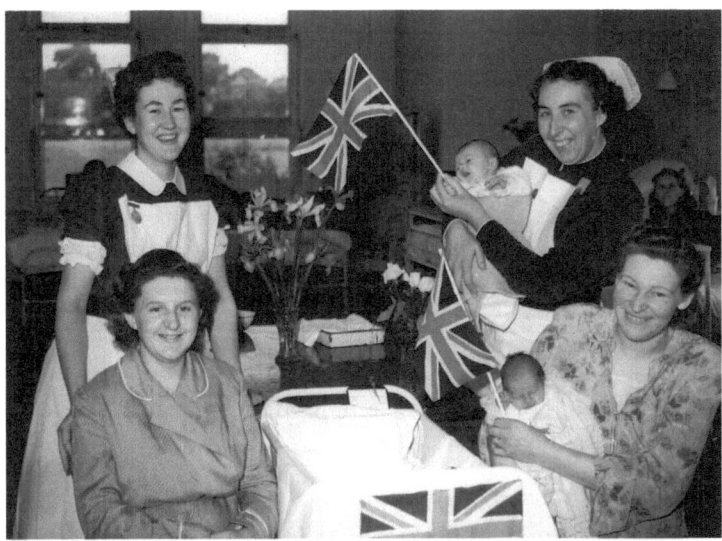

Figure 7.1 Coronation Day at Derby City Hospital, 1953. Courtesy of Muriel Chalkley.

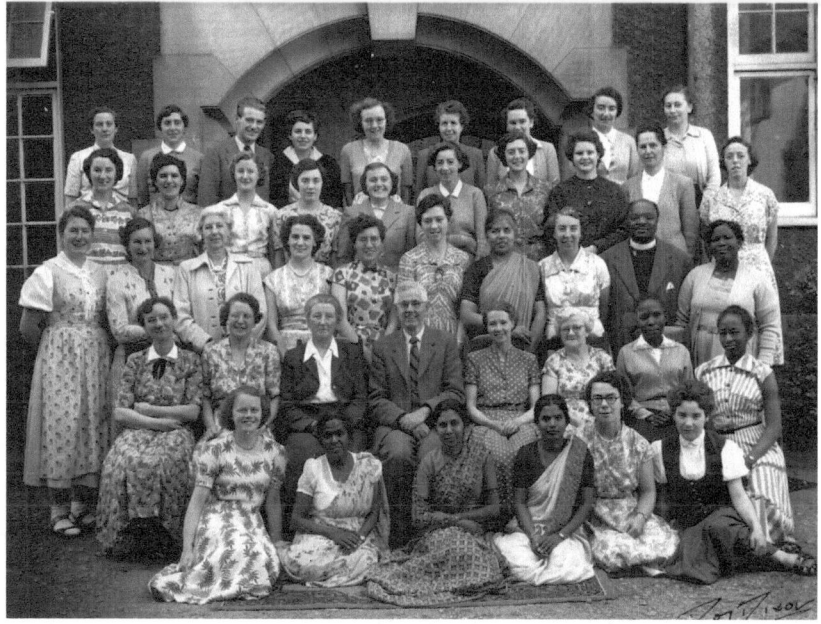

Figure 7.2 Muriel at Kingsmead College, 1955 (Middle Row, Third from Right). Courtesy of Muriel Chalkley.

a review of her suitability thereafter. For Muriel, this meant sorrowfully leaving her beloved job, breaking the heart of her doomed admirer and severely disappointing the Head Tutor who thought her quite 'mad' to go (Figure 7.1 and 7.2).

The Chantala

Kingsmead did not console, being dull fare, where the academic nature of Bible studies, to this practical Martha, was uninspiring and difficult. Expected to do three terms, her purgatory came to an end after two when informed of an urgent need to be parcelled off to Kenya to relieve a remote Methodist Mission Hospital where one of the two nurses was sick and the other on the verge of a mental breakdown. Muriel had only a fortnight to prepare.

MURIEL:[10]   So, I agreed to go. I had to go by train to London and said goodbye to my parents on the platform of Liverpool station and I had a little weep in the carriage. That was the last time I saw my dear father. I was very close to him.

At the London docks on 24 October 1955, Muriel boarded a cargo ship, the Chantala, to Mombasa, Kenya. The other passengers, numbering ten souls, were variously bound for Kenya, Tanganyika and the Seychelles; the men holding professions and the women housewives. Muriel was the only missionary among them, signifying the missionary decline post-war.

Unlike Audrey's experiences, Muriel's voyage was neither instructive, companionable or fun. The swimming pool was occupied by train parts, but there was deck tennis to play, partnering the ships' officers. Otherwise, there was no one much to talk to, and it was so very hot at times, especially going through the Suez Canal. Muriel felt distinctly awkward in the presence of these well-travelled passengers from the southern Home Counties. Yet despite or because of this the captain, on his swan-song voyage before retirement, took a shine to the homespun, badly dressed, plainly spoken missionary and every night at dinner insisted on seating her between himself and the purser, whilst the ladies bedecked in evening gowns had to content themselves further down the table. Muriel, no gourmand, needed to be tempted towards the exotic cuisine of asparagus spears and the like, coaxed along by the captain's jokes of 'Oh come on, you'll be eating zebra and all sorts soon'.

Three long weeks on board, Muriel was bored, fed up and suffering from heatstroke. At last, they docked at Mombasa where she was driven to coastal Ribe to spend the weekend with a Kingsmead colleague. An arranged sight-seeing expedition took in the Anglican graveyard where the graves of missionaries, their wives and infants, poignantly marked the short existences of those who stepped on African soil, clutching Bibles, only to die a few months later of tropical diseases. After this treat, disorientated Muriel was put on the train to Nairobi, beset by the usual traveller confusion of missed liaisons and lost letters of introduction – in this case boarding the right train at the wrong station, where she found herself sharing an overnight cabin with three European ladies, a-twitter at the smart and handsome young English policeman who had been searching the carriages in vain looking for a 'Miss Chalkley'. This, astonishingly, turned out to be a distant cousin now working in the Kenyan police force busily keeping a close eye on comings-and-goings.

Overseas missionary narratives, as Comaroff and Comaroff (1991) observe, offer travelogues of lengthy, strenuous journeys to remote destinations; and the more uncomfortable and poorly resourced, the better the tale of adventure. Muriel's journey was both more and less than these in the telling. Of duration, it certainly stood the test; of discomfort and danger, it had its shares; of pleasantries and wonder, it was not lacking, nor so the impact upon this weary traveller hailing not from the perilous North-West Frontier of India, but merely the provincial north-west of England. The ladies dined served by African waiters in long white robes while the wonderful sights of the Serengeti Game Park passed before Muriel's amazed eyes.

Dismounting at Nairobi station Muriel stood on the platform lost among the bustle and noise of many peoples: African Kenyans, the Indian bourgeoisie and displaced Europeans. Two of the latter detached themselves from the crowds; the chairman of the District Head of Mission in Kenya, Reverend Dr Bastin, and his wife, escorted her along the next leg of the journey in 'much too posh' a car for missionaries, thought Muriel. After this, came the local bus, riding with Miss Bertha Jones, an experienced missionary and headmistress of the Kaaga Girls Mission School in Meru, situated about thirty-five miles from Maua. *En route* Muriel received a basic language lesson in the Kimeru language from her, ad hoc compared to the in-depth tuition Audrey received in India. Muriel learned to speak a few phrases of tonal Kimeru but found it a difficult tongue and never approached the fluency Audrey acquired in Tamil.

Approaching the Central Highlands of Kenya stood the town of Nyeri, located not far from the tomb of the Boy Scout movement leader, Lord Baden-Powell. At Nyeri, a change of bus was required, Maua being still two hundred miles away. The second bus, in considerably worse shape than the first, broke down so often it was abandoned. Help was to hand, missionary couple John and Audrey Hattersley, volunteered to drive them onwards, with Muriel sat in front beside John at the wheel. Audrey declaring, 'I'd rather go in the back, then I won't see the road!'

MURIEL:[11]   I soon realised what she meant! As it was the rainy season the roads were muddy and we kept on skidding, and it was very hilly with more than one precipice at the sides. I was really frightened and imagined newspaper headlines saying 'Missionary killed on the way to her station!' But I didn't know then what a good driver (John) was – and eventually I had to drive myself on these roads. They were always a problem, but you got used to them: muddy and slippery in the wet season, and hot and dusty in the dry season.

They finally arrived in one piece at Meru Mission Station where Muriel was buttonholed by the very missionary whose nervous strain she been sent out to support. May Bennett poured out a litany of woes on weary Muriel over the long night ahead. The next morning, Harry Mills, an unseasoned, young missionary, unused to the road conditions, drove them onwards to Maua but within a mile his old Peugeot van broke down sinking into thick, oozing mud. All three got out to pull, heave and shove the stationary van, May Bennett receiving a mud bath for her pains. However, luck was on their side, it was Sunday and some African Methodist preachers stopped to help the trio, towing the car by rope until freed. Up and up, towards Mount Kenya in the distance, they then climbed. Hairpin roads and terrifying cliff-edge drops kept Muriel on the edge of her seat.

The vastness of the African terrain is said to have overwhelmed the British colonials' mindset for 'small-scale' tidy orderliness (Comaroff and Comaroff, 1991, p. 174). In fairness, perhaps not they alone, for according to Muriel, the name 'Maua' means, rather ominously, the place of no return in the Kimeru language. To her, it truly felt as though she had indeed travelled to the ends of the earth, it was so far away from everything she had known up to them.

Years after in Bournemouth on her wall hung a painting showing Maua as it had been. Depicted in a naïve, local style are round, pale-roofed huts, simple trees, men seated, a burden-bearing girl, cattle. Peaked hills form the sepia horizon. It was a good representation of Muriel's first glimpses of the locals:

MURIEL:[12]   Walking at the side of the roads a row of women, bent forward with huge loads of wood from the forest strapped to their backs and round their foreheads. Here and there a few scattered thatched, round, little houses. One little 'town-ship' Kangetta, ten miles from Maua had a market place with some little tiny shops (*dukas*) and women sitting on the ground in the centre selling maize, beans, yams. The scenery – green hills and extinct volcanoes was...beautiful but the area was very remote – and the road became narrower with many bends as we came to Maua.

The topography of Maua, high in altitude, is striking, sitting in a basin of the verdant Nyambeni Hills on three sides with one quadrant offering an incredible bird's eye view of a fall of thousands of feet across the plains (Gerrard, 2001, p. 62). Reverend Andrew MacKenzie,[13] the new missionary to Maua in the late 1960s, commented that Maua was set within the crater, highly inaccessible much of the time: chokingly dry and dusty or flooded and impassable. Altogether, a 'daft place to build a hospital', and for him, feeling at odds and alienated, Ikkadu felt 'claustrophobic'.

Dishevelled and muddy Muriel made an unprepossessing entry along the avenue of violet-bloomed jacaranda trees leading to the hospital. Her new quarters consisted of three small rooms serving as a bedroom, living room and a basic bathroom for washing; a primitive outdoor kitchen completed the 'cottage', consisting of a log fire and a rudimentary old, iron oven. There was no toilet, no running water or electricity. The midden, privy toilet was outside, to be shared with the Minister and the neighbouring dwelling. Going to the toilet was rather disagreeable, particularly at night, with only the company of a paraffin Tilley light casting shadows over the numerous spiders running up-and-down the walls. Her quarters were undeniably basic but manageable, and indeed Muriel made no complaints; although obliged to carry out her own bedding all the way from England.

Managing her little household would be 'Stephano',[14] a local Methodist preacher employed as 'houseboy'. Stephano's role was to do some light cleaning of the tiny home, shop and cook simple meals, but since Stephano could not cook at all and neither could Muriel, meals must have been interesting. Vegetables were provided from the tended 'shamba', the kitchen garden plot in the compound. Muriel had a poor opinion of the peculiar issue of avocado trees but bananas and other fruit were available in the market, along with eggs; although rice (outside of an English rice pudding), was definitely something she 'didn't bother with'.

Drawn from some formative folk memory of the good English housewife, Muriel, though, did teach Stefano the English tradition of the 'Sunday roast' (goat in this case), which was to last most of the week: roast on Sunday, cold on Monday, stewed on Tuesday, minced on Wednesday, desperation by Thursday and so on – all this without the benefit of a proper 1950s kitchen or refrigeration. Luckily for Stefano, Muriel was endlessly busy, relentlessly cheerful, enjoyed an undiscerning (and unadventurous) palate and had the constitution of an ox.

The sole and presiding doctor at the hospital for the past six months was Dr John Ware, May Bennett's bête noir, and it was he who took the cursorily scrubbed and more presentable Muriel for a tour around the hospital. The hospital itself boasted ninety beds divided across the usual male ward, female ward, a children's and a maternity ward. There was an outpatient's department, a very small operating theatre, a store room, a dispensary and two offices, one for the doctor and the other for matron's use.

The newly independent Methodist Church of Kenya in the early 1960s had promptly renamed the hospital built in the 1930s from the original, colonial name of Berresford Memorial Hospital (Gerrard, 2001; Pritchard, 2014), named in memory of the late son of a Mr Sam Berresford, a staunch Methodist from far off Chesterfield in Derbyshire. The handsome £3,000 presented by Mr Berresford for the building and equipping of the Methodist hospital in Maua poignantly represented the sum saved for his late son's training as a medical missionary, an ambition cut short by untimely death (Gerrard, 2001).

Close by the hospital stood a solid church, large for such a small community. This was built by Dr Ware's predecessors, Dr Herbert Gerrard, a Primitive Methodist by legacy, a graduate of the University of Manchester, and by all accounts a very energetic, dedicated and determined medical missionary, who, inspired by the example of Livingstone, had a clear sense of his Christian duty as a healer. Based at the Berresford Memorial

Hospital in the 1930s. Dr Gerrard and his wife, Doris (she who planted the jacaranda saplings years before) formed an effective marital missionary team, caring for the local people, other missionaries and their families. The extensive variety and range of Dr Gerrard's work involved the following tasks: to look after the dispensary, deal with medical and surgical emergencies, supervise the work of the schools, train teachers and preachers and to make regular surveys of the villages in his district in order to get to know and win the confidence of the chiefs (Gerrard, 2001, p. 45).

The Gerrards returned to England at the beginning of the Second World War but saw the erection of the new church at Maua, funded by the wider Gerrard clan and supporters, just before they left. The precious burden of the hospital fell to younger medical missionaries to continue. Maua Methodist Hospital had been previously extended by Dr Gerrard to provide a small maternity ward; while Dr Bastin added an oil-driven generator producing sufficient electricity to run an x-ray machine. Improvements had been made over time as and when funds were found. However, if Muriel had fewer qualms about her lodgings, her first sight of the hospital at this time made a distinct impression upon her. It was duly summed up in her 'Life Story':

> What a contrast to my hospital in the UK! ...I wrote in my diary my first impressions: 'FLIES -DIRT – SMELLS!' Especially on the Children's wards. There were just holes in the ground for latrines, potties for the toddlers but they didn't understand how to use them and just deposited their waste in little heaps everywhere on the floor! It was all such a contrast to having done four years in the UK, of course. But the African staff – mainly boys and young men – some now qualified, having done four years training were very welcoming to me. The beds were made of iron, with a wooden base and straw mattresses. Sterilising of instruments was done with Primus stoves, and at night theatre had an oil lamp fixed in the ceiling. But for all other procedures (including complicated deliveries) we only had Tilley (kerosene) lamps and torches.

The contrast between Maua and Nairobi would have been very striking. Even so, it is not hard to understand why Muriel might see Maua as literally being the 'back-of-beyond' (Figure 7.3).

As the Protectorate of British East Africa (BEA) in the late nineteenth century, Kenya held far less colonial importance than Uganda or Zanzibar, all of which made up the BEA. Nairobi began life as a train depot for the British Colonial Uganda Railway Company (Martin and Bezemer, 2020), the purpose of which was to open the interior to commerce; with mission work capitalising on this opportunity of access. The railway was completed

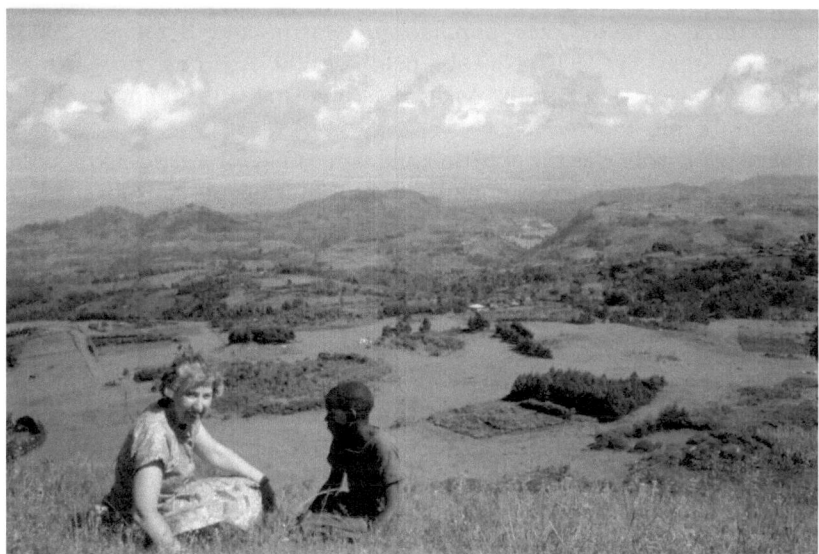

Figure 7.3 Nyambeni Hills, Muriel and Companion. Courtesy of Muriel Chalkley.

in 1903 at the staggeringly vast cost of nearly eight million pounds (Kyle, 1999). With this extravagantly expensive asset, upon which Nairobi was effectively founded, it could hardly fail to grow, and the watering hole area known to the Maasai as *Enkere Nairobi* ('the place of cool water'), was by the turn-of-the-century a main urban colonial conurbation (van den Bijl, 2017). Holding a mixed-race population of Europeans, Asians and African, Nairobi grew to a city fit for central colonial administration, as well as the less anticipated location of bolshy political activism and, so far as the Government was concerned, subversion.

These first European settlers were a mixed lot, comprising 'top drawer' British public school, officer types, would-be Afrophiles, opportunists and low-life too. As for location, Muriel placed in the far more remote highlands of Maua had instantly appreciated their beauty and coolness. Altitude in closer proximity to Nairobi, and equally delightful and fertile, formed highly sought-after areas for colonial occupation, involving due displacement of local people (Kyle, 1999).

Nairobi, providing entertainment, shopping and other civilised pleasures, was a popular destination for colonial rest-and-recouperation, although Muriel rarely had such opportunities. In the meantime, its population was rapidly growing, accelerating the need for effective urban planning, particularly given its strategic governmental importance in governing a mixed-race population. Martin and Bezemer (2020) enumerate that by 1920 Nairobi held 12,000 Africans, growing to 18,000 four years later, with 'Asiatics' composing 9,199 and European elites numbering a mere 2,665.

The new Nairobi was the experimental guinea pig for a series of modern urban planning movements, none being too injurious to Nairobi's urban glamour and convenience (Banyikwa, 1990). Yet as early as the 1920s, Nairobi received very positive endorsements from Kenyan-born Anglican missionary, Handley Hooper[15] for those back in England thinking of an African sojourn.

> I think the shops are one of the most remarkable features of Nairobi. We expected some fairly good Indian shops, and perhaps one or two with an English proprietor, but we found several pretentious building of two or three stories in height, with smart English assistants, and seemingly everything for sale which one could possibly desire. Of course, the prices range a good deal higher, but even so anyone coming out in ordinary times would do well to consider the advisability of getting more of the household goods here. Altogether it is a very English town, and the residential quarter on the hills which skirt the town, might be a garden suburb, with the additional advantage of a view over miles of level open country (the game reserve) out towards the green hill country north and eastwards of Nairobi. Nairobi is the hub of B.E.A. life and so one sees strange medley of native life, African and Indian, for the railway brought Indian labour into this country, and here it has stayed ever since, and increased. ... There is a large European population, from three to four thousand, and they employ a correspondingly large number of natives who have come from all over the country in search of employment.

Nonetheless, however materially convenient, Hooper did not regard Western civilisation and urban lifestyles, as paraded in Nairobi, being the way forward for African Kenyans.

Christianity, for Hooper, offered hope to Black Kenyans, who thereby empowered could own and shape their own future, for colonials failed to treat the African as a '"living soul"' (Cassons, 1998, p. 393).

The mission schools, of various denominations, provided a vital opportunity to educate African children towards self-improvement and to better their country, as exemplified by the towering political figures of Jomo Kenyatta and Nelson Mandela (Gerrard, 2001). Numerous political activists and future political elites gained access to sufficient western learning and literacy through mission school education to play colonial rulers at their own games, and to better it, if they could.

Hospitals too served two purposes, firstly and overtly, to provide much-needed health care for local people, most of whom lived in rural areas. Secondly, as medical training grounds, enabling Kenya to become independent of imperial resourcing in order to eventually meet the health needs of its population.

Muriel to her surprise at Maua, found that nurse trainees consisted of young men, rather than women, forming a contrast to Britain where nursing was very much a female-dominated profession. These youths, referred to as 'dressers' (connoting presumably the dressing of wounds) undertook a four-year nurse training programme under May Bennet. The few young women acting as assistant nurses received only two years' training owing to their limited school education. Third-year student Justus Gichungie throws insight on this anomaly writing in the first Maua Hospital magazine[16] in 1955.

> The education of girls was very rare. Those who were educated were stopped by their parents from becoming nurses. They believed that if they were nurses they would lose their sight and become blind. Even myself I was told this.

Bridget Robertson's 1993 coyly named autobiography, *Angels in Africa*, recalled her years of state colonial nursing in Kenya, describing being stationed in Nairobi from 1947 for several years, prior to being sent to the Rift Valley. She claims that the duties of a ward sister in the Nairobi European Hospital were not particularly onerous. Sent 'up-country' to the so-called African Hospital in Nakuru, in the Rift Valley, life was rather different. Patients were admitted with multiple fractures caused by agricultural and traffic accidents, but also weapon wounds inflicted by spears and *panga* machetes, together with crushing and mauling through wild elephant and leopard attacks. This was no exaggeration as Muriel would find out.

However, Robertson also complained that the local nurses required 'constant supervision' owing to their unfamiliarity with European standards of nursing (Robertson, 1993, p, 5). The only highly competent staff, she claims, were the midwives, and these had been trained in Nairobi.

Muriel confirmed in interviews with me that Nairobi was not just the best place for midwifery training but the only place providing midwifery training in northern Kenya. After gaining some Kenyan experience, and resisting the suggestion of relocating to Nairobi as a valuable Midwifery Tutor, Muriel took up the challenge to educate midwives at Maua. Three promising girls waiting keenly for that opportunity: Margaret, Leah and 'Deborah',[17] these would become Muriel's first midwife trainees in Kenya, and witnesses of her legacy.

Notes

1 Interview with Frank Biley, 2010. Ibid.
2 Workhouse Infirmary Nursing. *The British Medical Journal* Vol. 2, No. 1348 (30 October 1886), p. 831.
3 Workhouse Infirmary Nurses. Ibid.
4 Muriel Chalkley, interview with Fran Biley. Ibid.
5 Muriel Chalkley, interview with Author. Ibid.
6 Muriel Chalkley, interview with Fran Biley. Ibid.
7 Muriel Chalkley, interview with Caroline Ferris. Ibid.
8 Pat Tuffrey retired to the Bournemouth Nursing Home, remaining in contact with Muriel.
9 Muriel Chalkley, interview with Author. Ibid.
10 Muriel Chalkley, interview with Caroline Ferris. Ibid.
11 'My Life Story'. Ibid.
12 'My Life Story'. Ibid.
13 British Library 'Sounds'. Andrew MacKenzie, interviewed Moir Crockett, 8 December 1997. Methodist Church Oral Archive. **640/137/01-02.**
14 The biography of Dr Herbert Gerrard stationed in Maua during the interwar years also mentions a Methodist preacher by the name of Stephano. One presumes that this is the same individual in both cases.
15 Papers of the Hooper Family. Cadbury Library. Ibid.
16 Berresford Memorial Hospital Magazine, Maua, Kenya, 1955. Special Collection, SOAS. MMSL AF.LE 1088.
17 Anonymised by author.

References

Ashencaen Crabtree, S. (2021) *Women of Faith and the Quest for Spiritual Authenticity: Comparative Perspectives from Malaysia and Britain.* London/New York: Routledge.

Ashencaen Crabtree, S. (2012) *A Rainforest Asylum: The Enduring Legacy of Colonial Psychiatric Care in Malaysia.* London: Whiting & Birch.

Banyikwa, W.F. (1990) Signature of four generations of urban planning in Nairobi, Kenya. *Journal of Eastern African Research*, 20, 186–201.

Cassons, J. (1998) 'To plant a garden city in the slums of Paganism....': Handley Hooper, the Kikuyu and the future of Africa. *Journal of Religion in Africa*, XXVIII, 387–410.

Comaroff, J. and Comaroff, J. (1991) *Of Revelation and Revolution: Christianity, Colonialism and Consciousness in South Africa*, Vol. 1. Chicago, IL: The University of Chicago Press.

Davis, A. (2014) Wartime women giving birth: Narratives of pregnancy and childbirth, Britain c. 1939-1960, *Studies in History and Philosophy of Biological and Biomedical Sciences*, 47, Part Bm, 257–266.

Dingwall, R., Rafferty, A.M. and Webster, C. (1988) *An Introduction to the Social History of Nursing.* London: Taylor & Francis.

Gerrard, J.W. (2001) *Africa Calling: A Medical Missionary in Kenya and Zambia.* London: The Radcliffe Press.

Green, S. (1992) 'Spiritual science' and conversion experience in Edwardian methodism: The example of West Yorkshire. *The Journal of Ecclesiastic History*, 43(3), 428–446.

Hempton, D. (2005) *Methodism: Empire of the Spirit*. New Haven, CT: Yale.

Higginbotham, P. (2023) *The Workhouse: The story of an Institution*. Available at https://www.workhouses.org.uk/ [Accessed 17 March 2023].

Hogan, A. (2014) *Merseyside at War*. Stroud: Amberley Publishing.

Hopwood, D.A. (2007) *Streptomyces in Nature and Medicine: The Antibiotic Maker*. Oxford: Oxford University Press.

Hunter, B. (2012) Midwifery, 1920–2000: The reshaping of a profession. In Anne Borsay, Anne and Billie Hunter (Eds.), *Nursing & Midwifery in Britain Since 1700*. London: Bloomsbury Publishing, pp. 151–169.

Irvine, E.D. (1960) Midwifery Services. *British Medical Journal*, 23(1), 280. https://doi.org/10.1136/bmj.1.5168.280

Kyle, K. (1999) *The Politics of the Independence of Kenya*. Houndsmill: Palgrave Macmillan.

Leap, N. and Hunter, B. (2014). *The Midwife's Tale: An Oral History Form Handywoman to Professional Midwife*. Barnsley, S.Yorks: Pen & Sword.

Leachman, C. (2020) Birth at a time of national emergency: from the second world war to coronavirus. *The Conversation*, 3 August. Available at: https://theconversation.com/birth-at-a-time-of-nationahol-emergency-from-the-second-world-war-to-coronavirus-140488 [Accessed 6 October 2022].

Lesch, J.E. (2006). *The First Miracle Drug: How the Sulfa Drugs Transformed Medicine*. Oxford: Oxford University Press.

Martin, A.M. and Bezemer, P.M. (2020) The concept and planning of public native housing estates in Nairobi/Kenya, 1918–1948. *Planning Perspectives*, 35(4), 609–634. https://doi.org/10.1080/02665433.2019.1602785

Parker, J. (2023) *Analysing the History of British Social Welfare: Compassion, Coercion and beyond*. Bristol: Policy Press.

Prichard, J. (2014) *Methodists and their Missionary Societies, 1900-1996*. London: Routledge.

Pritchard, A.C. (2017) *Sisters in Spirit: Christianity, Affect and Community Building in East Africa, 1860–1970*. East Lansing: Michigan State University Press.

Robertson, B.M. (1993) *Angels in Africa: A Memoir of Nursing with the Colonial Service*. London: The Radcliffe Press.

Timmins, N. (2017) *The Five Giants*. London: William Collins.

Van der Bijl, N. (2017) *Mau Mau Rebellion: The Emergency in Kenya, 1952–1956*. Barnsley, South Yorkshire: Pen and Sword Military.

Wilson, K. 2011. *Methodist Theology*. London: T&T Clark International.

Worth, J. (2002) *Call the Midwife*. London: Phoenix.

8 The *Mutani* and the Mau Mau

Mission in Maua

Dr Gerrard's interwar casework at the Berresford Hospital was replete with cases of pneumonia, gastroenteritis, malnutrition, malaria, measles, leprosy and injuries (Gerrard, 2001). Little changed, for in the summer of 1958, Muriel wrote an airmail letter[1] to Bertha and Audrey (on furlough), describing some of her many and varied duties: setting fractures, dealing with *panga* wounds, including 'one, a small child, with his hand almost completely severed'. Generally, the children's ward was filled with patients sick or dying of tetanus, septicaemia and *kwashiorkor*, a severe form of malnutrition brought about by protein deficiency. Respiratory illnesses and a host of other ailments were common, including burns from open fires.

The greatest hazard to infants, however, was the risk they shared with their mothers – birth. Across the different accounts, Muriel left, childbirth was the dominant theme, unsurprisingly given her profession. Unlike England by then, childbirth in Kenya was often associated with danger and tragedy. Untimely death and lives snatched from the brink of eternity by the skill and devotion of the medial staff at the Maua Mission Hospital were recalled. It is to these stories that we will shortly turn.

Medical anthropology

Muriel had no doubt that Mission Hospitals and allopathy generally played a critical role in the preservation of lives. From our personal communications, I knew that Fran Biley was more sceptical. In an unpublished paper based on the sisters' history, Fran unambiguously critiqued the missionary enterprise. This was not in any way ameliorated but compounded, if possible, by the mission affiliation with 'Western' medicine. He questioned Muriel closely about her attitudes as a colonial midwife/nurse and her role in the hegemonic machinery of Imperial allopathic medicine. Exploring

DOI: 10.4324/9781003359746-8

Muriel's crusade to bring Maua women to colonial medical settings to be delivered by Western-trained midwives, her honest responses did nothing to defuse his suspicions,[2] discernible in the following interview extract:

FB: So how about our second subject then, which would be the medicalisation of childbirth.

Muriel: childbirth?

FB: So, childbirth becomes less of a natural function taking place in the outskirts and more of a hospital based…?

Muriel: Yes, oh absolutely, yes, I think the majority of people would now all go to a hospital.

FB: Is that a good … [clarifying] we're talking about in Kenya?

Muriel: In Kenya, yes

FB: And that's a *good* thing?

Muriel replied in the unambiguous affirmative, followed by lengthy explanations. To wit: the later innovation of establishing medical clinics close to remote villages, staffed by local and locally trained midwives with access to hospitals, like the Maua Mission Hospital, if complications occurred.

Listening to these interviews is to eavesdrop, not so much on what is said but that which is not: an unstated position of polarities shaping assumptive 'givens' surrounding the contentions of healing and treatment. Contrasting discourses like these form colliding bodies of 'authoritative knowledge', which Jordan (1997) defines as particular knowledge upon which decisions are made and justifications provided; the performance of superior knowledge of the recognised expert as opposed to the inferior lay. Fran proceeded from an assumption that traditional birthing practices were egregiously disrupted by the introduction of allopathic models, backed by the strong encouragement of persuasion, propaganda and government policy. Innocently damning herself by outmoded semantic infelicities, Muriel referred to traditional births as taking place in 'the bush'. Such terms smack of geospatial, moral parameters, marking out some areas as civilised by a colonial understanding of duly ordered processes and procedures, and those of the situated 'other'. The unwelcome but then commonly used term 'the bush' was fully exposed to critiques of imperialist connotations of an unregulated place of ignorant, Darwinian survival beset by benighted views and practices. Fran could have asserted that not only were these colonial medical practices unfamiliar to the Ameru people, but they were probably antithetical to their beliefs, thereby dismissive of local knowledge and ultimately disempowering. He could, moreover, have reasonably questioned the greater safety of these medicalised births, and with good reason, given that it was colonialist expansions and impositions, of which medicine was part, that was implicated in the introduction and spread of unknown diseases (Etherington, 2005).

So far as Muriel was concerned, medicine and trained medical staff saved lives. Proudly stamped by nursing and midwifery she believed both were essential to that outcome. Life, both mortal and eternal, were the twin enterprises medical missionaries chose to advance. Simply put, local women and their babies were less likely to die during childbirth or from post-birth trauma and infections in a hospital setting. They were, by the same token, more likely to die away from hospital care. Thus, for Muriel, women and their male guardians should be encouraged to preserve valuable lives by embracing the gifts that modern medicine brought. The efficacy of allopathy, regardless of its alien importation, could at least be assured as better than most others. The idea that unfamiliarity in healing paradigms might render them less effective than for populations accustomed to them was not immediately apparent. This conceptual disputation arose from the later interdisciplinary subset of medical anthropology with its focus on cross-cultural comparisons, providing insights into how allopathic

> diagnosis and therapeutic successes are limited because in practice its concept, outlook and institutional features lack the necessary 'goodness of fit' with those of the local culture.
>
> (Good, 1987, p. 14)

Later the presumed 'wonders of modern medicine' would be humbled under scholarly scrutiny problematising its premises and practices. Medicine's claims have been treated with scepticism, the arcane knowledge of its qualified priesthood questioned, and its pre-eminent status undermined. In the Internet age, despite or fuelled by international health crises and pan-national health inequities, there has been a return to the acceptability, if not entirely the respectability of, competing treatments; which in respect of the United States, Jordan (1997) finds it again replete with barber surgeons, alterative practitioners, home remedies and folk healers.

Muriel would have been dismayed by this wider loss of faith in medicine, regardless that John Wesley was equally sceptical of its efficacy in his day (Hardiman, 2008). She wholeheartedly believed in the Methodist mission, so usefully and appropriately attuned to the practicalities of health care. The question of the inappropriate displacement of indigenous healing practices by the purported usurpations of colonial medicine was one to which Muriel would probably have given short shrift; particularly because the cases that she saw were often desperate ones and the hospital a last resort when other means had failed.

Muriel was still at Maua when the Alma-Alta Declarations of 1978 were articulated, framing health as a physical, mental and social state of being. Recommendations followed regarding the incorporation of indigenous practitioners into healthcare system's general policy (Ties Boerma and Baya, 1990). Compatible with Good's (1978) position of complementariness this proposed ethnomedical approaches created syncretic models bringing together philosophies, practices and approaches in a democratisation of healing care.

Partnership rather than competing paradigms of healing are now the progressive way forward; in the Kenyan context, this may include the services of the *mganga* (traditional healer) and the 'traditional birth attendant' (Hillier, 2003). These two roles are distinctive: the *mganga* is not normally a traditional birth attendant; and between the two clear differences of status, education and practices exist, which are not shared or interchangeable bodies of knowledge across Indigenous healers (Ties Boerma and Baya, 1990). Traditional birth attendants are exclusively women (Thomas, 2003), largely illiterate and possessing of differing degrees of skills. In Ties Boerma and Baya's (1990) study of coastal groups in Kenya, antenatal and postnatal care were not offered by them, although some could recognise and sometimes correct abnormal foetal presentations.

In the 1930s, Dr Gerrard displayed genuine medical anthropological interest in *mganga* practices; although Muriel herself never sought out them out from any personal and professional curiosity, despite it being a topic Fran regularly returned to. She did witness the burns or cut marks of *mganga* treatment on admitted patients, but for Muriel, such healers were 'witch doctors'. Some, she recognised, as benign in intention, but others were not:

> I remember one young man brought to the hospital, who said he had had a spell (put) on him to say he was going to die. He really believed this, and although our doctor could not find anything wrong with him, he did in fact die after a few days.

She must have met birth attendants though, while actively pursuing public health initiatives through antenatal outreach care. Obliged to master, the hospital's old Bedford van Muriel weekly slithered or bumped painfully along the impossible tracks to the remote villages to administer antenatal care and basic treatment, giving health talk and demonstrations. If birthing fistulas were a common risk, Muriel appropriately had her own to contend with. Her reward for many long hours driving in atrocious conditions navigating mud, floods, ruts and landslides was to develop a rectal abscess that unobligingly erupted into an excruciating fistula; all matter-of-factly recorded unblushingly by her for posterity.[3]

Birth and death

The demographic context of childbirth in Kenya carries a maternal mortality rate of around 488 deaths per 100,000 births, with a neonatal mortality rate of 30 out of 1,000 live births (Bryne et al., 2016). This mortality rate may not yet compare favourably with those of Europe, but is considerably better than many neighbouring African countries, particularly Central Africa and the Horn (WHO, 2022). Negotiating medicalisation and cultural incongruences in contemporary Kenyan medical settings, patient preference for traditional birthing attendants over medical staff is noted' (Rono et al., 2018). A disincentive is the indelible inscription on women's bodies of socially-endorsed femineity, reframed as of questionable social status nationally, and a gendered practice of notoriety in the international health community.

Thomas (2003) throws more light: traditional childbirth was entirely managed by experienced neighbours, mothers themselves. Of these senior women, one was selected to attend the labouring woman as the *mwijukia*, whose duties include encouraging newborns not to return to the domain of the ancestors (the dead). The labouring woman takes up a similar position to the one she was placed in years before at her rite-of-passage, the *mwijukia* sitting before her open legs, another supporting her from behind. At the moment of birth, a cut may be made enabling the child to be born, after which the umbilical cord is severed. The liminal status of the immature young girl is replaced by the social status of maturity, conferred by ritual focus on her female genitalia, for childbirth bestows the next stage of woman's status and authority once again via the ordeal of her vulva.

> Whereas initiation situated a girl-turned-woman within the female hierarchies of her natal home, childbirth, particularly with a woman's mother-in-law serving as *mwijukia*, situated her within the female hierarchy of her marriage home.
>
> (Thomas, 2003, p. 64)

The rite-of-passage initiation Thomas refers to is a topic we shall return to. Birth, has until recently symbolised and actualised the essentialising division of the sexes; a view regarded in 'progressive' Western quarters as highly contentious, where 'culture wars' rage over the mutability or otherwise of gender versus biological sex. Even so, in most cultures birth is unchallenged as woman's defining unique contribution to human survival; even if motherhood is often 'more honour'd in the breech' as an abstract, hygienic concept rather than a lived, messy reality (Wadud, 2007). Birth is positioned in the interstices of the life-death continuum and the vital reforging of the ancestral nexus of generation. It is existential in meaning as well as visceral, bloody ontology. Accordingly,

> medical anthropologists have long considered matters of reproduction to be uniquely complex, in that bringing new members in to society is as social as it is biological, as dangerous as it is mundane.
>
> (Spengler, 2011, p. 438)

So much was evident to Muriel. The maternity ward had been endowed by past missionary superintendents with thirty beds, based on optimistic assumptions of increasing hospital deliveries, given the greater safety it afforded over village home births. Yet on arrival, Muriel found that half of these beds had been put into general nursing service, for few routine births voluntarily took place in the hospital over the emergency cases brought in from remote communities, often far too late, as Muriel, recalled in her 'Life Story':

> Therefore, often the poor women would eventually arrive at the hospital having been in labour for days, and often the baby was already dead and the mother exhausted or sometimes nearly dead if her uterus had ruptured. It was also not uncommon for a husband to arrive with a new-born baby, saying the mother had died of a haemorrhage. This was so tragic as one injection of ergometrine would probably have saved her.

Just as Dr Gerrard had visited local chiefs to plead the case of the Mission Hospital, vouchsafed by the good Stephano, Muriel plied her influence, accompanied by 'Mr Henry' a well-respected elder among his people, a Christian and qualified nurse with a side-line in dentistry and male circumcision. Sitting with one chief ('a real character') in his spacious, smoke-dimmed hut, surrounded by the nine smaller huts of his various wives and children, Muriel put forward her mission of mercy: to advise men to encourage their womenfolk to come to the hospital. Muriel and Mr Henry were graciously permitted to meet a large crowd of local men, arriving in obedience to the chief's summons, where shrouded in blankets they sat listening to a strange litany on the risks of childbirth, acted out with props: a model pelvis and the demonstration doll. After some confusion, with the men stating they were personally agreeable, but it was their women who baulked at hospital births, and the women saying precisely the opposite, Muriel was finally permitted to care for three pregnant women whose earlier labours delivered stillbirths. Duly following success Muriel's good reputation was slowly spread by word-of-mouth (Figure 8.1).

Over time one problem replaced the other: eventually, the numbers coming for delivery created such overcrowding at the hospital, that women

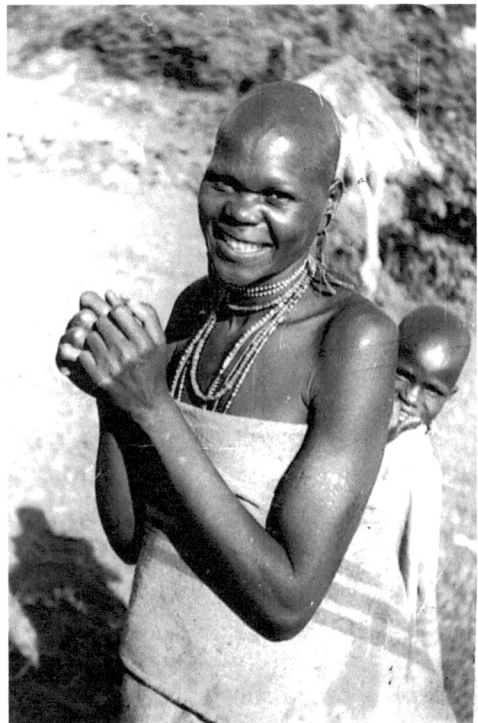

Figure 8.1 Mother and Child, Maua. Courtesy of Muriel Chalkley.

literally had to embody the role of 'outpatient', lying on the grass under the jacaranda trees waiting patiently for their turn to enter. Eventually, patients were 'topped-and-tailed': two shared one bed. This serendipitous arrangement arose from the fact that Muriel, no mathematician, had inadvertently ordered simple hospital beds to be constructed that were overly long for their original purpose, but ideal for space saving on overcrowded wards.

Finding Kimeru very difficult to acquire although examined in it, Muriel learned enough to issue simple directions to her patients: 'I'm going to examine you'. 'Turn on your side'; 'lie on your back'; 'the baby's coming; push'; 'stop pushing'. Anything more complicated relied on staff interpretation. The drama of birth was also greatly heightened given the prevailing rudimentary conditions, particularly at night, where for many years, in lieu of mains electricity, Muriel and her staff had little choice but to help deliver infants by lamplight or torch. Yet, although she adapted to the significant challenges of a poorly resourced, under-staffed and over-crowded mission hospital in one of the most remote parts of Kenya, Muriel, as Fran noted, inevitably brought with her, as expected and mandated, the ways of the West in terms of her training, management and care of patients. Truly, the sun never set on Imperial midwifery!

We know, for example, that in the 1950s at Maua, Muriel favoured the conventional British position for labouring women: lying on the left-hand side with a leg raised and supported to make way for the emerging baby. Later, after a few years back in England, she returned and used the supine position for labouring mothers, then popular with Western medical staff for the greater convenience it afforded them at the mother's expense. The late British childbirth guru, Sheila Kitzinger (2003), and other proponents of natural and active childbirth criticised this as an unnatural and harmful birthing position, narrowing the pelvis compared to upright and squatting positions. One wonders how it was received by birthing women at Maua.

Muriel was regularly the most senior person in charge and the responsibilities could be crushing at times, particularly when there was no doctor available to refer to. The consequences for women if complications set in without a doctor present were potentially very serious.

> One time when the doctor was away, I had a patient having her first baby, a primi (*primigravidae*) ... and it was a big one and I couldn't get it out. And there was no doctor. She was pushing and pushing and I did an episiotomy. I did all I could to get it out but I couldn't and it was a stillborn. I was very upset about it. So, when the doctor came back, I said 'if you're going to go away sometimes, you're going to have to teach me how to do forceps deliveries. So, that's what he did.... from then on, I did all the forceps deliveries as well.[4]

Obliged to do the best she could, Muriel undertook procedures that would normally have been regarded as beyond the level of a midwife's competence. She later mastered the ventouse suction cap for deliveries, a less traumatic procedure than the use of mechanical forceps. To avoid caesarean sections in obstructed labours, which, however enterprising or desperate the situation, she did not attempt, Muriel performed a symphysiotomy: cutting the cartilage dividing the frontal meeting of the pelvic bones, thereby opening the pelvis a further couple of centimetres. This now outdated procedure was risky and painful, and no longer practised. But as Barbara Dickinson,[5] Maua Hospital's current missionary nurse says, if all else failed, and where no caesarean could be carried out, at least it worked.

One of the greatest perils for was the distances between villages and the hospital, for transport was rudimentary for villagers and for some, particularly those most ill, it was a hellish journey.

Muriel: They (villagers) used to make a stretcher out of rope and leaves and they would carry her for miles, because there was no ambulance or anything.

For other women, hardly much better off, finding help meant several miles on foot while in labour. I can barely imagine what endurance that must have taken, thinking of my own experiences of childbirth, and how even a few paces down a corridor in the midst of painful contractions seemed interminable. Of those women who did suffer that tremendously arduous journey Muriel recalled one poor soul birthing on the road, burying the subsequent dead infant, and walking on bleeding to the Hospital to have her placenta removed. Another walked many miles in labour, birthing her newborn en route, and continuing on with her chilled, naked baby, umbilicus dangling, in her arms. This lady was actually producing triplets, says Muriel, but where the remaining unborn proved to be a living jumble of arms, legs, heads and protruding parts that were a complete impediment to normal birth. Muriel managed to save all four lives from an almost inevitable death and took a photograph of the happy family during their stay in the hospital (Figure 8.2).

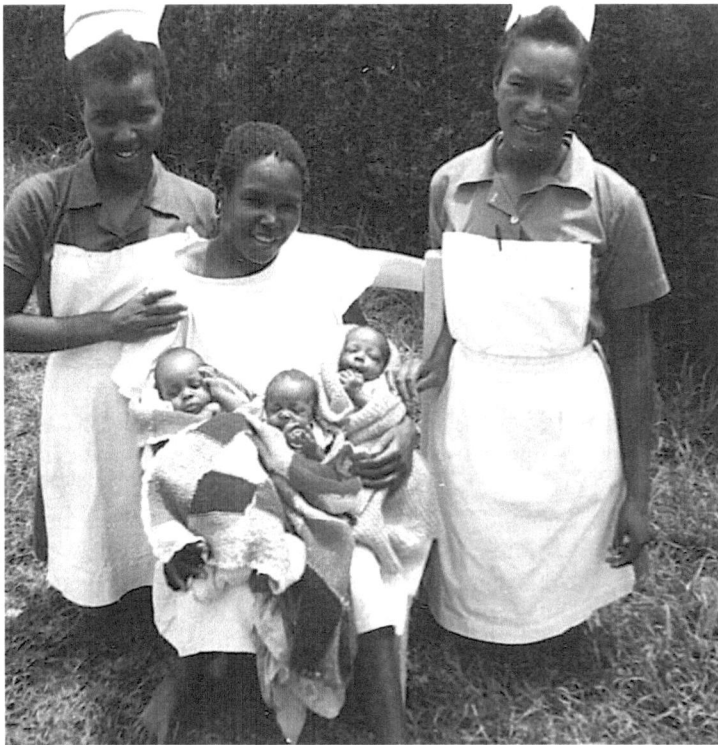

Figure 8.2 Mother and Triplets with Sisters Mary and Florence. Courtesy of Muriel Chalkley.

There were many awful cases, like the sixteen-year-old village girl discovered after three agonising days of labour, resulting in infant death and a terrible tear between vagina and anus. Another poor woman from the valleys was admitted not yet at term but very ill with cerebral malaria. While dealing with another tricky delivery next door, Muriel heard that the feverish patient had suddenly aborted the entire, unruptured, amniotic caul enclosing a small, dead infant, followed by the placenta. The junior midwife duly placed everything in the waste sluice for later disposal. Checking up later Muriel found to her amazement a living baby girl weighing just 3lbs inside a rubbish sack. She was revived and the mother eventually recovered sufficiently to return to her lowland home with her tiny but healthy, suckling baby. It was a miraculous escape for them both.

Despite all help, women sometimes died and so did their babies. One arrived 'bleeding to death' with placenta praevia. The baby was completely dead and the mother's life hung in an unequal balance. Muriel's ingenuity and determination was required in full measure. Praying earnestly while she scrubbed her hands, she grasped some Willetts forceps (a type of toothed forceps, later outmoded) and forcing this through the protruding placenta grasped the baby's head.[6] A rapid wrapping of bandages around the forceps handles which were then looped over the hospital bedframe created weighted pressure from the infant's head sufficient to stop the haemorrhage and stimulate contractions. Two hours later the mother pushed out the placenta followed by the dead child.

Other horrible necessities were required of midwives. One lady was admitted after labouring for hours at home. The unborn baby had died within her and the doctor unable to extract it decided to crush the skull with forceps.[7] Blood and brains poured on the floor and the broken body of the child followed. It was a hideous sight and Muriel not wanting her young nurses to have to deal with such a terrible job, quickly started to clean up with a mop and bucket. But 'Deborah', one of the midwife students, stepped forward and gently took the mop from Muriel's hand, saying 'You shouldn't be doing this, Sister' and proceeded to quietly clear up the gory mess herself.

The Mutani

It was rare to get a night's rest with junior staff tripping down the dark path to rap on the shutters of Muriel's little house calling: 'Sister, Sister, we have a *primi* making no progress!' Twins were common and the high rate of obstructed birth complications was a mere reflection of the general physical condition of many women in Maua, Muriel said, attributing this to two main factors. The first were pelvic malformations, a consequence of girls and women carrying extreme loads on their backs, tipping their postures forward unnaturally. Dr Gerrard took a number of photographs of Kenyan women in his time, later reproduced in his biography (Gerrard, 2001). These depict women loaded with heavy burdens containing water, firewood and straw, or balancing tiers of gourds on their heads. Robertson also attests to the high maternal-infant mortality rate in reference to

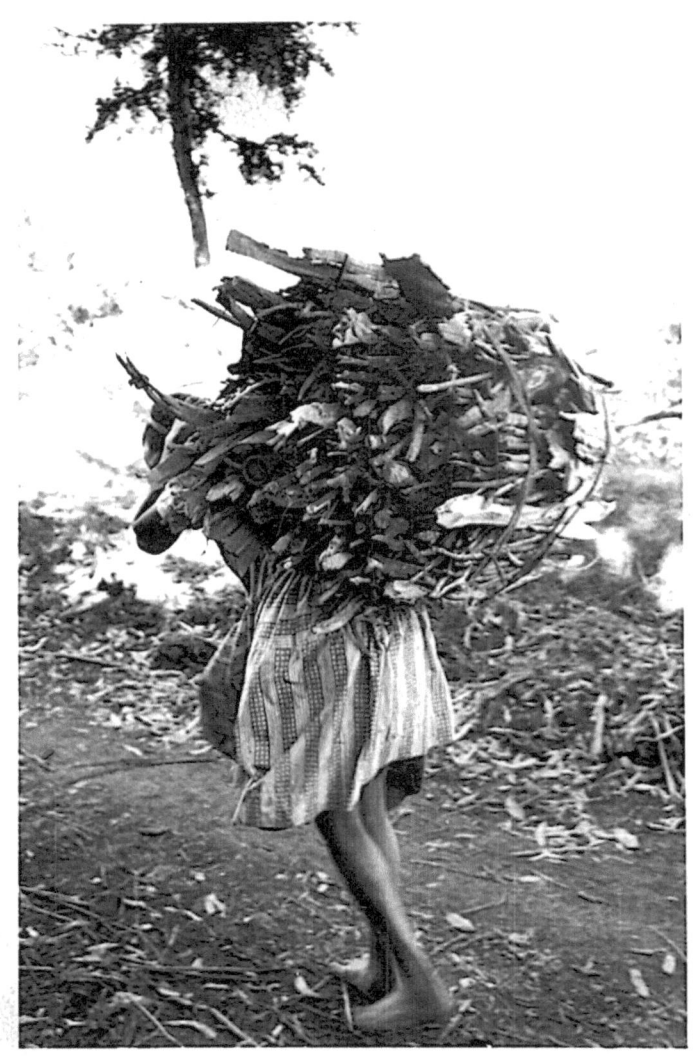

Figure 8.3 Girl Carrying Firewood, Maua. Courtesy of Muriel Chalkley.

Kikuyu women and the common problem of a contracted or flattened pelvis, caused:

> by carrying huge bundles of firewood, weighing 100 lbs (45 kilograms)
> or so, on their backs supported by a scrap around the forehead. Children
> of eleven or twelve years of age, whose bones were not fully developed,
> were compelled to this, thus starting the deformity early in life.
>
> (Robertson, 1993, p. 7)

The resulting attrition rate was noted by Europeans. The retired coffee
planter, Mr Wolfenden, wrote indignantly to the newspapers in 1933, stating Kikuyu women were much to be pitied in their community, where not
only did they suffer from high mortality rates but also although 'under-
sized', they 'do all the world on the reserve *shambas* and, with loads,
which I could not personally carry, strapped to their heads, act as beasts of
burden to their "Lords and masters"'. This a condemnatory reference not
to the colonials themselves but to their own Kikuyu menfolk (Figure 8.3).

Conditions in Maua for women were different. Barbara Dickinson
explains that the hilly contours at Maua prevented loads being balanced
on women's heads and instead everything needed to be carried on backs;
considered to be far more damaging. This point noted, we return to
Robertson's account where, strangely, little is said of the second major
cause of obstructed labour, something Muriel was continually confronted
by, the impact of so-called 'female circumcision'.

Muriel stated that every local woman she cared for at Maua had under-
gone the procedure and that, so far as she knew, this was true of nearly all
the female nursing staff too, or so they told her. Her unusual acquaintance
with the effects of the procedure in Kenya led to her being interviewed by
the historian Lynn M. Thomas on reproduction issues in Kenya. This opportunity arose not so much from any deep knowledge of the procedure by
Muriel, but rather the insights she indirectly brought to a continuation of the
practice in Kenya, after being ineffectively outlawed in the 1960s. Thomas
(2003, p. 73) points out that reformation of the practice was far more difficult to achieve when midwives themselves had been subjected to it.

Thomas (1996, 2003) notably employs the cautious term 'excision' for
the euphemistic, earlier term 'female circumcision' or the more contemporary and graphic 'female genital mutilation'. Her choice of nomenclature
avoids stigmatisation of gendered practices that were culturally normalised
to such a degree in Maua that a patient with a non-excised vulva, seen in
recent memory[8] was first treated as exhibiting *abnormal* genital growths.

The question of terms and semantics has presented me with some moral
and authorial dilemmas, where I fully recognise that the term 'female
circumcision' is a feeble misnomer, for this practice is not in any way
comparable to male circumcision. However, where it is cited by others,

I retain the term for historical authenticity. Meanwhile if 'female genital mutilation' arguably smacks of ethnocentric insensitivity, it also undisguisedly evokes the nature and the lifelong impact of this initiation procedure. Genital excision, preferred by Thomas (2003) may be precise and factual, bearing little or no moral overtones, or cultural bias, but it is also clinically antiseptic, non-judgemental and does not, on the face of it, engage with the repercussions of female genital cutting in the lives of girls and women. The prevalence of the rite among Muriel's colleagues, friends and patients in Kenya, as adolescent rites-of-passage did not obviate the serious consequences. Florence Mutiga,[9] Muriel's colleague, commented on the psycho-physical cultural and physiological connections between female genital mutilation and childbirth.

Florence: A custom – it was painful, you were told to be brave. The circumcision left a very small (hole), so need to make a large cut with scissors (during childbirth). There was terrible suffering, for when the baby comes. They were very brave, normally, Meru women. You are taught by the older ladies, no shouting, no crying, no screaming.

The question I return to as a biographer is what Muriel could have felt as a European midwife faced with the consequences of excision in her work with Kenyan women? She never witnessed the ritual itself, but saw and heard the loud celebrations on the day of the cutting of the excited girls going to their initiation. This noise, Muriel thought, served to drown the sounds of screams. She was mistaken: the cries she assumed must accompany such an assault, were culturally prohibited as unlucky cowardice, writes Jomo Kenyatta.

(Icy water) is thrown on the girl's sexual organ to make it numb and to arrest profuse bleeding as well as to the shock the girl's nerves at the time, for she is not supposed to show any fear or make at audible sign of emotion or even to blink. To do so would be considered cowardice and make her the butt of ridicule among her companions. For this reason she is expected to keep her eyes fixed upwards until the operation is completed.

(Kenyatta, 1965, p.140)

Dr Gerrard observed the coming-of-age initiation into manhood of adolescent boys' and duly described it as a swift and skilfully performed deed. Only his wife, Doris Gerrard witnessed the initiation to womanhood of girls' by the *mutani* (cutter) (Thomas, 2003):

There was much singing and dancing by girls and women before the operation. The girl then cast off her garment, sat down on a clean banana leaf, and was held very tightly by two other girls, and the circumciser did her deed with an axe head taken from a filthy bag. The girl was not allowed to cry or look sad. She was given just about a minute after the operation to sit. She was then made to stand up. Her legs were quivering, and blood trickling down them. She showed herself to the company, and then walked off to her own hut where she would be confined and fed for about three months. When I asked some of the women if she wouldn't have a lot of pain, they said she would be all right again in five days. One wonders how such a strange custom originated.

(Gerrard, pp. 40–41)

Muriel held genuine admiration for the remarkable stoicism of the Ameru women, comparing their childbearing endurance most favourably in comparison with Anglo-Saxon tolerance. Pain, indeed, agony, was an experience these women suffered with little complaint, if any. Muriel never expressed racist opinion that Africans experienced less pain than Europeans, rather she thought their ability to endure suffering patiently was remarkable and commendable. It must also have made day-to-day midwifery care more manageable given the midwifery emergencies and limited resources to hand.

The pain of childbirth, nonetheless, is particular and pregnant with meaning: symbolic as well as visceral; one that, Kitzinger (2003) insists needs to be understood, honoured, endured *with* rather than eliminated *by* medical impatience (Kitzinger, 2003). Hillier argues that modern obstetrics render the meaning of pain in childbirth redundant and irrelevant in the automatic control of pain through analgesics. Humane obstetrics notwithstanding, the greater part of such motivations, she believes, connects to a continuing Cartesian mechanistic view of the body – machines do not, *should* not, feel pain (Hillier, 2003). In short, pain gets in the way of the preeminent role of the medics: to work on the passive body. Nevertheless, racist associations of the Black body as predominantly physical and thereby robust, of baser animal rather than loftier, cerebral nature, are certainly implicated in scandals of assumed higher pain thresholds and resultant reduced analgesia and attention in Western medical settings towards non-White women, not to mention higher mortality rates (Redshaw and Heikkilä, 2011; Rios, 2022). For women of Maua, childbirth, as elsewhere in Africa, was both highly dangerous but valorising; courage and steadfastness in suffering was their gendered and honourable calling for which female genital mutilation at a tender age had prepared them.

Muriel saw the results of 'female circumcision' repeatedly and had to work with the effects of it. Having spoken to different people on different occasions about 'female circumcision', Muriel developed a certain narrative repertoire on the topic (Thomas, 1997, 2001): here the details are coloured in for Fran's benefit:

Muriel: Have I not mentioned female circumcision? Oh, I thought I had. Well, all the women had been circumcised with female circumcision. This was done as a routine when they were about twelve, thirteen years of age. They would be done in groups and I can remember seeing a group come near my home and they were singing and dancing and all dressed up and with bells on their ankles and all that kind of thing, and they would all be done in a group by a woman who was called a circumciser. And she had a little, I was told, kind of triangular-shaped razor blade and they had no anaesthetic. (The girl) was held down. It must have been terribly painful, and she (circumciser) would cut off the whole clitoris, in some areas they even cut off the labia as well, but in our area they just removed the clitoris. But, nevertheless, they often bled a lot, they often damaged the urethra.

Her view of the rite, discussed privately with me, was that it was simply 'awful'; and admitted to shock when she first encountered the results on her patients' bodies. The impact of genital cutting on childbirth was clearly and overwhelmingly apparent to her. While the impact on women's bodily integrity was one that she far from insensitive to, the rite's crude assault on women's sexual being and the reasons for it was one, she, the most chaste of women, characteristically did not dwell on and had little personal experience of.

Interestingly, as well, although Muriel referred to the cut as clitoridectomy, Barbara Dickinson's claimed that cutting was far more extensive, resulting in 'huge scars', which Muriel also attested to. This suggested far more extensive cutting than clitoridectomy, supporting the observation of women Methodists, among other trained nurses, of this in the Meru region in the late 1930s (Thomas, 1996). Doris Gerrard's account additionally affirmed that cutting involved the amputation of the clitoris, labia minora and part of the labia majora among Maua girls (Gerrard, 2001).

The inability of scarred tissue to stretch during birth led to medical episiotomies, adding of necessity a new mutilation to the old (Kitzinger, 2003). But at least here village women experienced much of the same at the hands of the *mwijukia*. To aid labouring women in her care Muriel devised her own system of creating a small cut into the scar tissue itself, which did not bleed and hurt less than a cut into healthy flesh. Her compassionate policy was to leave the vulva unsutured, so that it was, in her own words, 'slacker' for subsequent births.

Female genital mutilation as a phenomenon has unsurprisingly been subject to a considerable amount of voyeuristic horror; and it is not difficult to find diagrams and close-up photographs of excised vulvas on the internet, forming a kind of medicalised porn of indigenous female torture. More poignantly autobiographical accounts like Hibo Wadere's (2016) account of her agonising and devastating experiences in Somalia at the age of six, make for unbearable reading. However, the revulsion the procedure has drawn from shocked Westerners is certainly far from new. Protestant missionaries in particular were both disgusted and disturbed by the practice, which brought politely unmentionable female genitals into sharp and unwanted focus; whilst the suffering caused to indigenous girls and women could be only too well guessed at. The whole thing seemed grossly barbaric to missionaries, although there were historical accounts of clitoral amputation practices in Ancient Greece as well as in Victorian England (Lister, 2020). Unsurprisingly, some missions attempted to stamp it out as an ungodly, benighted practice. The Church of Scotland, a most vociferous opponent to the procedure, insisted that church members would be suspended from services if they subjected their daughters to female circumcision (Strayer, 1978).

The effects of missionary opposition to 'female circumcision' were calamitously sharp reductions in church membership. The CMS were similarly concerned but avoided banning membership as deterring conversion and church attendance. The Methodists in Meru had been badly bruised by the plummeting loss of congregations when they opposed the rite. Dr Gerrard in Maua, himself surely no stranger to the physical repercussions of the practice, preferred to look the other way rather than risk Methodist mission work and decant churches of congregations. Yet this was merely following the lead of the General Superintendent, Reginal Worthington, and his successor, Arthur Hopkins, who led the Methodist mission in Kenya, both preferring to ignore the practice (Prichard, 2014). Indeed, Hopkins attempted to elucidate matters to appalled Western critics by explaining how it was viewed from the local point of view.

> It is a simple fact that girls in Meru look to this rite as a dignity which gives them a standing in the tribe, which otherwise they would they would not possess.
>
> (Prichard, 2015, p.144)

The rite transformed immature girls of social inconsequence into responsible and capable women of recognised community status, whose role were to ensure the fertile productivity of the people and the land (Fiona and Mackenzie, 2000). Indeed, cutting was intended as preparatory for these rigours in demonstrating a girl's ability to endure hardship as well as suffer the extremes of pain and fearlessness in facing these womanly trials (Thomas, 2003).

Nonetheless, to the missionaries, it was an ordeal that served little purpose, except to perpetuate female suffering lifelong; and in the view of plantation owners, to weaken the African workforce (Wolfenden, 1933). In a stern letter to the *British Medical Journal*, Dr John Arthur (1942), having earlier resigned from the Kenya Legislative Council over the matter (*Truth*, 1930), uncompromisingly argued that the major variant of this 'permanent mutilation' destroyed 'physique and vitality'.

> The most disastrous results of the operation occur at times of childbirth, especially with *primiparae*. Labour is always delayed and mother or child or both, often die in consequence of the unfavourable conditions caused by the operation. When mission hospitals were established it was found necessary to make incisions, sometimes several, to enable a child to be born.

However, an 'uncircumcised' woman was not only held in light regard in her community, but was deemed incapable of giving birth to 'persons', but only to non-human 'dogs' (Thomas, 2003, p. 25). Of all the local Kenyan women that Muriel worked with, she knew only of one who had escaped the rite. When it came to her turn, 'Deborah', an Ameru Christian girl had run away in fear from the ceremony and remained unmutilated. Married later, Deborah's case was particularly and tragically ironic, giving birth to a profoundly disabled daughter, embodying the very prediction that the custom sought to prevent. Deborah was quickly abandoned by her husband, who married a woman regarded as fit to bear normal children. Muriel kept in touch with Deborah for years from England, often telling me about her periodic telephone calls, where in the background she could hear this pitiful adult child, her mother's stigmatising burden, loudly mouthing not human speech but indistinct noises.

The attempts by Protestant missions to ban 'female circumcision' to the extent of meddling in Kikuyu political membership (Natsoulas, 1998) were more than a public relations disaster for the missions. So enraging were the Mission efforts at curbing the ritual that on one occasion a violent attack by locals resulted in the death of an elderly foreign missionary in the attempt to genitally mutilate her (Anderson, 2005). Protestant mission influence, however, was not altogether unsuccessful, where a ban on the practice introduced by one distinct commissioner was supported by 1956 by one district commissioner supported by some Black Kenyans. However, the ban proved ineffectual for, defying the ban, local girls took up the rallying call of *Ngaitana* ('I will circumcise myself'), using razors rather than the *mutani*'s triangular knife to emulate the practice (Thomas, 1996).

In fact, Muriel recalled five girls being admitted to Maua Hospital with self-inflicted genital injuries. Wryly, Thomas (2003) notes that such injuries caused far less damage, owing to girls' physiological ignorance, than a competent *mutani* would otherwise have inflicted on them.

Yet, if by the 1970s, an uncircumcised woman was still regarded in her community as incompetent and socially questionable then to abandon a time-honoured practice at the behest of missionaries must have seemed an unimaginable infringement of custom and tradition (Strayer, 1978). Accordingly, the scene was set to frame custom as the great cause célèbre of African nationalist politics against the colonisers in Kenya (Thomas, 2003). The driving centrifugal force of Kikuyu politics in particular revolving around this issue of the right to 'female circumcision'; and indeed, Kenyatta, a Kikuyu himself, describes 'clitoridectomy' as the fundamental basis of the moral and religious order of the people (Natsoulas, 1998). One wonders then what he made of the presumably intact body of one of his eventual three wives, an English schoolteacher, Edna Grace Clarke, whom he married and produced a son with during his fifteen years of self-imposed exile in bucolic Sussex.

The emergency, the Mau Mau – and Muriel

The resentment of Africans towards the colonial government exploded into the Mau Mau insurgency to forcibly reclaim land for the landless (Angelo, 2017). The government responded; and Muriel stepped off the Chantala's gangplank in 1955 right into the middle of the pronounced State of Emergency.

The background to indigenous land dispossession began at the end of the nineteenth century in East Africa, when African communities were corralled in small areas, designated 'Reserves', while former territories were now held by white settlers. For the nomadic, cattle-wealthy Masai a treaty was drawn up in the early twentieth century persuading them to move their cattle out of the desirable Rift valley, now occupied by white settlers. The end of the Great War exacerbated land loss through reparation to British war veterans for their suffering, at the expense of Africans, by allocating a million acres for settlement in the desirable Central Province area under the Soldier Settlement Scheme (van den Bijl, 2017).

African poverty was exacerbated by heavy taxation introduced in the early twentieth century in the form of Hut and Poll taxes, amounting to two months' annual wages (van der Bijl, 2017). To generate further African manpower, forced labour was introduced through the Registration of Natives Ordinance and Northern Labour Circular in 1910 (Fiona and Mackenzie, 2000). Human labour and productivity became commodified under colonialism. Freedom of labour movement was made extremely difficult where African men were controlled and degraded by the enforced wearing of the *kipande*, the 'cowbell', where their employment record was held in a container hung around their necks (Kyle, 1999). Labour enforcement of men meant that women's farming labour on Reserves needed to be intensified, yet farming was also subject to the experimental and disastrous interference by the Colonial State attempting to increase local yields by providing unsuitable and unfamiliar, non-native seeds to approved 'progressive' African *male* farmers (Fiona and Mackenzie, 2000), thereby damaging food production. Colonial patriarchal assumptions stood at odds with the gendered normativities of African culture in completely overlooking that the land's fertility was, as Thomas (2003) explains, linked implicitly to women's fertility; and in turn premised upon female status of gendered maturity through 'female circumcision'. Colonial efforts to increase production through the reflexive response towards men, marginalised women farmers holding mother-to-daughter hereditary knowledge of indigenous agriculture (Fiona and Mackenzie, 2000).

The fuelled resentment led to protests against the use of the *kipande* and the forced labour of women and girls in the 1920s. The organisation behind the protests was the East African Association founded by the able and active, Harry Thuku, a Methodist, Mission-educated individual from the Kikuyu community, who was also a co-founder of the Young Kikuyu Association (and future leader of a dominant political party, the Kikuyu Central Association in the 1930s (van der Bijl, 2017).

At this time, the colonial government was operating a divide-and-rule policy of granting political authority to local indigenous communities through recognised chieftainships (Swainson, 1978), earning alliances. However, the government was also pressed by the bolshy white settler community for further control (Kyle, 1999). Thus, British policy walked a teetering line attempting to strike a balance between competing demands from white settlers demanding greater representational power and government control – and African demands for greater freedom and equality. By 1923, the Colonial Office was sufficiently exasperated to set down the following principles that the Indian minority should have elected representation; that the interests of the Africans were paramount; and where they conflicted with the settlers, the interests of the Africans took precedence (van der Bilj, 2017). Nonetheless, African demands were viewed by colonials as unhealthily encouraged by Indian 'agitators' whose presence in East Africa, had, ironically, been marshalled by British Imperialism, as policy encouraged migration of useful skills deemed peculiar to ethnic groups for distribution across different parts of the Empire (Ashencaen Crabtree, 2012; Ashencaen Crabtree and Wong, 2012). The Indian contingency had been valuable in the construction of the Uganda Railway (Martin and Bezemer, 2020). So too were they useful in developing mercantile industries in

Nairobi and even the outback, like Maua, where local shopkeepers were Indians serving Africans and the odd European, like Muriel. Yet Indian colonist rivalry with Europeans for prime land ownership was begrudged, and thus it was expedient to articulate that African interests took precedence (Kyle, 1966). Equally aggravating, the Indian intelligentsia in Kenya of the early twentieth century mixed with emergent African activist politics, exemplified by the concord between Jomo Kenyatta and Gandhi in London. These political accords resurrected stereotypes: wily, politically savvy Indians manipulating amiable, gullible Africans. Such unwelcome alliances profoundly disconcerted missionaries like Reverend Handley Hooper, in apparently usurping their cherished role of spokesman and advocate of the native underdog (Kyle, 1966).

Capitalist hegemonies commodifying African ways of life predictably encouraged the seeds of indigenous entrepreneurship towards goods, such as coffee (Swainson, 1978). This homegrown, African commercialism met with disapproval from white competitors, like Mr Wolfenden, cited earlier, expressing his strong opinion of how unsuited Africans were to the responsible business of growing coffee. Yet, even those sympathetic to Africans in Kenya measured the people by their Western work ethic, albeit here, via their ability to navigate the capitalist world successfully. In one letter Handley Hooper[10] compared two ethnic groups he was familiar with: the Kikuyu and the Kavirondo. Kikuyu men were viewed by Hooper as fundamentally idle, but the male Kavirondo was applauded as

a cheerful, self-confident person, seemingly with the genius of the cuckoo for ousting other natives out of employment. He means to get on, and already one can see the effects of his pushing qualities in the number of Kavirondo boys employed in Nairobi.

Nevertheless, the Kikuyu were deemed a very capable people, if overly interested in politics and noted for their 'commercial astuteness', their religiosity, together with their competence at clerical and stewardship jobs (Greene, 1999, p. 188).

By 1940, among the Kikuyu, one out of every eight was an indentured tenant 'squatter' of an acre of land on European-held farms (Anderson, 2005). The worldviews of the white farmers and their African squatters were entirely incongruent at the latter's expense, with the squatters believing that their right to *githaka*, customary ownership of land for themselves and their descendants, would still be honoured. However, colonial law provided the farmers with the right to evict squatters at will. A change in economic fortunes provided the opportunity. Van Bijl notes that the resultant inequity was horrifyingly stark with over a million and a quarter Kikuyu squashed into 2,000 square miles of land, and 30,000 colonials spread out over 12,000 square miles. The grotesqueness of the situation piqued gallows humour among the Africans

> When Europeans arrived in Kenya they had the Bibles and the Africans had the land, but now it is the reverse.
>
> (Van Bijl, 2017, p. 33)

The post-war period brought in further demands from Africans towards independence. In 1947, a huge general strike was held in Mombasa, bringing in the formation of the African Worker's Federation in its wake, spreading from dockers and railway workers, to sugar plantation workers and domestic staff (the so-called 'houseboys') (Durrani, 2018).

By the 1940s into the 1950s, Nairobi was disputed territory: no longer a colonial playground but one that held the heating cauldron of nationalist politics. Squalid overcrowding in the African shanty quarters of the city, holding 80,000 people living cheek-by-jowl, provided 'rich recruiting ground for the militants' (Anderson, 2005, p. 35). The pell-mell of politics was afoot, and political parties mushroomed in Nairobi, whether promiscuous in dealings, oppositional or internecine in their conflicts, they conspired, clashed, morphed and melded, struck alliances and enemies, threw up potential leaders and cast them down (Kyle, 1999, 2008). Ethnic supremacy among African tribal groups was a potent part of the political mix, with the Kikuyu occupying an elite position, later maintained throughout postcolonial Kenyan politics (Swainson, 1978). Anderson (2005) summarises the three factions of internecine Kikuyu conflict: firstly, the conservative chiefs and tribal Christian, Kikuyu leaders bolstered up by colonial rule. Secondly, there were moderate nationalists from privileged backgrounds, mission school educated, besuited and Westernised, articulate and metropolitan, typified by Jomo Kenyatta. Finally, the militant nationalists, affiliated with the Mau Mau; these were also for the most part mission educated but from poorer backgrounds, whose targets were both the conservatives and the moderates (Anderson, 2005).

Thousands of African Kenyans had fought for the Allies in the Second World War and what they learned there would soon prove useful in the coming political ferment of guerrilla warfare during the State of Emergency (van der Bijl, 2017). Post-war, saw British troops, fighting on two home fronts: tackling the alarming communist insurgence in Malaya and dealing with the Mau Mau in Kenya. Their experience of guerrilla warfare under the dense rainforest canopies in Malaya against a very determined and capable enemy would provide essential training for the Kenyan situation against experienced and hostile African ex-servicemen. Yet, as van Bijl (2017) comments, the British military command in Kenya were correct in refusing to draw close comparisons between the two insurgencies, one being a major regional threat and the other, a rebellion. A very nasty uprising, nevertheless, whose victims were more than the disembowelled, white settler-owned cattle and sheep (van den Bijl, 2017).

Durrani (2018) argues that those initially turning to the Mau Mau were the disenfranchised, drawn by ideologies of anti-colonialism, anti-imperialism and the proletarian struggle against capitalism. Muriel would probably have sympathised with that for those principles were not discordant with her own – had they remained unsullied by violence. Personally, she rejected colonial arrogance and carried little in the way of class pretensions: either towards social snobbery (putting on 'airs-and-graces') or the inverted snobbery of inflating the claims of an aristocracy of labour. The Mau Mau, however, had other goals, and if strenuous political activism with the cut-and-thrust of eloquent argument and debate did not displace the colonials, then force was justified.

How far Muriel was aware of the extent of the Emergency turmoil in Kenya when she waved goodbye to her parents is unclear. It seems unlikely that the Methodist Mission Society or Kingsmead would not have provided her with a certain amount of necessary information as part of her orientation. It may merely have reflected the cautious government line that this was no more than 'civil disturbance' (Anderson, 2005). The Methodist Church typically remained relentlessly strong in faith despite (or even because of) the bloodshed of Christians.

> The Church in Kenya has indeed been a Church under the Cross and those who remained faithful in the darkest days shared something of the sufferings of Christ. Yet the sufferings have brought a new surge of spiritual life and the persecution of a new purity of purpose.
>
> (MMS, 1956, p. 28)

Interestingly, in a letter home dated 1959, Muriel does not refer to the State of Emergency. Nor did she discuss this in interviews with the Methodists or Fran, but they were discussed with me. This represents a curious earlier silence, for on her arrival Kenyatta had already been imprisoned for two years of his sentence for suspected association with the Mau Mau. Later, as long-serving president of Kenya from 1963 onwards, his disavowal of the Mau Mau and ready adoption of pre-Independence laws banning the Mau Mau movement, gave credence to his assertion of denial of any association with the movement (Angelo, 2017).

During the 1950s, however, Nairobi in particular was steeped in political militancy, and inevitably subject to close scrutiny by the colonial government of the various comings and goings, benignly spotting Muriel's name in the crowds. One might imagine the topic of the Mau Mau was foremost in the minds of colonials, but if so, perhaps it was a conversation *non grata* for the European ladies Muriel found herself tucked in with on her first Kenyan train journey. Then again, maybe it was subject to such cautious (fearful perhaps) reference that the topic, if alluded to, went over the head of the nonplussed missionary. Certainly, however, the Mau Mau was a name striking terror in the heart of many and for good reason. Victims, whether African or European, were slaughtered with horrific brutality sparing neither man, woman or child. The Mau Mau turned on loyalist Kikuyu chiefs and Christian Kenyans generally, with terrible and merciless ferocity. Thriving Kikuyu villages like 'Lari' were subject to wholesale massacre. Details were widely reported across the British media.

> Altogether 150 men, women and children met their deaths in the Uplands, hacked to pieces by the three Mau Mau gang which descended on them. Some truly terrible stories have been told by survivors. One woman was forced to watch a terrorist as he hacked off her child's head with repeated blows; another woman saw her son's throat cut and the terrorists drink the blood. Chief Maikmei himself escaped the massacred, flying from the scene after shooting one terrorist, and he is now rallying loyalist opinion among the Kikuyu in the Kiambu area. The loyal Africans are violently incensed at what has happened and are indeed retaliating...It clearly represents a new and even more savage phase in the struggle in Kenya and indicates the extent of Mau Mau organisation.
>
> (The Sphere, 1953)

The article commented on the extremely violent assassinations of other chiefs; and carried an additional eye-catching headline indicating growing siege mentality: 'NAIROBI HOUSEWIES AND BUINESS GIRLS PRACTISE SMALL-ARMS FIRING'.

Graham Greene fuelled by a restless, adrenalin-fuelled, journalistic inquisitiveness, travelled pre-war and post-war across troubled international borders, including the British and French Imperial landscapes of Asia and Africa that were filled with danger and precarity, writing acerbic essays on what he found. Both Malaya and Kenya were visited in turn and as cited, his observations of each were sharp and cinematic in a graphic display of literary portraiture.

The terror that Greene describes is qualitatively different from the extreme danger posed by the Communists in Malaya: strangers ambushing colonials outside in daylight with modern automatic weapons. Even more terrifying, if possible, the Mau Mau attacked victims in their own home, by stealth, suddenly, and primarily at night. The means of murder was particularly hideous: victims were hacked bloodily to death by multiple blade wounds, and subjected to further mutilations even after death.

There seemed to the authorities an ecstasy of violence and lust for gore that defied conventional humanity and reason (Anderson, 2005).

Solidarity and commitment to the cause was forged by the taking of a sworn oath of secrecy, sacrifice and dedication to cause of *Uhuru* (translated as both 'freedom' and 'Independence') (Durrani, 2018). Although thousands flocked to take the oath, voluntarily and idealistically, it soon acquired ugly features of menace and intimidation meted out by thugs (Durrani, 2018, p. 21). The penalties of refusal to take the oath on the grounds of personal conscience were severe.

Muriel: I heard of one woman who refused to join the Mau Mau. They wanted women to join because they were hiding in the forest and women would cook and take them food. They dug a grave and showed her the grave and said, 'if you won't take this oath, this is your grave'. But she refused to take it because it was against her Christian faith. So, she was murdered and put into it.

A comparable account is offered by Ndubai (2012): a devout Christian woman named Cio-Muguru was mysteriously murdered in the Kathiranga village in 1952, several miles from Maua; where it is rumoured, but not confirmed, that the cause of her death was refusal to take the Mau Mau oath.

This matter of the oath, however, was particularly sinister. The elaborate, bizarre, visceral and perceived depravity of the most serious one was swathed in secrecy and dire portents, that bore a decidedly occult overtone – from a European perspective at least. Certainly, although uncharacteristically stiff-lipped on this matter, Muriel regarded the whole business as nothing short of devilish stuff. Louis Leakey, the anthropologist offshoot of the famous Anglican Kenyan missionary family, was brought in by the colonial authorities to provide helpful insights into the Mau Mau movement. Connections were drawn between the KAU oath, Kikuyu membership and the Mau Mau, the latter being regarded as essentially a religious cult; the ritualised covenant in blood an obscene inversion of the Holy Communion (Leakey, 1954). Muriel was very clear in her mind, correctly so, that Christians were overtly targeted by the Mau Mau and particularly if African.

Muriel: Three of our young men had been to a Christian meeting and met the Mau
Mau on the way home and were killed.

Robertson (2003, p. 41) shares the general impression of the persecution of Christians, commenting on the martyrdom of many 'true and dedicated African members of the Christian church'. Ndubai (2012) offers a different perspective by mentioning the lamentable killing of three young men, but these, he says, were shot by the colonial forces as Mau Mau suspects.

With the aim of rehabilitating Mau Mau oath-swearers under government auspices, Louis Leakey spent time deciphering the fearsome magic of their sacrament, conjuring up another to counterbalance it as ritual cleansing (van der Bijl, 2017). This, as London newspapers noted, was administered by high status 'witch doctors' in government service, using an unsavoury rite with a dead goat's blood and entrails, designed to cause initiates to vomit up the toxicity of the Mau Mau (*The Sphere*, 1952).

The cultural signifiers and ritualisation of the Mau Mau movement had, however, been sufficient to damn another famous Kenyan anthropologist by association: Jomo Kenyatta, stood accused of being the lynchpin of the movement (Kyle, 2008). Anderson (2005, p. 57) comments that the Leakeys regarded the Mau Mau as 'a backward and atavistic revival of ancient tribal practices in the face of the challenges of modernity and 'civilisation'. They were well qualified to offer useful interpretations of Mau Mau beliefs and practices, for Louis as a boy, like his cousin Arundel Gray Leakey, was initiated into the Kikuyu community (which, one presumes involved undergoing the ritual circumcision along with other Kikuyu lads). Opposed to the Mau Mau, the Leakey family would pay a terrible price. In October 1954, Mau Mau fighters broke into the farmhouse of Gray Leakey, throttling his wife and disembowelling the Kikuyu Catholic cook; following which Leakey was forced up Mount Kenya and there in the forests buried alive, head first (Anderson, 2005).

The hideous events of these years were shockingly hard to reconcile with the intelligent, helpful, piously inclined and largely innocuous Africans that the settlers thought they knew.

> It was as though Jeeves had taken to the jungle. Even worse, Jeeves had been seen crawling through an arch to drink on his knees from a banana-trough of blood: Jeeves had transfixed a sheep's eye with seven kie-apple thorns; Jeeves had had sexual connection with a goat; Jeeves had sworn, however unwillingly, to kill Bertie Wooster 'or this oath will kill me and all my seed will die.
>
> (Greene, 1999, pp. 188–189)

The Bertie Wooster at one point was Jim, Jack's debonaire, elder brother, who came to Kenya in the 1950s to work as a meteorologist. It was here where he met his future wife, a hearty Women's County cricketer from the Wirral, as coincidence would have it. The sunny, good life in Nairobi was a far cry from the draughty, dismal boarding rooms of wartime Liverpool and the couple enjoyed it considerably. All went as merry as a wedding bell, until, that is, their affable African houseboy confessed to them that he had taken a Mau Mau oath to despatch them both one night. But being fond of Jim and Betty he had arrived at an excellent solution, which was to swap his assassin's duty with the houseboy's next door, equally under oath to slaughter his employers. It was an ideal solution, except that his conscience still pricked him. The couple felt highly motivated following this little revelation to hotfoot it back to England with all speed; and fortunately lived to tell the tale. What happened to this honest houseboy I do not know, but hope that Fortune looked kindly on him; for those Africans who broke silence to offer information about the Mau Mau were considered traitors by them, with dreadful penalties meted out.

In Malaya, the enemy was identifiable and external, and the Malay houseboy was at least on the colonial's side, as Greene (1999) quips. Whereas, in Kenya, the enemy was the treacherous everyday member of the daily household or the benign farm hand in the field.

The Ruck family murders of 1953 completely unsettled the settlers who staged a large and vociferous protest at Government House in Nairobi demanding decisive action to stamp out Mau Mau activities (Aberdeen Evening Express, 1953). Ruck was of a breed Greene disliked: an outspoken, racist farmer and a keen member of the Kenya police reserve. He, his pregnant wife, and small child were slashed to death and their bodies mutilated one fine night by their own servants (van Bijl, 2017). A couple of years and very many murders later, 1955 saw the killing of two British schoolboys (Liverpool Echo, 1955); and an eleven-year-old girl and her mother murdered by their gardener (Coventry Evening Telegraph, 1955). As was recognised though, of all the Mau Mau victims, African Christians suffered the most, if not in terms of terms of sheer savagery, certainly numerically.

The end of the Empire seemed mired in civil and political conflict, a drain on resources and a waste of lives. The Westminster Government was eager to shed it, with, nominally, imperialist ambitions. Two British novels published within a twelve-year period captured the mood of anomie caused by the shattering of faith in Enlightenment progress. The Nazi atrocities still fresh in the public's mind represented the polarity of hideous extremes in otherwise civil society. This, the diverse children of Imperial Rule were purportedly allied against. Consequently, it is hardly surprising that an apparent reversion to the atavistic, represented by the Mau Mau rebellion, would be viewed as holding distinctly satanic allusions (Maloba, 1998), in the minds of a shaken but still predominantly Christian West. It is perhaps no coincidence then these years of dreaded moral collapse were realised in the publication of William Golding's portentous and contemporaneous 1954 novel *The Lord of the Flies*, the diabolic descent led, significantly, by a Cathedral Choir School product. By 1966, the mood had changed, England had won the world cup, the NHS was a success, and the Imperial load was being removed to general relief despite patriotic deflation. The public were now ready for the pathos of the tragi-comedy by Leslie Thomas (1966), *The Virgin Soldiers*, a very British tale of green and bewildered National Service recruits shipped out to fight the battle-hardened and experienced Chinese communists in the Malayan 'jungle', with the help of some loyal, post-Empire Nepalese Gurkhas, famed for chopping the enemy up into the size of stock cubes with their lethal kukris.

Thereafter revisionist histories keenly condemned the imperialist response during the Emergency period. Stuart (2011), for one, sharply criticises the colonial police machinery which detained and maltreated many Mau Mau suspects, these being mostly men with a few women besides. Such critiques point to the unequal numbers of victimhood: while there were three score European victims, the number of African victims of the Mau Mau numbered in the hundreds. Anderson (2005) in turn deplores the methods used in crushing the rebellion with 2,609 African suspects charged on Mau Mau offences, of which 40% were acquitted, 1,574 received capital sentences, and a final 1,090 subsequently hanged, in addition to those killed in direct armed conflict.

The harshness of the colonial government response did not fade into historical impunity. In 2011, the High Court in London ruled that compensation claims brought by a small group of Kenyans, on the ground of torture during the State of Emergency of the mid-1950s, could proceed. The BBC covering the story interviewed individuals on both sides of the conflict. Wamahio Kabugu from Nyeri was reported as saying

> I feel this decision is justice for Kenya as it is our fathers who were the ones who were tortured and killed. The court's ruling is only a good thing but now they should give compensation to every Mau Mau and any families who have been affected.
>
> (BBC, 2011)

Not everyone agreed and there was some bitterness among Britons that the victims (or their descendants) of the Mau Mau atrocities received neither an apology nor compensation.

Muriel never conveyed that she had felt fear during these years, downplaying any sense of personal threat by saying that the crisis was dying down by the time she arrived, which indeed in some ways it was. Danger, however, was very close to home. Meru, some miles away, was the location of the sole post office with the designated local 'postman' trudging the journey by foot. It was perilous, for Meru was also where active pockets of Mau Mau resistance held out the longest, refusing to capitulate (Angelo, 2017); and they were supplied with weapons, food and information (Maloba, 1998).

Warned that the Mau Mau were in the forests close by Muriel was given a police whistle to go to bed with for protection. Armed with this, even with a police station close by, she would have been in great danger had anyone been out to harm her. One might think that at least immunity from murder would have been granted to useful and altruistic colonial medical staff working with African communities, but this would not have saved Muriel, for among their previous victims were two European women doctors: Dr Esme Ruck, she of the Ruck murders, with a practice patronised by African villagers; and Dr Dorothy Meiklejohn who despite injuries survived, although her husband did not (Anderson, 2005).

If no gangs of murderers entered the Mission Hospital grounds, the grisly evidence of the conflict was before them, as one of Muriel's former midwifery students (now a celebrated Kenyan academic) remembers:

Leah:[11]   Yes, it was hard, because apart from being almost pioneers in the area it was also during the Mau Mau rebellion, and we were working there risking our lives, not knowing when we can be subjected to the people who were fighting. And we were also nursing them, the casualties, (those) would come who had been attacked. We were all young – teenagers – taking care of the people from deliveries to old age, including the people who were attacked. I remember one day I had delivered a stillborn and I was taking that little baby to the mortuary and there I met, I had no idea, that someone had been burned at night and the whole body was so swollen, and on the bed, I saw a charred body and I was screaming in front of postnatal mothers. They knew what I was carrying and they knew! I remember dropping that baby down because I was so scared. Muriel was so caring, [she] put my emotions together.

Muriel herself took the precaution of wearing her whistle and putting up with being escorted by a police officer, bumping along beside her in the Land Rover on her regular (painful) trips to the remote villages. The Mau Mau fighters by then were being rounded up in large numbers and imprisoned in large camps to await their fate, and they too deserved compassion. With her missionary hat on, Muriel went to take a service there, seeing hundreds of prisoners dressed only in blankets as their clothes had been confiscated; although she said at the time she knew of no additional maltreatment. Perhaps her urge to bring Methodist comfort to the prisoners was not particularly eccentric; it was after all, her perceived Christian duty and prison was where the Methodists had first started out as 'The Holy Club' (Hattersley, 2014). Incarceration and religion often go hand-in-hand, and conversions to one faith or another are not uncommon (Ashencaen

Crabtree et al., 2016). Greene (1999, p. 202) records that many Mau Mau converted to Roman Catholicism in prison and those that were executed made their confessions willingly and went quietly to their deaths, as the Padre said then, 'like angels'.

Muriel sympathies were always meted out to those that needed them, for she had witnessed some appalling racism in Kenya. One such case was of a woman in labour whose care required her to be urgently transferred to the larger Meru Hospital thirty miles away. It probably occurred during one of those stressful times with the doctor away, a dire emergency to deal with and Muriel professionally unable to perform a caesarean. The colonial police officer she had appealed to for ambulance assistance initially refused to drive the patient, saying that he was low on petrol and had the woman been white it might have been different matter altogether. This scandalised Muriel so much he backed down in the face of her angry determination and two more lives were hopefully saved. She also saw how those with policing powers could maltreat Africans with impunity. She described seeing one man accused of theft, being verbally abused and kicked around. Muriel was horrified: 'the way he spoke to this African was awful!' These, in fact, were not the rank-and-file police, nor the more liberal-minded of white settler-types Greene (1999) found he liked, but those, like Ruck, that dubious breed of colonial police reservists. As for Muriel, she judged that not only were Africans often appallingly badly treated but how much 'ill feeling and resentment' it caused. The outcome of which the colonial community had already discovered to their cost.

She returned to England in May 1959 to care for her now widowed mother, taking up a post at Clatterbridge Hospital once more, but was back in Maua again in February 1962 in time for momentous events. The Mau Mau were defeated, Kenyatta was free and about to found a political dynasty, *Uhuru* was coming – everyone knew it, but how it could be wrought and into what shape was far from clear. Westminster policy was to divide perceived moderates from extremists, the identities of which tended to shift with the prevailing currents. Kenyatta for example was viewed at one time as a moderate and then an extremist (Kyle, 2008). The insidious influence of Cold War politics was thought to be implicated in the complexities of the Kenyan situation, with some African leaders cosying up to the USSR and Communist China and others 'thick as thieves' with the Americans. Matters, from London's point of view, did not look promising:

On 1 February 1962, when Kenya's independence was less than two years away, Harold Macmillan's Deputy Private Secretary, Michael Cary, summed up the prospects grimly: 'Already in fact bankrupt but with worse to come, wholly lacking in political, cultural, social and economic cohesion, threatened with internal tribal strife and external attack from the north but lacking both funds and forces to maintain adequate security services, an independent Kenya presents the least hopeful prospect of all the Colonial territories to which we have given or contemplate giving independence'.

(Kyle, 1997, p. 42)

As with India, a particular individual of a certain relentless ability was required to see Independence through in Kenya. This was Duncan Sandy, Winston Churchill's former son-in-law and the current Commonwealth Secretary. A man, Kyle describes, as insensitive, detail-driven and armoured with ruthless stamina (Kyle, 2008). Relentlessly he went on bulldozing until the job was done.

In May 1962, Muriel, happily back in Kenya, was writing a letter to the Methodist circuit[12] back home with updates. KADU (Kenya African Democratic Union) and KANU (Kenya African National Union) are, she wrote, making unrealistic promises,

to get the vote from simple, village folk...and people believe them and do not know any better – but the poor folk will of course be sadly disillusioned! They have big political meetings from time to time and Jomo Kenyatta is in Meru only this weekend and crowds of people gather to listen to these leaders speaking...Our staff are very sensible to it all. They take a keen interest – especially the boys, and listen to the wireless, and love to talk politics – and yet they sincerely long for a peaceful settlement, and realise that Kenya is not yet ready for independence.

But Muriel, the midwife, certainly got her dates wrong on this one, for over six months later, *Uhuru* was born and Kenya would become feted as an exemplar of African post-colonial success.

Notes

1 Dated sometimes between May and September 1958. Frank's health seriously compromised, the letter, addressed to Mrs & Miss A, Chalkley c/o Mrs Wicks, 65, Rydal Gardens, Wembley, Middlesex, England, suggests a respite from care duties.
2 Muriel Chalkley, interview with Fran Biley. Ibid.
3 'My Life Story'. Ibid.
4 Muriel Chalkley, interview with Fran Biley. Ibid.
5 Author's interview with Barbara Dickinson, 2 November 2022.
6 The use of Willetts forceps for placenta praevia was described in an article from Hong Kong in the British Medical Journal in 1945. I do not know if Muriel read it or whether it entered midwifery orthodoxy, but she was perfectly capable of hitting on this idea herself.

7 Herbert Gerrard records a similar event of dismembering of a dead, unborn infant's skull in Maua in order to save its mother's life.
8 Barbara Dickinson, interview with Author. Ibid.
9 Author's interview with Florence Mutiga, 25 October 2022.
10 Papers of the Hooper Family. Cadbury Library. Ibid.
11 Author's interview with Professor Leah Marangu 16 November 2021.
12 Carbon copy letter without name of recipients, dated 13 May 1962 from Muriel Chalkey recording her address as The Berresford Memorial Hospital, P.O. Maua, via Meru, Kenya, E. Africa.

References

Aberdeen Evening Express (1953) Europeans demand to see Governor. *Aberdeen Evening Express*. 26 January 1953.

Anderson, D. (2005) *Histories of the Hanged*. London: Phoenix.

Angelo, A. (2017) Jomo Kenyatta and the repression of the 'last' Mau Mau leaders, 1961–1965. *Journal of Eastern African Studies*, 11(3), 442–459. https://doi.org/10.1080/17531055.2017.1354521

Arthur, J.W. (1942) Female circumcision among the Kikuyu. *The British Medical Journal*, 24 October 1942, p. 498.

Ashencaen Crabtree, S. (2012) *A Rainforest Asylum: The Enduring Legacy of Colonial Psychiatric Care in Malaysia*. London: Whiting & Birch.

Ashencaen Crabtree, S. and Wong, H. (2012) 'Ah Cha'! The racial discrimination of Pakistani minority communities in Hong Kong: An analysis of multiple, intersecting oppressions. *British Journal of Social Work*, 43(5), 945–963. https://doi.org/10.1093/bjsw/bcs026.

Ashencaen Crabtree, S., Husain, F. and Spalek, B. (2016) *Islam & Social Work: Islam and Social Work: Culturally Sensitive Practice in a Diverse World*. 2nd ed. Bristol: Policy Press.

BBC (2011) Kenya's Mau Mau Uprising; Your stories. *BBC*, 21 July 2011. Available at: https://www.bbc.co.uk/news/uk-14233738 [Accessed 28 January 2020].

Byrne, A., Caulfield, T., Onyo, P., Nyagero, J., Morgan, A., Nduba, J., and Kermode, M. (2016) Community and provider perceptions of traditional and skilled birth attendants providing maternal health care for pastoralist communities in Kenya: a qualitative study. *BMC Pregnancy and Childbirth*, 16(1), 43. https://doi.org/10.1186/s12884-016-0828-9.

Coventry Evening Telegraph (1955) Mother and daughter murdered in Kenya. *Coventry Evening Telegraph*, 3 November 1955.

Durrani, S. (2018) *Mau Mau: The Revolutionary Anti-Imperialist Force from Kenya. 1948–1963*. Kenya Resists No.1. Nairobi: Vita Books.

Etherington, N. (2005) Education and medicine. In Norman Etherington (Ed.), *Missions and Empire*. Oxford: Oxford University Press, pp. 261–284.

Fiona, A. and Mackenzie, D. (2000) Contested ground: Colonial narratives and the Kenyan environment, 1920–1945. *Journal of Southern African Studies*, 26(4), 697–718. https://doi.org/10.1080/713683602

Gerrard, J.W. (2001). *Africa Calling: A Medical Missionary in Kenya and Zambia*. London: The Radcliffe Press.

Golding, W. (1954) *Lord of the Flies*. London: Faber and Faber.

Good, C.M. (1987) *Ethnomedical Systems in Africa: Patterns of Traditional Medicine in Rural and Urban Kenya*. New York/London: The Guildford Press.

Greene, G. (1999) *Ways of Escape*. London: Vintage Books.

Hardiman, D. (2008) *Missionaries and their Medicine: A Christian modernity for tribal India*. Manchester: Manchester University Press.

Hattersley, R. (2014) *John Welsey: A Brand from the Burning*. London: Abacus.

Hillier, D. (2003) *Childbirth in the Global Village*. London: Routledge.

Jordan, B. (1997) Authoritative knowledge and its construction. In Robbie E. Davis-Floyd and Carolyn Fishel Sargeant (Eds.), *Childbirth and Authoritative Knowledge*. Berkeley: University of California Press, pp. 55–79.

Kenyatta, J. (1965) *Facing Mount Kenya*. New York: Vintage.

Kitzinger, S. (2003) *The Politics of Birth*. Edinburgh: Elsevier.

Kyle, K. (2008) The politics of the independence of Kenya. *Contemporary British History*, 11(4), 42–65.

Kyle, K. (1999) *The Politics of the Independence of Kenya*. Houndsmill: Palgrave Macmillan.

Kyle, K. (1966) Gandhi, Harry Thuku and early Kenyan nationalism. *Transition*, 27, 16–22.

Leakey, L.B.S. (1954, 2004) *Defeating the Mau Mau*. London: Routledge.

Lister, K. (2020) *A Curious History of Sex*. London: Unbound.

Liverpool Echo (1955) Two British schoolboys murdered by Mau Mau Gang. *Liverpool Echo*, 21 April 1955.

Maloba, W.O. (1998) *The Economics of Rebellion Mau Mau and Kenya: An Analysis of a Peasant Revolt*. Bloomington: Indiana Press.

Martin, A.M. and Bezemer, P.M. (2020) The concept and planning of public native housing estates in Nairobi/Kenya, 1918–1948. *Planning Perspectives*, 35(4), 609–634. https://doi.org/10.1080/02665433.2019.1602785

MMS (1956) *Beneath the Cross. The Annual Report and Accounts of the Methodist Missionary Society*. London: Methodist Missionary Society.

Ndubai, G.K. (2016) *The Ameru in the Mau Mau, 1945-1965*. Unpublished Masters of Arts. Department of History and Archaeology. University of Nairobi. Kenya.

Natsoulas, T. (1998) The politicization of the ban on female circumcision and the rise of the independent school movement in Kenya. *Journal of Asian and African Studies*, 33(2), 137–158. https://doi.org/10.1163/156852182X00011

Prichard, J. (2014) *Methodists and Their Missionary Societies, 1900–1996*. London: Routledge.

Redshaw, M. and Heikkilä, K. (2011) Ethnic differences in women's worries about labour and birth. *Ethnicity & Health*, 16(3), 213–223. https://doi.org/10.1080/13557858.2011.561302

Rios, E. (2022) 'Birthing while Black' is a national crisis for the US. Here's what Black lawmakers want to do about it. Available at: https://www.theguardian.com/us-news/2022/apr/19/black-mothers-birth-maternal-mortality. *Guardian*,19 April 2022 [Accessed 2 December 2022].

Robertson, B.M. (1993) *Angels in Africa: A Memoir of Nursing with the Colonial Service*. London: The Radcliffe Press.

Rono, A., Maithya, H. and Sorre, B. (2018) Experiences from a rural community in Western Kenya. *Sociology and Anthropology*, 6(1), 56–63. https://doi.org/10.13189/sa.2018.060105

Spengler, S. (2011) To open oneself is a poor woman's trouble: Embodied inequality and childbirth in South-Central Tanzania. *Medical Anthropology Quarterly*, 24(4), 479–498. https://doi.org/10.1111/j.1548-1387.2011.01181.x

The Sphere (1953) Mau Mau enters upon a new phase. *The Sphere*, 18 April 1953.

The Sphere (1952) Witch-doctoring to combat Mau Mau. *The Sphere*, 6 December 1952.

Strayer, R.W. (1978) *The Making of Mission Communities in East Africa: Anglicans and Africans in Colonial Kenya. 1875–1935*. London: Heinemann.

Stuart, J. (2011) *British Missionaries and the End of Empire: East, Central and Southern Africa, 1939–64*. Grand Rapids, MI/Cambridge: Wm. B. Berdsman Publishing Group.

Swainson, N. (1978) State and economy in post-colonial Kenya, 1963–1978. *Canadian Journal of African Studies / Revue Canadienne des Études Africaines*, 12(3), 357–381.

Thomas, L. (1966) *The Virgin Soldiers*. London: Constable.

Thomas, L.M. (2003) *Politics of the Womb: Women, Reproduction and the State in Kenya*. Berkeley: University of California Press.

Thomas, L.M. (1996) 'Ngaitana (I will circumcise myself)': The gender and generational politics of the 1956 ban on clitoridectomy in Meru, Kenya. *Gender & History*, 8(3), 338–363.

Ties Boerma, and Baya, M.S. (1990) Maternal and child health in an ethnomedical perspective: traditional and modern medicine in coastal Kenya. *Health Policy and Planning* 5(4), 347-357.

Truth (1930) A new controversy in Kenya. *Truth*, 22 January 1930.

Van der Bijl, N. (2017) *Mau Mau Rebellion: The Emergency in Kenya, 1952–1956*. Barnsley, South Yorkshire: Pen and Sword Military.

Wadere, H. (2016) *Cut*. London: Simon & Schuster.

Wadud, A. (2007) *Inside the Gender Jihad*. Oxford: Oneworld Publications.

WHO (2022) Number of maternal deaths. *World Health Organization*. Available at: https://platform.who.int/data/maternal-newborn-child-adolescent-ageing/indicator-explorer-new/mca/number-of-maternal-deaths. [Accessed 4 March 2023].

Wolfenden, A.M. (1933) Kenya Coffee – Natives as Growers. Letters. *The Scotsman*, 4 January 1933.

9 New Jerusalems

The end of mission

The aim of overseas mission, declared Henry Venn, the Secretary of the Church Missionary Society in 1844, was nothing less than 'euthanasia' (Pass, 2014, p. 185). If European missionaries left their bones in foreign fields, permanent Christian legacies were the goal, not permanent individual residencies. Obsoletion was the marker of mission success, reflected in a later change of name from missionary to 'mission partner' (Figure 9.1).

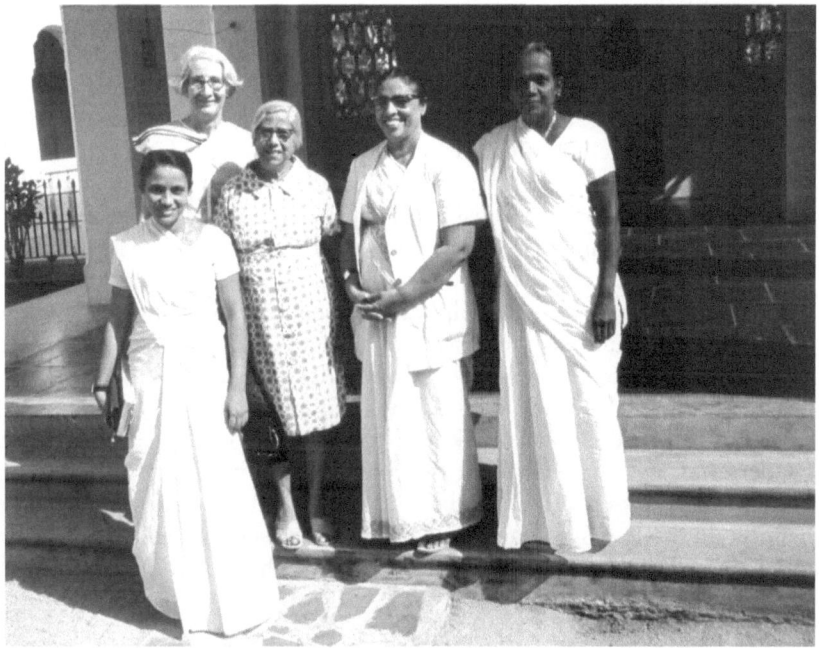

Figure 9.1 Audrey and Ikkadu Hospital colleagues. Courtesy of Muriel Chalkley.

DOI: 10.4324/9781003359746-9

Writing on the day that Muriel would have reached her 101st birthday, I ponder on the tracks the sisters laid towards this destination of dispensability, wondering too how they were perceived by others? Would we find a rehearsal of Paul Scott's (1966, 1975) novels: Muriel, an absurd, garrulous Barbie Bachelor? Audrey, a remote Edwina Crane manqué? What of the humanity of our sisters, their wishes, their pleasures, their sorrows? Was their inner self-hood entirely subjugated to their godly labours?

The mission trinity

The goals of twentieth-century Methodist mission were three-fold. Foreign missionaries were directed towards urgent needs affecting local communities and the sustainability of mission work, whether in education, medicine, administration, welfare or community work. While never to be neglected, the strengthening and nurturing of the implanted Christian faith. Resultant expectations of missionaries were therefore extensive in remit and demanding of proficiency (Figure 9.2).

Needs

Of the first goal, the sisters' immediate impression of the task ahead has been described ('FLIES – DIRT – SMELLS!'). By 1972, Muriel remained troubled by the dangers of childbirth: 'many must just die and be buried there in the village'.[1] By 1981, she[2] notes the 'very primitive conditions' communities endured, ameliorated by 'harambee' (participatory grassroots action). In India, Audrey's teaching still addressed the continuing epidemics of cholera, smallpox and plague (Chalkey, 1974). Terrible famines in South India had been regularly reported in British newspapers since the mid-nineteenth century at least, continuing with tragic monotony a hundred years later. Audrey describes a particularly bad drought-scourged famine in the mid-1960s, requiring emergency mission help, above their regular feeding of the malnourished many. In Kenya too, drought brought crop failure, triggering two extreme episodes of famine in 1961 and 1970 (Mbithi and Wisner, 1973).

The Methodist minister on the Maua Circuit from the 1960s onwards was the Reverend Bernard Jinkin, a former East End Methodist Youth Leader; and, by coincidence, in the rough-and-tumble neighbourhood of Poplar (beloved of all BBC 'Call the Midwife' fans). Whatever challenges he faced in the East End paled into insignificance compared to the unfolding tragedy in the arid north of Maua in 1970, where no rain had fallen for three years. Jinkin tells the story.[3]

> Everything was dying, cattle, giraffes, elephants, people. We were feeding the children one kilo tin of boiled maize just to keep them alive.

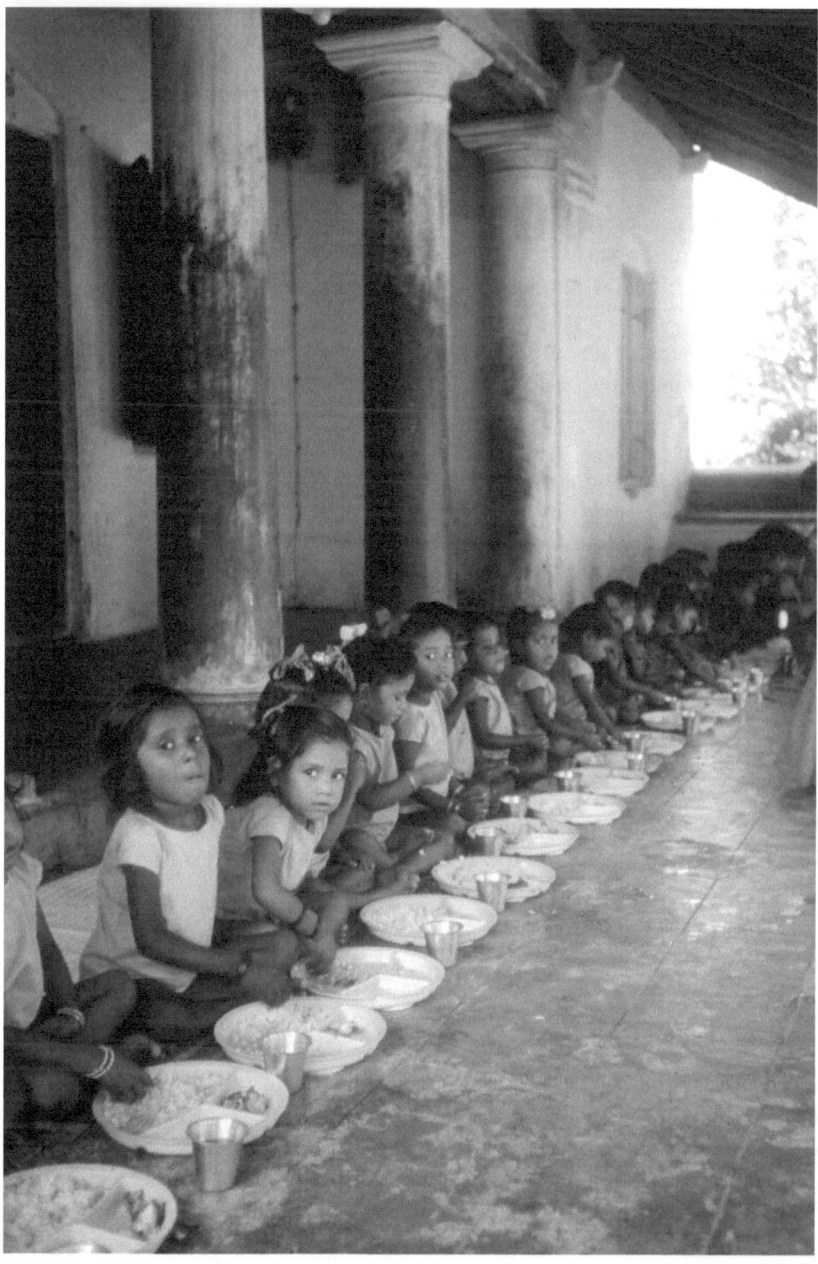

Figure 9.2 Feeding Ikkadu waifs. Photograph by Audrey Chalkley. Courtesy of Muriel Chalkley.

Three youngsters, now wizened husks, so far gone in starvation they could not even eat soup, were gently laid in the back of Jinkins' Land Rover and driven slowly to Maua Hospital one hundred rough-road miles away. Only two of the teenagers survived, where, after much care, were finally fit enough to be discharged home again:

> I took them back to Murti, this place. They slept out in the open. There were no buildings. By this time hyenas were ravenous and one of those two surviving children was eaten by a hyena *alive*!

So cruel was the famine and so inadequate the resources frontline missionaries could muster in the face of overwhelming need that they too became the target of others' despair:

> (Christian) Ministers used to come out …to these feeding centres, and nearly always used to weep. I remember one wept and turned to me very angrily: 'what's your God doing about this?!

Jinkin never recovered from these horrors. As for the Chalkleys, they tackled emergencies more extreme and terrible at times than they would have otherwise encountered in any conventional nursing careers, away from the battlefield (Figure 9.3).

Deeds

While Muriel recorded some of these events in an incomplete cache of preserved letters to the Methodist circuit in England, Audrey's narrative turns towards the second of their roles: the sustainability of mission work, involving the continuing survival of Methodist-fostered services in South India.

Rising swiftly in the field from hands-on nurse to supervisory roles, Audrey became variously a hospital supervisor and manager of nursing, an examiner and inspector of hospitals, the All-Indian Secretary for midwives and leader of training for the Auxiliary Midwife Nursing organisation. Regularly on the road and still unable to afford a car, she made do with a rickety motor scooter with dodgy brakes. One day the inevitable happened, rounding a corner she encountered a dozy calf in the middle of the road. A fall and fractured arm ensued but it could have been so much worse. The Hindu deities protected the calf, and as for Audrey, she sung as she rode: 'The Lord is my Shepherd'.

A recognised national expert of nursing in India, Audrey took a scholarly path towards training, publishing a popular nursing textbook in 1968 on auxiliary nurse midwife education. It was updated when the WHO's 1978

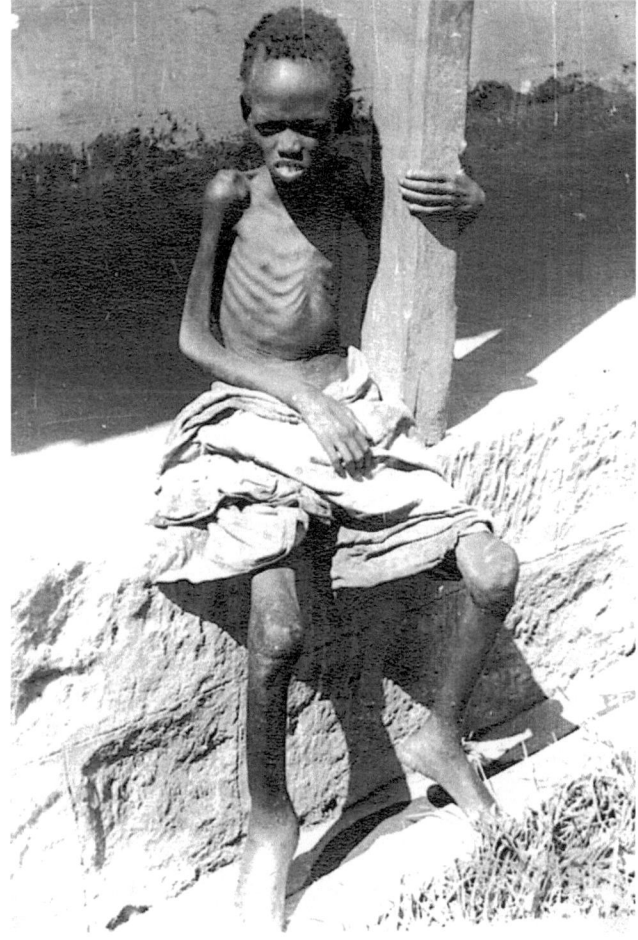

Figure 9.3 Famine. Courtesy of Muriel Chalkley.

call 'Health for All' by 2000 was announced. This consensually changed the focus of international health strategies of member countries (Mahler, 1988). The WHO impact in India and Kenya encouraged wholesale over-hauls of nursing-midwifery and training syllabi to meet changing times.

The Indian Nursing Council decided that the resultant broader focus on community needs were best met by the creation of new primary health worker roles able to negotiate and apply medical skills in both clinical and remote community settings. The gendering of the new health workers' roles demarcated professional territories: nurse-qualified women would concentrate on children and families, and male counterparts on disease prevention.

The Christian medical mission influence is discernible in the revised textbooks' prefaces, where Audrey thanks the Board of Nursing Education and the Nurses' League of the Christian Medical Association of India, specifically the South Indian branch (Chalkley, 1986, 1987). The revised books gained favour, becoming a standard textbook for all health workers across India, translated into four languages and still in print. My own well-thumbed, second/third/fourth-hand copies lie beside me as I write. These were discovered by Fran on a trip to India who sent a triumphant photograph back of his exciting acquisition.

In Kenya, the new government-approved (WHO-inspired) three-year syllabus took up much of Muriel's time, offering a generic skills-based union of general nursing, midwifery and community health, with the similar intentions of producing multiskilled primary health care workers able to turn their hand to a variety of health needs. For Muriel, this involved tutoring female and male students in midwifery; a somewhat suspect innovation, she felt, which predated similar initiatives in Britain by years.

Muriel was proud of the standards of nurse training at Maua, and kept abreast of developments by undertaking external examiner roles for the higher-grade nursing programmes at the big teaching hospitals in Nairobi. At Maua, almost eternally in the financial 'red', there were always more student applications than places to offer, for these additionally offered a small allowance, free accommodation and meals. Every six months there would be a new cohort to train. Being a dedicated and determined teacher ('a battle-axe' she chuckled), Muriel expected her students to be punctual and keen to learn. She found them diligent, eager, hardworking students, education being much respected among African Kenyans.

MURIEL:[4]   Even our nurses... loved their lectures, a punishment
              would be to stop them going.

The cultural significance of dance and song in Maua was not lost on Muriel. Not only was she familiar with these performances but inventively adapted it to her teaching – creating *performative tuition*, as it were. The following description is taken from some scribbled, handwritten fieldnotes on the back of a used envelope when Muriel unexpectedly launched into an irresistible anecdote one afternoon, just after I was packed up and ready to leave.

Fieldnotes. Pedagogy Muriel-style.

1 Muriel arranged the 'boys' and 'girls' in groups. Girls form a ring around 1 in the middle – the ovum. The boys, sperm racing down the corridor towards the ring of girls, the corridor being the fallopian tube. They try to get to the ovum, repelled by the other girls. Once inside, they take the

girl to a seat that Muriel draped a red cloth over, this being the symbolic uterus.

2 Muriel divides students into four groups to teach them about contractions. They all chant 'This is how contractions are'. Then group 1 slowly and quietly chant: 'we are weak, we are weak, we are weak and irregular'. The second group chants 'we are stronger, we are stronger, we are stronger and more regular now'. Group 3 chants 'we are strong, we are strong, we are strong and regular now!' The final group chants 'we want to push! We want to push! We want to push the baby out!'

In her seventies, Muriel was given a glitchy CD of miscellaneous videos and photographs compiled for her in Kenya. This was a video clip of her post-retirement return visit back in 1991, recording what seems to be a very happy and welcoming occasion, the hospital staff partying in celebration of her return to Maua. Muriel is shown warmly greeting old colleagues and comrades, beaming matronly sisters critically inspect the student nurse choir. Stephano is there, shrunken with age but grinning happily. To cheers, Muriel is presented with her 'old friend' the classroom 'baby', a threadbare demonstration doll; maybe the same one she showed the Chief's men all those years before. Much dancing, singing and eating ensues. The video hiccups – but there she is again joining in the hand-clapping, circle dances.

Faith and fellowship

The final arm of this mission trinity is its quintessential raison d'être. Audrey earned her place within the CSI ecclesiastical hierarchy as a devoted and trustworthy servant of the unified Church, receiving supervisory guidance from Bishop Leslie Newbigin, espousing a powerful belief in the purpose of the Church as fundamentally engaged in mission (Goheen, 2009). She also enjoyed an excellent relationship with Bishop Sundar Clarke sharing his interest in Charismatic Christianity. This tradition, inspired by Methodism, makes spiritual space for the gifts of prophecy, miraculous healing, dreams and glossolalia, as commonly associated with American religious revivalist Pentecostalism (Hempton, 2005). Yet these spiritual manifestations were established in India long before the first Pentecostal missionary set foot on the subcontinent (McGee, 1999, p. 648). In the mid-nineteenth century, Tirunelveli and Travancore missionaries were already reporting ecstatic phenomena among local Indian Christians (McGee, 1999).

A flowering of spiritual sorority emerged within the CSI. Clara Clarke, Bishop Sundar's wife, was heavily involved in the women's fellowship movement. CSI Deaconess Carol Graham established a women's spiritual treat in India: 'Vishranthi Nilayam'; the forerunner to her later women's religious Farncombe Community in Surrey (Graham, 1980). There were also the Indian diocesan Bible women, single women all; some educated at a Kingsmead equivalent, a women's Christian college in Madras. 'Super-chastity' was demanded of Bible women, who might otherwise be taken for some kind of Christian temple prostitute (Kent, 1999, pp. 146–147), an insult occasionally levied at foreign women missionaries (Pass, 2011).

One Bible woman, named after pealing church bells, was a qualified school teacher who rejoiced in prayer, preaching to the people and hymn-singing accompanied by percussion 'clappers'. Now elderly, ill with tuberculosis and rejected by her family, Audrey found her alone, neglected and homeless, so took her in. 'Rebecca' was an illiterate woman preacher, teacher and healer of the sick (much in the early Methodist tradition). Rebecca became a dear friend, unfailingly delivering a monthly tithe of the tenth of her earned pittance for Audrey to deliver to the CSI.

Forging Christian Fellowship among their nurses, strengthening faith and vocation was an intrinsic part of the sisters' work and working week. A much-faded photograph shows Audrey strumming a guitar to a grave group of sari-clad nursing devotees clustered around. It is an intimate, gentle and even maternal scene: Audrey with her 'daughters'.[5] In Maua, *conjubilant* rejoicing involved the energetic harmonies of a percussion 'orchestra....a drum, tambourines, shakers, and small cymbals and two sets of bells – so we make plenty of noise when praising the Lord'.[6]

Africa carried a Christian potential that missionaries struggled to find in Indian caste society. In Kenya, religious observance was well-entrenched, and if once admittedly heathen, there were rich roots of belief from which the Tree of Life could 'strike' and flourish. The indigenous people worshipped a Creator God (Mogai/Ngai), possessing a Genesis creation story of a first man and woman with dominion over the Earth (Kenyatta, 1965). This was an encouraging start compared to the bewildering cosmological, complexities and paradoxes of Hinduism. As in India, customary practices experienced as oppressive lead some Africans to embrace Christianity and the mantle of indigenous evangelist. In her unpublished memoirs of twentieth-century mission work (1925–1955), Dorothy Ross neé Jewett, describes a young woman of the Niger delta giving birth to twins: a taboo: the babies are drowned in the river and the mother set adrift towards exile. Offered sanctuary with a CMS missionary, she eventually chooses to be baptised into the Anglican faith, taking the name of 'Rachel'.

> She found peace in the love and friendship of Christians, and eventually was impelled to tell her husband and friends of God's love and goodness to her, and to offer it to her own people.
>
> (Ross, no date, p. 28)

There were other distasteful tribal habits offending Christian propriety, like the lack of funeral rites among the Kikuyu, where the 'unclean' dead were left out to be eaten by hyenas, and the dying abandoned beyond village walls in preparation of their demise and dismemberment.[7] Nevertheless, even these perceived ungodly practices changed. Mission schools mushroomed and disseminated the Good News message, while Handley Hooper exalted Christ's pre-eminence and living spirit in indigenous people (Strayer, 1978). The Methodists were typically dauntlessly optimistic about the working of Christ in people's lives, where the 1956 Women's Work Annual Report (MMSWW, 1956, p. 44), confidently announced:

> As the darkness recedes in Meru, Christ will rebuild and we believe the best is yet to be seen. Suffering has brought a new surge of spiritual life and the persecution has brought a new purity of purpose.

Mission schools had been effective in offering education to many, but if the Jesuits claimed otherwise, it was clear that such schooling did not always mean Christianity was absorbed along with the '3 Rs'. Nor could mission hospitals boast that all staff were committed Christians, although many were or became so. Accordingly, Muriel[8] sadly tells Methodist supporters in a 'round robin' letter how some Kenyan staff in the hospital were becoming cold towards Christianity. Attributing this in part to Satan's wiles, she was surely also aware that grievances towards colonisation implicated mission in an increasingly common accusatory refrain.

Nevertheless, the inherent ardent religiosity of African Kenyans welcomed the emanations of the Holy Spirit, the Paraclete; where workings of the Spirit were central to African Methodists together with the postcolonial independent African Churches (Anderson, 2004). Muriel repeats the testimony[9] of a 'glowing' European missionary minister who came to pray with her when her robust health collapsed and she was acutely ill in Maua with tick typhus. She describes how an African schoolboy, acting as the Minister's Swahili interpreter, accompanied him to a Sunday Service in Mombasa. The boy asking permission to preach himself invited the audience to give their lives to Christ. The response from the congregation was so immediately impressive that the astonished missionary questioned him. 'The young lad replied "It is the power of the Holy Spirit" and then went on to say '"you can have this also". So then, Alan said he knelt down and this lad prayed for him to receive this gift of power and he did!'

Muriel was also bestowed with grace, uttering the mystical speech of angels: *glossolalia*, otherwise known as 'speaking in tongues' (Ashencaen Crabtree, 2021), a holy gift esteemed by both Early Christians and Pentecostal movements alike (Gooren, 2004). On one extraordinary occasion, Muriel rose to the occasion for my own particular benefit when she felt, with good reason that I needed an injection of spiritual succour and holy strength during a time of intense personal hardship that was making me miserable and ill (academic life, regrettably, attracting at times not only rational and generous attention, but banditry and derangement as well). Her glossolalia performance seemed entirely fluid and as authentic as any supranatural gift can be. It was strange, uncanny even, but so far as I could hear, entirely fluent, seeming neither forced nor artificial. I do not know if Audrey shared this gift of glossolalia, but one evening musing out loud, Jonathan sitting beside me, whimsically retorted, 'And did Audrey use rupees to ride the bus in India?' Well, I suppose she must have – and duly then I suppose that she did.

Just like Audrey in Ikkadu, forging Fellowship was another priority at Maua. Muriel's support was evidently successful where by 1955, her first year in Maua, the MMS report of 1955 (p. 27), commented approvingly on increases in the training of nurses: 'their spiritual life is maintained in regular prayer meetings'.

MURIEL:[10]   Our day would start... seven o'clock in the morning the bell would go and we would all meet in the church for a short time for prayers. We would take it in turns to lead. And then we would all go to our wards and the nurse in charge of each ward would lead prayers in the ward as well, because it was a Christian hospital. The whole idea was to show (that) God cared about bodies as well as souls, and our nursing was all linked to the spiritual side of course, although we didn't stress it all the time....Prayers were also always said before anyone had an anaesthetic because they (patients) were very fearful of that.

There are parallels to be found here with Galvin and Todres's conceptualisation of open-hearted nursing as encompassing 'head, heart and hand' (2009, p. 146). Framed as an exercise in existential (potentially secular) meaning-making in nursing, within medical mission service, care of patients could not be desegregated from the grace of a far greater Authority moulding the healer to the task. No human skill could affect any healing whatsoever without that higher mandate that directed all human activity, so Muriel believed.

The Holy Spirit was a surprisingly late arrival in Muriel's life. It had been little mentioned in her religious upbringing. The mature Muriel embraced the power of the Holy Spirit fully thereafter; this breath of God reaching into Christian hearts, lighting yearnings to be ever closer to absolute perfection and love. She had felt it during her youthful crises, but it was through Charismatic Christianity in Africa that Muriel discovered herself to be a veritable conduit through which the Holy Spirit moved. Christian Fellowship created those blissful moments when It was felt to be most present within a communion of shared understandings of God-energy powering and nurturing this remote African Hospital. Forging, what Pritchard describes, in an interesting historiography of women's evangelism and mission congregations in East Africa (2017, p. 4), as an 'affective spiritual community': a self-sustaining, reproductive Fellowship of shared beliefs daily translated into ubiquitous, faith-inspired medical practices.

In 1975, Muriel's faith was further reinforced by attending a 'Unity in Christ' Charismatic conference, accompanied by nursing students and Audrey, who had long saved for a reciprocated trip to see her sister. The event attracted a multitudinous and varied flock of a thousand people, culminating in an ecstatic Christian rally in Nairobi's Uhuru Park. The Fisherfolk, a transnational Christian band played at the conference, teaching the audience new songs, elating musical Audrey. Overtures of love (agape rather than eros) were issued and invitations offered. Muriel described an incredibly festive mood, with people dancing around together, their hands joyously raised high to the heavens, much to her initial discomfiture:[11]

> I can remember thinking – at the beginning – I'm not going to raise my arms for anybody....and before the end my arms were raised – and ever since I have had a job to keep them down anywhere there is good, real worship!

For Audrey too, it was spiritually transformational:[12]

AUDREY: And it seemed to me that the heaven was opening and we were worshipping with the angels in Heaven and it was a wonderful experience to me. ...And it was so lovely.... when I walked home after this service, I was walking as though I was on air. It was a great thrill. ...that night I couldn't sleep...like waves washing over me of love and joy and peace; and I just felt ...a new love for Jesus and assurance that he loves me and I was his child. And so after that experience I went back to India rather a different person...

The communal participation in the body of Christ is *the* Christian creed, although the Indian theologian Kaj Baago, noting the thousands of Indians in Madras without an obvious connection to Church life, asks 'Must Buddhists, Hindus and Muslims became Christians in order to belong to Christ?' (Hunsberger, 1998, p. 112). I hazard the guess that Muriel would probably have answered 'yes'. This seemingly provocative query touches on the far greater question of how far Christian witness can be meaningfully entwined within the religious frameworks of other faiths, highly relevant to multicultural contexts (Hunsberger, 1998). This certainly has been realised for some, the American Roman Catholic ordained priest and theologian, Paul Knitter (2011, p. 53), for example, describes himself as Buddhist-Christian, stating that 'without Buddha I could not be a Christian'; with other examples beside.

Yet theological syncretic sophistication was not Muriel's strength, nor was solipsism her vice. Being a gregarious philanthrope, she needed to rejoice in the shared company of fellow Christians. To me, she admitted how hard it was to commune with God sometimes in an increasingly isolated old age, where she was too physically infirm to join the live congregation, and too technologically antiquated to go online. One happy irony arose: Muriel's ancient terrestrial television, unworkable for satellite networks, tuned happily into the BBC's forgotten weekly programme 'Songs of Praise' (the 'God-slot'), now disconnected from secular digital primetime. With that for company, she prayed often and hard from her reclining chair, but was increasingly bewildered to find herself alone and unheld by a Christian commonwealth of companions. Muriel's faith could be construed as naïve and unnuanced, but it was also pure in simplicity, reflected in an expressed 'longing' to become a 'channel for the Holy Spirit to manifest Himself in my life at Maua'.[13]

Hardiman (2006) points to the independent African churches performing Pentecostal-type healings of the sick to missionaries' disapproval. Their alleged reluctance to indulge in African frames of spiritual reference of exorcisms, religious charms and the laying on of hands inhibited missionaries' abilities to relate to local people. While this may have been true for some, for Muriel, miracle healing was entirely compatible with her own Christian beliefs and practices, evolving through her spiritual experiences in Africa.

MURIEL:[14]   Another interesting case we got, which I'm sure was an answer to prayer. We had this girl, another one with eclampsia, having fits, and she had a cerebral haemorrhage as a complication and she was completely unconscious and we had two doctors at this time. They both said they thought she would die. It was hopeless. We put her in the side ward and I remember the baby was ...perfectly alright. We used to put the baby to the breast and yet she (mother) was unconscious and I can remember I ... looked at her and I thought it so sad: the baby's perfectly healthy. And I really prayed and I really felt God telling me to lay hands on her. And I didn't know whether to call one or two of the other nurses in, who I knew were keen

Christian, or not. And then I thought, well, I better not in case nothing happens and they'll be let down, you see. But I laid hands on her and I prayed, I prayed in tongues actually and as I was praying, she blinked and opened her eyes and looked at me and from then on she began to recover. She made a complete recovery and went home with a live baby. And I'm sure that was an answer to prayer, which I was very thrilled about, and then of course I wished I had called them in.

Miracles by their very nature are not everyday events, a trite self-evident truism. The philosopher Hume, followed by Swinburne (1968), posits miracles as witnessed and non-repeatable transgressions of the laws of nature. This leads to questioning the veracity of miracle witnesses and a presumption that the inexplicable awaits a future logical explanation. Within the bounds of what a miracle may be, they are by their nature exceptional, following a certain script: succour is desperately hoped for, directed through extraordinary intervention from (a) supreme being/source, responding to specific and absolutely pressing human need. As Hempton (2005, p. 37) says, whilst John Wesley ruled out some events as miracles he certainly believed in 'a strange chain of providences'. The Scriptures, of course, are full of miracles of Christ's healing ministry; and thus, while we might casually regard a remarkable change of fortunes that saves someone unexpectedly from say, bankruptcy, deportation or prison, we might also think these are merely the prosaic extraordinary, removed from extreme life and death matters. The dying woman Muriel felt impelled to pray over and lay hands upon, could, possibly, (a sceptic might argue) have drawn back from the brink naturally and spontaneously at that very moment. Yet, I doubt I am the only one that feels that often the so-called 'rational explanation' is one that stretches the credulity quite as far as any belief in miracles.

Those of us who believe that these occurrences are indeed the result of direct, supernatural intervention must be reminded of the admonition of Franz Werfel, 'For those who believe, no explanation is necessary; for those who do not believe, no explanation will suffice'.

(Diamond, 2008, p. 351)

Having, I think, witnessed and experienced miracles myself, which during my atheist years I might have labelled 'magic', I find my credulity tips towards accepting the odd 'miracle'. Perhaps Muriel was indeed divinely used on this exceptional occasion.

More moving is that which sceptics might point to: Muriel's doubt. How she must have kicked herself for her quavering resolution to permit others to witness what befell. That hesitancy, so human, so prevalent, so understandable stirs my compassion. Yet doubt, is part of the Christian tradition. To grapple with doubt, as Reiss (2016) expresses, is part of the journey of faith that is repeatedly tested; each step a struggle, demanding of the thoughtful believer, continual re-examination and re-commitment, of which doubt is the essential component of that measure (Ashencaen Crabtree, 2021).

Unmasking the missionary

Edens: raw and refined

Muriel's letters to British Methodists spanned two decades. They were important for tapping donations for the Hospital and keeping supporters abreast of news in Maua and beyond, supplementing media reports of terrorism, *Uhuru* and postcolonial governance (given government crackdowns on civil unrest and Jomo Kenyatta's tarnishing halo) (Angelo, 2017).

British readers had long become used to dramatic headlines concerning Kenya. Of less actual harm but symbolically inflammatory, was the Mau Mau's burning down of 'Treetops' in 1954. This was the unique, prestigious safari park hotel in the Aberdare Range near Nyeri, which, sensationally, two years earlier had hosted a particular Royal honeymoon couple where a Princess ascended a giant fig tree to descend thereafter a Queen. By 1959 the hotel had been rebuilt and entertained British royalty again, with Elizabeth, the Queen Mother, described by the *London Illustrated News* of 7 February 1959, as enjoying thrilling spectacles from the viewing platforms: great beasts, baboons swarming the balustrades and eyes gleaming in the dark.

'K*eeny*a', as British colonials then pronounced it (Kyle, 1999), was not only the province of visiting VIPs, the displaced European planter, the city 'Happy Valley' hedonist and their terrifying nemesis – the night-time assassin. It was also a favourite location for cinematic portrayals of a metaphorical, imaginary Africa, an Africa of nature in the raw. Here, for little-travelled audiences was the thrillingly unfamiliar terrain of the feral and untamed. If the enlightened privileged enjoyed sighting Kenya's 'big game' with the aid of binoculars, the white game hunter and trophy hunter remained a trope still actively celebrated, exemplified by the absurd 1953 'movie' *Mogambo*, featuring a smug Clarke Gable polishing his rifle, atwix a luscious love triangle composed of Ava Gardener and Grace Kelly. Much later in 1985 came the more nuanced, 'epic' film 'Out of Africa' (1985), featuring another white game hunter played more sensitively by Robert Redford, as the lover of the real-life Danish aristocrat-cum-plantation owner, Karen Blixen. The opening scenes portray huge elephant tasks being loaded onto the train carrying the elegant Nordic naïf to her new life in BEA. The backdrop to the action is the First World War in Europe but the politics of the mass killing of people and the plundering of nature remained unexplored.

Drama apart, Africa nature films were in their nascence. Before David Attenborough, by the 1950s Armand and Michaela Denis were already shown in early colour films shooting nature with a camera rather than a gun. Armand brought European, middle-aged, bespectacled mansplaining gravitas to proceedings. and Michaela, an understudy to Deborah Kerr, alluring in safari trousers, was deliciously vivacious. Apparently travelling nowhere in the bush without her trusty box of cosmetics, Michaela, tossing her strawberry-blonde locks and fetchingly fearless, brought glamour to proceedings.

Later in life after Armand's death, Michaela became an aristocratic dowager by wedding Sir William O'Brien Lindsay, the former chief justice of Sudan – followed by his funeral a mere three months later. It was in her later incarnation as Lady Lindsay that Michaela was befriended by my own glamorous, widowed mother, Elvira, and became a raconteur at our family home in West London, retelling her many adventures, conquests and the shock of finding poor Lindsay dead as a dodo. On her oscillations between England and Kenya, Michaela bestowed on us a very nice upright piano she had no longer had house room for and a ravishing, pink satin, wasp-waist frock she no longer had the figure for. It is easy to imagine her modelling it, towing her pet cheetahs through Nairobi's high society, stunningly defiant of Mau Mau menaces.

Michaela and Armand were contemporaries of that other famous nature-loving Kenya couple George and 'Joy' Adamson, although there was no love lost between them. The Adamsons' fame was founded on Joy Adamson's published story of the couple's adopted lion cub, Elsa the lioness. In 1966, this was turned into the film 'Born Free', after the book of the same name; featuring the ever-popular, wholesome British actors of their day, Virginia McKenna and Bill Travers.

Muriel never mentioned meeting the Denises, and indeed many of their safari adventures, like those in the Serengeti in Tanzania, lay far beyond Muriel's stamping ground. Twenty miles downhill from Maua, where forests were being cleared for coffee and tea plantations, was bush teeming with wildlife. Muriel loved her mini-safaris and to her English correspondents. she writes[15] of seeing black rhinos, giraffes, buffalo, bush pigs, elephants, ostriches, lions, buck deer and the monkey brethren. Bird spotting, she particularly enjoyed and had some amusing tales to tell about alarmingly close encounters with prowling lions (Elsa's cubs, she felt sure) and being chased by angry, ear-flapping, 'big tuskers', while the Bedford coughed agonisingly along.

Later on, the area was turned into a 'game park', an interestingly anachronistic choice of words, suggestive of an appreciation of wildlife as being primarily destined for sport. This became Meru National Park, its warden, George Adamson. Having 'taken the pledge' in childhood, and as simple and ascetic in her habits as a hermit, Muriel was unlikely to bump into Adamson, a regular at the Pig and Whistle Hotel in Meru, unlike vacationing nurse Bridget Robertson (1993) dining on fresh trout and guinea fowl. However, Muriel did mention bumping into Joy Adamson sometimes, and it was quite clear that this celebrity lover of lions left Muriel with a poor impression. In reality 'Joy' was not cinema's archetypal animal-loving Englishwoman but the (possibly ironical) nickname of the aloof, aristocratic Austrian-born Friederike Victoria Gessner. Despite Joy Adamson knowing the old Beresford Hospital well and even writing an endorsement for its fund-raising efforts, she cold-shouldered Muriel with snubs.

George Adamson was murdered in 1989 by Somali bandits along with his two African assistants (Schanche, 1989), some nine years after Joy Adamson was also murdered. At first, it was thought a lion attacked but soon after came confirmation that she had been multiply stabbed. A young man, Paul Nakware Ekai, convicted of her murder, years later stated that rather than stabbing Adamson, he shot her in self-defence. More credibly he claimed that she often behaved in a despotic and tyrannical fashion towards her African staff, where a quarrel precipitated her murder over a pay dispute (Vasagar, 2004). Certainly, Adamson's conduct towards her employees did not bear close scrutiny from Africans or Europeans alike. Michaela Denis's obituary claimed she disliked Joy Adamson intensely owing to unconscionable conduct towards her African staff (Boucher, 2003). Karen Blixen won no approval either in her disdain of conservation. If Michaela confided these enmities to my mother, then regrettably it was not in my hearing. Instead, we rely on Muriel's memories of Meru National Park and seeing Joy Adamson forcing her African staff to sit precariously on the bonnet of the jeep she drove, rather than permitting them to sit more safely in the cab beside her. A paradox of polarities could spark dangerous resentments, for Elsa, the Lioness and her kin occupied a status and regard denied to Adamson's African staff, an ugly truth belying the pictorial, fictionalised gloss.

In 1980, Muriel enjoyed a few minutes of fame when she was invited to have a short walk-on part in a BBC programme, 'A Long Way From Home', interviewed by the Methodist minister, missionary writer and BBC broadcaster, Dr Colin Morris. Seen as a controversial figure, Morris had accused the British Conservative government in the 1960s of devising a draft policy for immigration deemed so severe that Christ Himself would have been an unwelcome migrant. What Morris would have made of the far more draconian Conservative government's immigration policies in the twenty-first century would be worth hearing. Under this policy, 'illegal immigrants' could be deported to Rwanda in Central Africa, a nation paid handsomely for guarding human unwanted flotsam and jetsam washed up on British shores. The brainchild of successive British Home Secretaries, we may reflect on their interesting personal legacies of migration through Asia, Africa and Europe. Former Home Secretary, Priti Patel's family were members of the Asian Ugandan community later expelled in 1972 from Uganda under the demented diktats of the dictator, Idi Ami. I remember as a child seeing these new classmates utterly bewildered, homesick and shivering knock-kneed under the onslaught of their first British winter.

Patel's successor, Suella Braverman's father came from the Kenyan Asian community. Both Conservative politicians worked with or under the Premiership of Rishi Sunak, whose own parents were migrants from Kenya and Tanzania respectively. Under these policy architects Africa, which endured the diasporic waves of colonials from Imperial shores, was now identified as a suitable dumping ground for unwanted migrants post-imperialism.

The apologist tone of Morris' documentary brought critical humility to re-examining mission in Kenya, interspersed with footage of working missionaries. Muriel, in her Nursing Sister's 'blue', is shown teaching attentive students, but nothing substantial is said about the hospital unfortunately. Probably in response to a question off-camera, she is drawn into explaining that once European missionaries in Maua lived in a big house away from African staff, but now a more egalitarian relationship between overseas and local staff existed. While undoubted true, viewers may have received a rather skewed impression of her life in Maua as more segregated and privileged than it actually was. Audrey's early missionary experiences were a closer reflection of that.

AUDREY: It wasn't *quite* what I expected. The 'bungalow', which sounds like a small building, was enormous, with very high ceilings and we were sort of living in luxury. I had seen on the train so many very poor, small huts of the poorer people. And other things that surprised me were that I was expected to have visiting cards and was taken out by the senior lady missionary, the chairman's wife, in a car with a chauffeur to visit other senior missionaries in the area and also for tennis twice a week; and we were taken to dinner parties where we wore long dresses. We mixed with the embassy staff and ex-patriot businessmen... I felt rather awkward in this kind of society.

I was invited to the English Club for a swim, no Indians allowed were there except the waiters and it was difficult to get talking with any Indians it seemed. In the bungalow, we had servants, such as the butler, and the *chota wallah* who was also called 'the boy'. And we had sweepers and someone to pull the *punkah* for our meals, because it was very hot and there were no electric fans in those days. I was rather glad when that kind of attitude of looking up to the British came to an end, a bit later than that, but it did. The attitudes did change for which I was much relieved.

Back in the mountainous backwater of Maua, Muriel did not mix in the same exalted circles as Audrey's. Bashing around the bush in the Bedford van and camping out was more her style. Then again, as missionary Christine Macqueen[16] says, in Africa, there were no charming hill stations for reviving exhausted colonials from the scorching and enervating summer heat of the valleys, as there were in Asia. Although the famous colonial hill station resorts, such as Murree in Pakistan or the supreme Simla, the summer capital of the British Raj, were many miles away, British Methodist missionaries, along with their American cousins, could still bask in the comparative cool of these highland retreats.

Somewhat frustratingly, Audrey[17] fails to specify exactly where her designated refuge, 'Wiseman Cottage' stood (evidently named after the Methodist grande dame, Caroline Meta Wiseman herself). We know it 'was in this beautiful place. More like England' in offering gently rolling verdant vistas, where Audrey, a strong walker, strolled through 'country lanes' and 'forest places', with her enchanted fellow missionaries.

In her account of the colonial Hill Stations of Asia, Crossette (1999) spends time surveying a number of these former resorts, noting their state of preservation, ossification, deterioration and vulgarisation, depending on the circumstances, indifference or protection afforded to them. In reference to Simla, some tired old tropes are trotted out: the British Raj's preoccupation with starched-collar rank versus the more relaxed, social unbuttoning at Kodaikanal in Tamil Nadu, a resort developed and colonised by American missionaries and their fellow countryfolk. It is therefore interesting to learn that English missionary, Ruth Ansty[18] also frequented Kodai, and Audrey may have too.

Or she may have followed Mary Spear's example[19] resting at the other Tamil Nadu retreat at Meghamalai. This, built to entertain Queen Victoria's heir 'Bertie', the portly, if racy, Prince of Wales, and future Edward VII, his wish at Meghamalai was to bag the biggest of game – elephants. Using 'coolie' (Outcaste) labour, a route to the top was carved out in preparation for the Prince's hunting expeditions. Thankfully for the elephants he never went; instead, the hills were discovered to be the ideal place for growing tea. Spear recalls how in her day the 'coolie catcher' would come to the mission asking 'have you got any coolies to work on the tea estates?' Those that were recruited were given a weekly bag of rice, a doled proportion of their wage, accruing the final sum at the end of an eleven-month contract. Tea-picking was such a lucrative business, at which Outcaste women excelled, that colonial plantation owners willingly built accommodation, crèches and day schools to accommodate their women workers and their families.

Religious leadership, says Spear, was provided at Meghamalai in the form of Mr Levi, a clergyman brought in to cater for the Outcaste Christians. Sadly, the poor fellow did not last long: Blackwater fever finished him off only two years from taking up his hilltop ministry. Influenza hit the community at the same time and the Methodists rushed in to help, with one even laboriously cycling up a terrific incline carrying 'masses of quinine and other drugs' to help the labourers. This so impressed the plantation owners they vowed to give the Methodists land to build bungalows and a church.

The final contender for Audrey's pleasure was also the closest to Ikkadu: 'Snooty Ooty' (Ootacamund), the summer home of the Madras colonial government (Crossette, 1999, p. 114). Not entirely immune to their charm, Pradhan (2017) critiques the value-laden cultural aesthetic of British imperialism the hill stations evoked, of which Ootacamund was a notable ornament in its ornately 'dignified' civic buildings, as J.B. Priestley might say (1934), where these sumptuous hill stations boasted museums, theatres, preparatory schools, libraries, botanical gardens and parks, Anglican Churches, around which nestled quaint homes, in handy proximity to the ubiquitous colonial 'Club'. Ooty was parodied by Scott, as the fictional hill station of 'Pankot', a high altitude, claustrophobic enclave of increasingly irrelevant, besieged colonial lives. Yet, it was precisely these cultivated virtues of civilised bourgeois suburbia in Britain that had improved the lives of the lower classes via the 'garden city' movements and the worker villages of Nonconformist corporate philanthropy. The grandly twee architectural vernacular of the Hill Stations must have seemed immensely evocative to Andrey: for here in India was another Port Sunlight.

Today the hill stations attract a different visitor. There are plenty of 'cottage' holiday rentals to be found as tourist attractions; although sadly no trace of 'Wiseman Cottage' in any. Maybe it was demolished or had its name changed to something more pseudo-pastoral and would-be English: 'Briar Rose', 'Lavender Lawns', 'Raj's Repose' perhaps.

Audrey correspondingly became more independent and adventurous. On 2 March 1968, she wrote to Dorothy and Bran to tell them of her fiftieth birthday treat, trekking towards Mount Everest's base camp. This trek, rigorous now, was then far less attuned to tourists. She and the shepherding sherpas camped in an abandoned 'cosy' ruin in the sheltering lea of boulders. To make it even partially habitable overnight, the so-called walls and roof need to be patched with clumps of leaves, a little warmth and illumination provided by a candle; mackintoshes draped over sleeping bags kept the worst of the damp out. Audrey thought it a simply marvellous holiday.

Opinions and observations

A year before *Uhuru* Muriel[20] was commenting on the improved relationships between Europeans and Africans, with old prejudices and superiorities dissolving and a new spirit of cooperation and friendship in the air. Yet a decade later, Muriel was lamenting froideur at Maua.[21] Reverend Andrew MacKenzie's[22] smarting from unfair traducement at Maua, noted the whipped-up neighbourhood hostilities directed towards the Hospital, staff and clergy, in ways that were 'very hard and unnecessary'. Such astringent correctives sharpen any tendency towards saccharine sentimentality of Methodist mission harmony.

Digging deeper, I sought answers to the question of how the sisters had been perceived. Helen Cooper and Susan Dutton, Mary Rathbone's daughters, the friends from Muriel's Macclesfield days remembered her with deep affection and respect.[23]

HELEN: She was a role model, her faith was so strong, she was so exuberant, she was so kind, she was so jolly. I started to have a heart for Africa from 'Aunty' Muriel. She was what a Christian ought to be, a whole rounded person, joy in her faith, joy in life, joy in person.

All well and good, but what might those who had worked with Muriel have to say? Barbara Dickinson, whose service overlapped Muriel's by four years, considered the question:[24]

The staff loved her... because she was very fair to the staff, and supportive; and the students loved her because the staff loved her and the patients respected and loved her too. She loved them.

This accolade from one British missionary to another must be weighed against the testimonies of African Kenyans who had known Muriel and her methods far better, as former students and later professionals in their own right.

One who had travelled very far from her early days as a young midwifery student in Maua is Leah Marangu. Hers has been a 'stellar' career of the highest academic kudos where she served Kenya in many prestigious roles, breaking barriers of gender and ethnicity in her meteoric rise upwards. Steeped in a transnational Methodist legacy, she draws from Kenyan, British and North American traditions.

I knew of Leah before I met her. Muriel proudly showed me a formal photograph of her splendid, former protégé in a glossy graduation 2009 brochure. Leah was resplendent as vice chancellor of the Africa Nazarene

University, founded on Wesleyan Methodist principles. It was clear what Muriel thought of Leah, but what in turn would Leah make of her old mentor?

LEAH[25]:   She was very humble; down-to-earth. Willing to help others in a selfless manner and truly wanting to transform the lives of people, both the students she taught and the patients she took care of. She was very passionate. Actually, for us we accepted her and she accepted us...It worked very, very harmoniously. At times she was learning from us and we were learning from her – there was no friction.

Muriel did not manage to stay in touch with all her students. Some like Leah travelled far beyond the immediate constellation that Muriel was still in communication. One who remained in close contact was Margaret Aritho,[26] whose contact I traced through Leah. Margaret was not unlike Muriel, a hearty, good-humoured lady, whose genial son, John, helped us with an IT rescue every time the Zoom connection faltered, which it did frequently. Together Margaret and John had many memories of Muriel and the Mau Mission Hospital to share.

MARGARET: She was a very cheerful person....Muriel was so easy to get on with. She was invited to our houses for evening meals (as) she visited the homes surrounding the hospital to check on health care. She was like a sister to me. she particularly loved me and I loved her *too* much.

Muriel, like soon-to-born, *Shilling Itano*, was renamed in Maua. The foreign missionaries were known to the African staff by secret names; some may have less complementary but Muriel's was well chosen: *Kagwira*, the 'Happy One'.

In the last few years of her work at Maua, Muriel's load was considerably lightened by the Kenyan colleagues taking forward the work of which she was now feeling the weight. Accordingly, I was delighted to be introduced to one of the two 'Florences' who worked closely with Muriel in these final years of her service in Maua. Florence Mutiga[27] turned out to another effusive, assertive lady, magnificent in colourful turban and robes.

FLORENCE: I came to Maua in 1969 and that was when Muriel was going back to England, so I was new coming to start training in Maua Hospital. Then in 1977 that's when I was working with Muriel in the maternity. Muriel came to understand me, a person we can work with. She loved

me so much, so much, so much... She loved us and we
loved her. I take it as a favour of God that I worked with
such a wonderful person, a wonderful Christian.

Such assertions of affection flowing unchecked from these participants in
response to a simply framed, starting question, 'Can you share any of your
memories of Muriel?', seeming almost extravagant in the abundance of
praise for an Englishwoman who once worked at Maua and had not been
seen for many years thereafter. One would expect memories of Muriel to
fade; particularly given the great changes that swept away the last ves-
tiges of colonialism in Kenya as a functional structure and ideology. One
might expect a certain objective and critical revision to have occurred, an
emotional-intellectual demotion through fainter praise. I anticipated this
in relation to Muriel so was taken aback by such an extravagant display of
attachment from each interviewee, which exceeded what one might expect
in terms of politeness and respectful affection. The word 'love' was offered
time and again in these narratives. Love that had been given, returned,
shared and multiplied between Muriel and staff, the students, the birthing
women, and their little babies. Love unbounded, unmeasured, unqualified and unforgotten in its regeneration through memory. It was all rather
overwhelming and easy to see why Muriel had cherished them so much,
treasuring the words of her farewell, retirement song, written and performed by the Maua Hospital staff.

The fruits of sister Muriel are openly seen.
In many of our hospitals here in Kenya.
Many are students that have been trainees by her.
And many are patients those whom she has helped
And of you nurses, many of whom are Muriel's children
We request you to take up her example
You do your work with dedication and a loving heart
And truly you'll get many God's blessings.

What then of Audrey? In the family, her memory was unequivocally
burnished not only by Muriel but younger relatives too. 'Patricia', one
of Audrey and Muriel's surviving kin was forgivably partial to one aunt
over the other, summing up Audrey as 'very generous and *more* amazing
than Muriel.... She was dedicated to everything she did in a quiet and
calm way'. Audrey 'was 'nothing but kindness'. Unlike tone-death Muriel,
Audrey could play the violin, the piano and guitar. Moreover, she had a
'wonderful voice too, very sweet'.

Audrey was clearly a most remarkable woman, but whether she was
more so than her younger sister is something the reader must decide for
themselves.

As mentioned in Chapter 1, it was disappointingly difficult to hunt down those who knew Audrey in South India. However, Dalit theologian and CSI pastor, the Reverend Dr Gnanavaram Masilamani,[28] recalled Audrey vividly.

> She loved us and we loved her, she was a very, very great personality... She was the Head of the Nursing Dept at the Ikkadu CSI ...she was also involved in the Church Ministry along with the Hospital Ministry, where I am really, really happy to note she became the treasurer of the local Church at CSI Ikkadu. I was talking to an elderly person this morning. He was saying she did the treasurer ministry very diligently and her accountability was so much there. It was model for the local ... leaders both in the Church and in ...Society.

This probity is corroborated in Audrey's effects by an undated, hand-written farewell letter in lurid green ink from the 'members of the hospital staff and nurses', praising Audrey's merits:

> We take pride that you have excelled many of the missionary ladies who have come to India on our Lord's mission. Your total involvement in people and projects, and your absolute trust worthiness in matters of finance speak louder than the words of Christ's love for us.

A folder is entitled 'Poem read to felicitate Miss A.M. Chalkley on behalf of church congregation of the occasion of her visit to the Goudie Memorial Church, Tiruvallur during the harvest festival of 14.09.1997'. The enclosed eulogy was written by the faithful Ratnam Jacob of the Ikkadu Cottage Industries celebrating Audrey's return visit to South India some years after her retirement. It is an epic of a poem. Audrey is compared to Florence Nightingale 'She stressed Nurses to serve with love and dedication'. Moreover, she is like saintly Mother Theresa in identifying with 'the downtrodden; as a Guardian Angel in the hours of Suffering and Pain'. The poem ends with the final flourishing stanza:

> We thank the Lord for her Glorious example
> Who exemplified Christ in her life ample
> May you be blessed with a life of Long Span,
> And may God be with you till we meet again

I turn to a poignant and mildly comic letter in copperplate type from the Ikkadu's Boys' Home comparing Audrey again to the 'Lady with the lamp', adding the memorable words:

> 'We the people of Ikkadu and the C.S.I Home for Boys, Ikkadu, owe to you much for your kind gesture. Your helping gesture is unparalleled.

Your love of discipline is unique. By your generosity of spirit, your chummy behaviour, you have endeared to one and all. You have distinguished yourself with your commendable tact and impartiality even beyond the capacity you have been holding. Above all you speak your heart without fret or fear and you proved to be a true Christian in thoughts, words and deeds...'. Signed 'The manager, staff and children'.

I 'deplore', as Miss Freethy might have said, a lamentable insufficiency of greater, more varied testimonies by which we might judge Audrey's character, disposition and habits further. But sometimes, folks, that's just the way it is.

Intimacies

Photographs of Muriel in her prime mostly depict her in uniform on the ward, typically cradling an infant. Apart from some faded family photographs none depict Muriel in any kind of romantic folie-à-deux situation. Only two show her enjoying recreational fun with a man. Here she is in monochrome in a summer dress on a spartan Methodist holiday retreat in England. The two photographs are dynamic action snaps, taken within moments of each other, showing frontal lobbies and back-handers. A good-looking, smiling youth in plaid shirt and slacks is Muriel's opponent; while she, a tall, ungainly figure is caught swooping in with buck-toothed, bat-wielding enthusiasm. All 'good, clean fun' – there is clearly no attempt to assail Muriel's stalwart heart going on.

Muriel was frank about her attitude to men and relationships with them. In her world, men were non-cohabiting relatives, colleagues or students with potential for promotion to friendship. The dire warnings Frank issued, to wit: no larking about with boys, she fully took to heart. Thereafter any association with males was regarded as posing a vague but serious threat and was the root of her great distress at the Leasowe TB Hospital, where the 'big boys' on the ward were 'a terror'. These adolescent patients, a menace and a misery to Muriel, a gauche, nervous girl, probably wanted no more than cheerful, flirtatious feminine attention to remind them they were indeed lads like others. It was a wish that went unmet for Muriel was simply terrified of them, sparking a certain desperate sadism in their teasing.

Playing matchmaker was not beneath Frank either, drawing Muriel's shrinking attention to a suitable lad from his Methodist Youth work interested in getting to know her better. Muriel not quick in the game of sexual politics found these convoluted, double messages confusing. But then, as she said, nothing came of it, for the boy drowned during the war as a young Merchant Naval recruit, when his ship was torpedoed by the Nazi U-Boats. I rather think that Muriel, never short of natural, spontaneous compassion, had no particular secret sorrows to overcome at this unfortunate youth's death beyond a generalised sadness for that generation's sacrifice. Instead, as she gained experience of the world, crude approaches replaced her fear with a deep repugnance of the male's blunt sexual pursuit of the fair.

MURIEL: I've never felt longing for a man and never been kissed, except once when I was about fourteen and this youth of about seventeen – we were playing Postman's Knock, he put his tongue in my mouth and it was *horrible*!

Another story, another man and another unpalatable memory. In her late twenties, she was suddenly propositioned, much to her surprise, by a man who was part of her friendship walking group.

MURIEL: It was in Macclesfield and I was moving to Stoke-on-Trent and then this fellow said 'don't go to Stoke, Muriel, stay here and marry me'. I didn't have the slightest inkling, but his mother had just died and I think he wanted someone to cook for him. He *smelt* of beer!'

The nasty, boozy breath of this luckless wooer put an end to any of his marital presumptions. But even if he had been the model of Methodist sobriety, I doubt he could have dissuaded Muriel from pursuing her nursing vocation, which offered so much more than marriage.

The gendered hazards of social disgrace lay behind Frank's warnings and matchmaking. Midwives regularly encountered illegitimate births as the consequences of feminine imprudence (Worth, 2002); the social repercussions of childbirth out of wedlock being very serious indeed for women and their children. The illegitimate baby with Down's syndrome that Muriel delivered as a midwife in-training was likely to have ended up in institutional care. However, this was not the only hazard awaiting unwanted children. Some 130,000 British children in institutional care were deported to the colonies between the 1920s and the 1960s[29] with the aim of turning them into robust colonials under the casual care of strangers. The unforeseen but terrible abuses many of these lost children experienced came to light in a major scandal in the millennium, forcing then Britain's Labour prime minister, Gordon Brown, to follow Australia's lead in issuing a public apology to survivors (Davies, 2017).

Jonathan was lucky not to have been among that number, for as Muriel knew, he was the adopted illegitimate offspring of an illicit union. With the privilege of his gender, the blameworthy youth fled the scene, while she, culpable poor girl, was not permitted by her family to bring the child home.

In-between her Kenyan years, Muriel returned to work at Clatterbridge Hospital. It was there that Jonathan was born during one of these serendipitous sojourns. Astonishingly Muriel was quite certain she remembered the case and that the child destined to become Jonathan entered the world into her waiting hands. Like so many in Maua, he was greeted as one of her own special babies.

Muriel remained a self-affirmed virgin her entire long life. In another age, she would have been celebrated for her dedicated chastity, a model of sexual continence to inspire others. In these contemporary times, such protracted celibacy might suggest either some psychological condition or an obvious sexual orientation away from men. How 'queer' was Muriel is an inevitable question. However, her distaste for heterosexual congress does not necessarily suggest desire for alternative adult intimacy. Although hardly unacquainted with the results of sex, to me, she seemed so innocently oblivious it was easy to fancy it beyond Muriel's 'ken'. Nonetheless, she did attract a genuine passion in her lifetime, albeit one that was ultimately unrequited. Hearts were broken, but not, in fact, hers.

Muriel donated to Fran[30] a heavy, racing-green photograph album with leather corners, expensive in its day, bearing the gold-lettered legend 'M. Chalkey'. This half-filled album yields some clues regarding Muriel's private life, where on the flyleaf, Muriel wrote in her large, looping hand the following firm disclaimer:

> I did not buy this album!
> It was given to me by M.P. (author's omission) one of my students who became a close friend and rather doted on me! She was also a photographer.
> She asked me to express my life through photos in this album, which goes from days of girl guides – nurse training – qualified working at Clatterbridge Hospital & training school. Macclesfield Infirmary & West Park Stoke on Trent – City Hospital Birmingham – Loveday Street (Midwifery Tutor Course)'.
> In Kenya as a Missionary Nurse – In charge of Maternity work and training and teaching Kenyan students.
> Then back to Clatterbridge after Father's death. Back to Kenya. Then retirement in Southbourne Bournemouth.

Several tea-tinted pages lie thick with glue displaying chronologically arranged photographs of Muriel: with sisters, parents, good chums, on the wards, at her desk, until finally, we come across three photographs of 'M.P.' – a young, German midwife trainee. A bespectacled young woman of oval face and regular features, irreproachable in her dark midwife's coat and badged cap appears. Another photograph: hair neatly pinned up but for a lolling, plump curl. In two more, M.P. smilingly bears the midwife's tribute of plump babies in her arms. At the bottom of one photograph Muriel has written 'She rather "doted" on me and was very upset when I went to Kenya!'.

To me, Muriel described M.P. as having 'a crush' on her. It was more than that for M.P. was really in love with Muriel, ascertaining correctly that she was not cut out for a conventional marriage. She was devastated when Muriel chose her missionary vocation over a life of unconventional love. Had Muriel remained in Derby, she would have kept the job she loved and the woman who loved her.

Yet if Muriel had reciprocated her suffering protégé's adoration, it would have overturned everything Muriel understood as sanctified by God. Conventional (heteronormative) marriage was an ideal, but easy sacrifice to make. That which marriage could bring was a harder one to bear, as she said.

MURIEL: I've never craved for a husband but I've craved for a baby.
MURIEL: I would have loved a baby. I wanted a baby more than a husband.

Muriel's passions were spent on mothers and children in her care. To bring forth life was all important to her; cradling the babies, particularly the premature ones lonely for their mothers, her comfort. Even so, temptations beset her.

A local man walked to Maua Hospital carrying a newborn baby and the saddest of tales. Returning from labouring in the fields, he had returned home to find his wife had given birth alone in the village. The young woman was quite dead, her body bathed in blood, but there with her lay the still attached, crying infant she had birthed. The father, burdened with other children and now no wife, promptly proffered up the baby girl to the Hospital along with five shillings, the cost of the Mission Hospital birth in the 1930s (Gerrard, 2001). The baby was taken in and nameless, promptly nicknamed 'Shilling Itano' (Five Shillings), for want of a better name, and there she stayed in the hospital, growing plump and delightful, cared for by Muriel and the nurses. One day thoughtfully looking over the thriving child, Muriel announced that *Shilling Itano* looked just like Mary, the nurse beside her, and should be renamed. Muriel grew extremely fond of little Mary, regularly taking her to her quarters to bathe, clothe, feed and play during her hours off.

Yet, although orphaned babies were often left in the hospital when their mothers had died, it would not do forever. Muriel was put under a lot of pressure by the resident doctor to decide what was best done with the toddler, now walking and talking. The necessary and painful day came when Muriel decided Mary had to be adopted by a 'good Christian family' locally with the birthfather's uninterested consent.

On 3 December 1972, Muriel updated the Methodist support circuit:

> Mary will be 2 years old on December 11th. She is quite settled and happy in her foster home, and running around and talking quite a lot now. I still see her from time to time and though she is a little more shy of me, she still seems to know me and will let me cuddle her. I keep her supplied with clothing from your parcels – so you can still feel a link with her.

Muriel's connection was life long, she never forgot Mary and spoke of her often with me. It had been a huge wrench to part with the beautiful baby that she secretly yearned to adopt, despite the practicalities of being a single, working woman in an extremely hectic vocation. But Muriel knew she would one day return to England and worried about dislocating Mary from her people and her culture. A prescient thought for British social work would come to frown upon international and inter-racial adoptions (Hayes, 2000; Parker, 2002).

A counter argument I refrained from saying was that Muriel's love, generosity and formidable character would have been a good shield and example to any child nonetheless. However, the main reason Muriel gave up the idea of keeping the beloved child was simply that she was an unmarried woman with no prospects of being any other. Her unshakeable belief was that a child should grow within the protective boundaries of a sanctified union of a father and mother. This is a view so at odds with contemporary understandings and lifestyle choices that it may seem to some as utterly preposterous. Had she known of it, Muriel might also have taken heart by the example of Mary Mitchell Slessor, a Victorian missionary teacher with the Scottish Presbyterians in East Nigeria, who from 1876 went on to give excellent Christian service there and despite spinsterhood became the mother of several adopted African daughters (Grimshaw and Sherlock, 2005) (Figure 9.4).

If Muriel had been less emotionally fixated upon Frank, and Bertha had been central to her childhood loyalties, she might have squared her need for motherhood with Mary's need to be mothered. But no other man could ever measure up to Frank's stature in Muriel's affections. Frank's decline through rapid onset dementia was something that she was thankful she never saw, for the awful irony of these diverse organic psychiatric conditions is that it often removes the strongest personality traits others knew them by. A famously difficult, cantankerous relative of mine was robbed of her long-lived spite to become a short-lived, bemused and sweet-tempered old lady; whilst tragically for great-hearted, pious Frank, the opposite

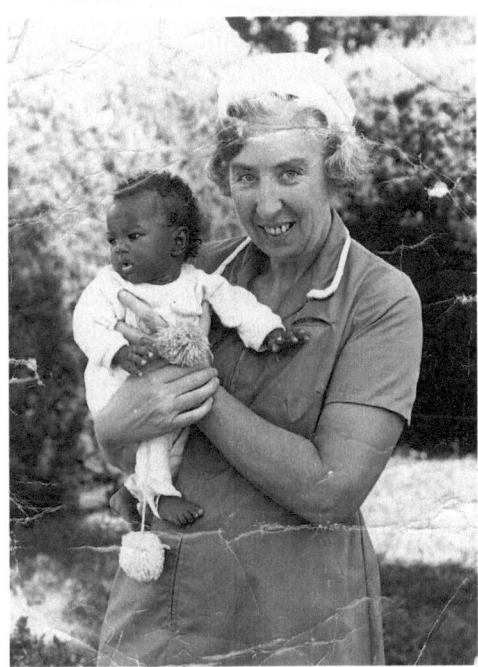

Figure 9.4 Muriel and orphaned baby, Maua. Courtesy of Muriel Chalkley.

occurred. He fell into a calamitous decline, where before long he knew neither wife, home, nor probably his God. Frank was transferred to a psychiatric hospital, ending his days in specialist residential care. Muriel could not have borne it, and so Audrey did, returning from India to care for both parents. Later, after Frank's death, the sisters swapped their filial duties and Muriel returned from Kenya to care for the parent she had loved less. Coming home from Clatterbridge Hospital, one evening she discovered Bertha dead in the bathroom. One had been 'Daddy' and the other only 'Mother'.

Later while Muriel said that she remembered Mary far more than she could possibly remember her, Mary proved faithful. The CD of Muriel's party shows her leaning over a gentle young woman, whose arms, like those of the smiling husband beside her, are filled with their children. Muriel is overheard asking earnestly, 'Mary, are you happy?' The girl's shy assent reassures.

Her childless state was Muriel's one real abiding regret. I once asked her if she thought Audrey had felt similarly, but Muriel could not say. This was a subject they had never tiptoed over, although confidences are the hallmark of women's intimacy. Audrey had not lacked for male admiration;

boyfriends she had known, and in addition to her passionate Irishman there was another handsome chap seeking her favours apparently. However, once Audrey felt the call to become a missionary in foreign fields matrimony was no longer a viable path for her. 'That's the end', says Muriel. 'You don't meet many men then'. This, whilst true of so many women missionaries, was far from the case for men for whom the missionary and married state were never viewed as incompatible choices (Prevost, 2008).

The candle that women missionaries carried was akin to that of nuns', demanding a spotless purity arising from abnegation of body and spirit. Muriel understood this chaste vocation well and what was given up for it: 'Audrey was so engrossed with her work, she would have liked a baby maybe, but you sacrifice that when you feel called to God'. For Audrey, the path she travelled, for which she had firmly resisted all romantic temptations, may clearly have carried the greatest of sought rewards. For Muriel, standing with heatsinking hesitation at the crossroads of a Call that refused to be muffled, the sacrifices it had demanded had been dreaded, but still she had stepped forward.

Notes

1 Letter to Methodist supporters dated 3 December 1972.
2 Letter to Methodist supporters dated 25 October 1981.
3 Reverend Bernard Jinkin interviewed by Caroline Ferris, 1993. Methodist Church Oral Archive. British Library 'Sounds', C640/003/01-02.
4 Muriel Chalkley, interview with Fran Biley. Ibid.
5 Audrey Chalkley, interview with Caroline Ferris. Ibid.
6 Letter to Methodist supporters dated 9 July 1977.
7 Papers of the Hooper Family, Cadbury Library. Ibid.
8 Letter dated 10 September 1975. Ibid.
9 'My Life Story'. Ibid.
10 Muriel Chalkley, interview with Fran Biley. Ibid.
11 'Life Story'. Ibid.
12 Audrey Chalkley, interview with Caroline Ferris. Ibid.
13 Letter to Methodist supporters dated 10 September 1975.
14 Muriel Chalkley, interview with Fran Biley. Ibid.
15 Letter to Methodist supporters dated 2 September 1972.
16 Sister Christine Macqueen interviewed by Caroline Ferris, 1992. Methodist Church Oral Archive. British Library 'Sounds'. C649/054 (1992).
17 Audrey Chalkley, interview with Caroline Ferris. Ibid.
18 Ruth Ansty, Interview with Caroline Ferris. Ibid.
19 Mary Spear interviewed by Alistair MacDonald, 1995 Methodist Church Oral Archive. British Library 'Sounds'. C640/024
20 Letter to Methodist supporters in England dated 13 May 1962.
21 Letter to Methodist supporters dated 10 September 1975.
22 Andrew MacKenzie, interview with Moira Crockett. Ibid.
23 Author's interview with Susan Dutton and Helen Cooper, 2 November 2022.
24 Barbara Dickinson, interview with Author. Ibid.

25 Leah Marangu. Interview with Author. Ibid.
26 Author's interview with Margaret and John Aritho, 29 June 2021.
27 Author's interview with Florence Mutiga, 25 October 2022.
28 ·Author's interview with Reverend. Dr Gnanavaram Masilmani, 16 November 2021.
29 British children being transported to the colonies was nothing new. Millions of readers have been inadvertently introduced to the idea through L.M. Montgomery's (1908) much-loved story of *Anne of Green Gables* (1908) set in nineteenth century Canada. 'Home' born Anne is seen as having a higher moral claim to be adopted by caustic, cautious Marilla, than the stigmatised, misused orphan migrant: the 'London street Arab'.
30 Fran's unfulfilled plans were to donate this and other documentary items Muriel gave him to the British Royal Society of Nursing for archival conservation.

References

Angelo, A. (2017) Jomo Kenyatta and the repression of the 'last' Mau Mau leaders, 1961–1965. *Journal of Eastern African Studies*, 11(3), 442–459. https://doi.org/10.1080/17531055.2017.1354521

Ashencaen Crabtree, S. (2021) *Women of Faith and the Quest for Spiritual Authenticity: Comparative Perspectives from Malaysia and Britain.* London/New York: Routledge.

Boucher, C. (2003) Obituary. Michaela Denis. *Guardian* 13 May. Available at: https://www.theguardian.com/media/2003/may/13/broadcasting.guardianobituaries [Accessed 16 December 2022].

Chalkley, A.M. (1987) *A Textbook for the Health Worker (ANM)*. Volume 1. New Delhi: Wiley Eastern Limited.

Chalkley, A.M. (1986) *A Textbook for the Health Worker (ANM)*. Volume 2. Madras: The Christian Literature Society.

Chalkley, A.M. (1974). *A Textbook for the Health Worker (ANM)*. Volume 1. New Delhi: Wiley Eastern Limited.

Crossette, B. (1999) *The Great Hill Stations of Asia.* New York: Basic Books.

Davies, C. (2017) Britain's child migrant programme: Why 130,000 children were shipped abroad. *Guardian*, 27 February. Available at: https://www.theguardian.com/society/2017/feb/27/britains-child-migrant-programme-why-130000-children-were-shipped-abroad [Accessed 5 January 2023].

Diamond, E.F. (2008) Miracles. *The Linacre Quarterly*, 75(4), 345–351.

Galvin, K.T. and Todres, L. (2009) Embodying nursing openheartedness. *Journal of Holistic Nursing,* 27(2), 141–149.

Gerrard, J.W. (2001) *Africa Calling: A Medical Missionary in Kenya and Zambia.* London: The Radcliffe Press.

Goheen, M.W. (2009) 'As the Father sent me, I am sending you'. Lesslie Newbigin's missionary ecclesiology. *International Review of Mission*, 354–369.

Gooren, H. (2004) An introduction to pentecostalism: Global charismatic christianity. *Ars Disputandi*, 4(1), 206–209. https://doi.org/10.1080/15665399.2004.10819846

Graham, C. (1980) *Between Two Worlds.* Madras: Selly Oak College.

Grimshaw, P. and Sherlock, P. (2005) Women and cultural exchange. In Norman Etherington (Ed.), *Missions and Empire*. Oxford: Oxford University Press, pp. 173–193.

Hardiman, D. (2006) Introduction. In David Hardiman (Ed.), *Healing Bodies, Saving Souls: Medical Missions in Asia and Africa*. Amsterdam: Brill, pp. 5–58.

Hayes, P. (2000). Deterrents to intercountry adoption in Britain. *Family Relations*, 49(4), 465–471.

Hempton, D. (2005) *Methodism: Empire of the Spirit*. New Haven, CT: Yale.

Hunsberger, G.K. (1998) Conversion and community: Revisiting the Leslie Newbigin M.M. Thomas Debate. *International Bulletin of Missionary Research*, 22(3), 112–117.

Kent, E.F. (1999) Tamil Bible women and the zenana mission of colonial South India. *History of Religions*, 39(2), 117–149.

Kenyatta, J. (1965) *Facing Mount Kenya*. New York: Vintage.

Knitter, P.F. (2011) The meeting of religions: A christian debate. In Gavin d'Costa, Paul Knitter and Daniel Strange (Eds.), *Only One Way? Three Christian Responses*. London: SCM Press, pp. 47–90.

Kyle, K. (1999) *The Politics of the Independence of Kenya*. Houndsmill: Palgrave Macmillan.

Mahler, H. (1988) Health for All – All for Health. *World Health*. Geneva: WHO.

Mbithi, P.M. and Wisner, B. (1973) Drought and famine in Kenya: Magnitude and attempted solutions. *Journal of East African Research and Development*, 3(2), 113–143.

McGee, G.B. (1999) 'Latter Rain' falling in the East: Early-twentieth-century pentecostalism in India and the debate over speaking in tongues. *Church History*, 68(3), 648–665.

MMS (1955). *The Changing Church*. The Annual Report and Accounts of the Methodist Missionary Society. London.

Parker, J. (2002) Adoption and loss: Implications for contemporary social work in the UK. *Practice: Social Work in Action*, 14(3), 15–30.

Pass, A. (2011) *British women missionaries in India c. 1917–1950*. PhD Dissertation. University of Oxford.

Pradhan, Q. (2017) *Empire in the hills: Simla, Darjeeling, Ootacamund, and Mount Abu, 1820-1920*. Oxon: Oxford University Press.

Prevost, E. (2008) Married to the mission field: Gender, Christianity and professionalization in Britain and Colonial Africa, 1865–1914. *Journal of British Studies*, 47(4), 796–826.

Priestley, J.B. (1934) *English Journey*. London: Victor Gollancz.

Pritchard, A.C. (2017) *Sisters in Spirit: Christianity, Affect and Community Building in East Africa, 1860–1970*. East Lansing: Michigan State University Press.

Reiss, R. (2016) *Sceptical Christianity*. London: Jessica Kingsley Publishers.

Robertson, B.M. (1993) *Angels in Africa: A Memoir of Nursing with the Colonial Service*. London: The Radcliffe Press.

Ross, D. (No date) *The Pattern of a Life*. Unpublished. (See Cadbury Library, University of Birmingham, CMS/ACC908).

Schanche, D. (1989) Conservationist slain by bandits in Kenya. *The Washington Post*, 22 August. Available at https://www.washingtonpost.com/archive/politics/1989/08/22/conservationist-slain-by-bandits-in-kenya/ee273f79-ebc8-46d2-9bce-28022b6e5eb1/ [Accessed 15 December 2022].

Scott, P. (1975) *A Division of the Spoils*. London: Heinemann

Scott, P. (1966) *The Jewel in the Crown*. London: Heinemann.

Strayer, R.W. (1978) *The Making of Mission Communities in East Africa: Anglicans and Africans in Colonial Kenya, 1875–1935*. London: Heinemann.

Swinburne, R.G. (1968) Miracles. *Philosophical Quarterly*, 18(73), 320–238.

Vasagar, J. (2004) Joy shot me in the leg so I gunned her down. *Guardian*, 8 February. Available at: https://www.theguardian.com/environment/2004/feb/08/kenya.conservation [Accessed 15 December 2022].

Worth, J. (2002) *Call the Midwife*. London: Phoenix.

WWMMS (1956) *Annual Report and Statement of Accounts for 1956*. Marylebone: Methodist Missionary Society.

10 Conclusion
An unfolding legacy

People, place and passion

Ethnographers bear responsibility for participant's confidence in the dicing, slicing and repackaging interpretative process where narratives form a fit to an analytic discursive frame. Biographies carry an additional representational responsibility, demanding a dogged authorial faithfulness to the facts of lives lived. This weight is even heavier when it concerns those personally known to the author, there being the rub. The obligations to intellectual integrity demand a tempering of sensibility through robust interrogation, if justice is to be done to the topic, and so I have tried to rebuke and restrain any creeping excess of bias for these sisters, English eccentrics in the best tradition.

Knowing Muriel personally generated a powerful motivation to write this book, yet inhibited its commencement. We stood on a bridge of mutual understanding balanced across time, generational expectations and life experiences; with gulfs of differing social meanings and discourses dividing the world she had inhabited from the one I navigated. Call it kindness or cowardice, but mindful that the usual scholarly deconstruction and general analysis of a faith (to which these sisters gave their lives) was fraught with potential hurt and offence, I procrastinated. By the time I began this book, Muriel was sequestered in institutional care and becoming lost to her own history. Fearing she was approaching the end of her life, as she was, I pledged myself to get on with fulfilling my promise to write.

However, I could not create a straightforward chronological account, often encountered in missionary autobiographies of endless events, each reasonably gripping, but tedious overall in lacking deeper contextual discussion. Breathless hagiography would not do either. Equally unwelcome was a post-colonial polemic of revisionist history exploiting the hapless figures of the Chalkleys, cruelly illuminated on a dusty, outmoded and unwanted Imperial stage set.

DOI: 10.4324/9781003359746-10

As Colin Morris saw in the 1970s, a critique of mission was essential for post-colonial nations and scholars in sorting wheat from chaff. Yet my work with Muriel changed me and my perceptions of Christian mission. While I have always been interested in the lives of women, academically, professionally and personally, this had not been extended to women missionaries. Once my thinking might have verged on callow, unnuanced and reactive, judging mission *per se*, as irredeemably contaminated by contemporary controversy. It's hard to remember if I ever thought that or not, but certainly the academic world I inhabited largely did. Thus, the extraordinary lives such women have been often overlooked.

We occupy *post* post-colonial times (Ashencaen Crabtree, 2012) where revisionist histories will continue to be subject to further revisions. There is no end point where an absolute judgement can be reached and no final conclusion stands unquestioned. There have been scholarly obstructions to fully appreciating the powerful, social momentum and incentivisation of faith (Billington Harper, 2000). Or that perhaps there was more to evangelism than hypocrisy and power-grabs (Strayer, 1978).

> A secular age is inclined to under-rate the importance of religious forces born in another era; an anti-imperialist scholar is repulsed by the generally unabashed cultural imperialism of nineteenth-century evangelists.
>
> (Etherington, 2012, p. 31)

A latent deep scepticism, if not hostility, continues to colour academia, I find, where Christian mission is still a byword for unforgivable bigotry, standing in undifferentiated bad odour. Thus, it is altogether too easy to dismiss all who participated in mission as not only culturally but scholastically irrelevant. This is particularly so when insufficiently explored connotations are compounded by the casual sexism of dismissing the narratives of ageing, single women, former missionaries, from often, very ordinary backgrounds, as merely irrelevant products of their unreformed times.

Not everyone agrees, especially those who actually encountered missionaries personally and were able to examine them and their motives at close quarters. Nonetheless, tutored in these sensitivities I personally did not expect much affirmation when I nervously tiptoed towards a discussion of mission legacies in conversation with Florence Mutiga,[1] acknowledging timidly how much the criticism missionary activities including mission nursing had aroused. Florence seemed frankly amazed and outraged by this statement: 'WHY?!' She boomed at me with indignant fury, provoking relieved chortles.

I reflect on an observation made to me, to wit that mission was decidedly passé: 'The world had moved on, but they (the sisters) hadn't'. To be fair, this is a true statement: the world had indeed changed. Intrepid women would no longer feel a hallowed compulsion to pack their trunks and bravely set forth to goodness knows what adventures and ordeals, trusting simply in God to keep them safe from harm. Otherwise, resignedly submitting to the Almighty's will, because they sincerely believed that in some remote corner of the little-known world, they were deeply needed (Prevost, 2010). Whether one regards that as delusional, hubristic or rather admirable, by heaven, it was undoubtedly brave.

Providence determined their path: Muriel was certain that God had picked precisely the right locations for them both. India was not for her and Audrey not for Africa. The places missionaries were chosen for, as much as their choices, generally shaped them so profoundly that forever after they carried the indelible imprint of deep religo-cultural richness (Graham, 1980; Pritchard, 2017). Equally, it magnified the importance of the very people missionaries served: new generations of Indigenous Christians shaping the future of their nations.

> And so many more,
> Years ago, my girls,
> My pupils, my 'daughters'
> Demure in their green school saris,
> In the classroom. In the hostel,
> Prayerful, sincere in the morning assembly,
> Or in the quiet of the prayer room,
> Singing and singing the Christian lyrics
>
> (Margaret James, undated, stanza 2)

In such places, of mostly forgotten peoples in the backwaters of Empires, foreign female missionaries could achieve a stature largely denied them back in their home countries. I do not refer solely to status, although of course that was often implicit to the roles they were expected to undertake; but to the whole person. Determination and robustness of character, not to mention physically, were traits deemed conventionally unfeminine, but faith emboldened women. Mission employment of skilled and educated labour, unusual qualifications among the majority of Western women, often demanded levels of initiative, responsibility and decision-making most unusual in the wider, conventional world of gendered hierarchies.

Here then I am conscious of attempting to raise Lazarus once more, by revealing the sisters to be vibrant, living, thinking, feeling, *real* people, not just flattened two-dimensional caricatures of eager evangelism, the unwitting instruments of colonial misrule. Or indeed, more benevolently, two dear old ladies, saintly and unworldly. Being committed to an active Christian life did not create an absurdly ecstatic blindness to life's problems, a myopic 'happy-clappy' euphoria. Their passionate faith was maybe little questioned, but it did not remove uncertainty and fear from their lives. It did provide a strong sense of guided meaning and supreme solace that we might all wish for. Audrey, for one, was often described as embodying peacefulness, tolerance and joy, yet her poems convey a more complex character, one grappling with her own demons (James and Chalkley, undated). Here, for example, are a few lines of her verse that reveal a vulnerability lighting kindred sympathy for her fallibilities.

> Lord you are my leader, I have all I need.
> You calm me down when I am moody,
> With your love and power you fill me,
> When in trouble you will lead me,
> Your protection makes me unafraid.
>
> (Audrey Chalkley, undated, stanza 1)

The thematic threads of people, place and passion affixed to the sisters' lives, words and companion, supplemented by scholarly commentary and speculation, have hopefully helped to cement them a little more firmly in the contentious and slippery history of modern Christian mission. Bringing, hopefully, a humanity to the polemical and humility to critique; as well, perhaps, as cementing the sisters further, if needed, in transient memory.

A diaconic legacy

Muriel retired at the conventional age then for British women, of just sixty. But this was not an easy decision to make; it gave her some sleepless nights, as the passing on of the spiritual leadership of Vishranthi Nilayam did to Carol Graham (1980). On the one hand, Muriel had been offered the chance of a nestling into a covetable situation, with a lovely stretch of beach effectively at the end of her road in the warm south of England. On the other hand, she agonised about whether it was the right time to relinquish all her responsibilities at Maua. Audrey, a few years older, also set an awkward example in having agreed to continue her work in India to revise the earlier volumes of the Auxiliary Nurse Midwives textbooks. For Muriel though the time had clearly come to terminate her own indispensability and realise the mission aim: obsolescence Her twin roles of ward management and midwifery tutoring, she decided to split between Florence Mutiga and Florence Mubichi, together more than capable of taking her work over. She resigned, to the regret of the Kenyan Church. Stefano inherited her coveted radio and 'comfy chair' with everything else she owned auctioned off to raise funds for the planned new maternity ward.

It took time for Audrey to join Muriel but eventually released exhausted from her duties she retired to Bournemouth, living across town until

Wesley's chains of Providential care fortuitously linked her to Muriel just a few paces away across faded carpeting of an upstairs hall landing. They had long known that their shared spinsterhood in Christ meant setting up home together. Given their daughters' destinies, Frank and Bertha left their home in Brombourgh to Audrey and Muriel, on the paternalistic grounds that Dorothy was set up in life through marriage. The proceeds of the house sale the sisters put aside for future needs, continuing to generously bestow money on the Ikkadu and Maua Hospitals from, as Audrey said, 'a legacy',[2] by which she must have meant their joint inheritance, having no other money but their modest pensions.

It was a decided culture shock adjusting to life back in Britain.

AUDREY: I'd learnt in India to be very economical and to live frugally...And at first it was so difficult....the prices were so outrageous! I mean so high. It was far too expensive and so I was loath to spend and I really didn't know at first how much income I would be getting.

Reliant on Muriel's more practised help, Audrey could only bring herself to buy second-hand furniture with a strict tally kept on expenses. Each was entitled to triple pensions from the NHS, the statutory State Pension and the Methodist Church; and while in reality, this was but a humble total, to them it seemed more than ample. Most of this income was squirrelled away carefully, little spent the more to give to others.

AUDREY: I found that in this way of living I could still live a healthy life, as I'd been teaching the people in India, on only what is necessary. And so we got our bargains and we managed to live on a low income so that we can continue as far as possible to help people who are not so well-off in India and Kenya – and also help with good causes overseas.

This did not conclude their charitable giving to good causes, for well into her nineties when still independently managing her financial affairs, Muriel gave generous amounts to those that needed it back in Kenya, including 'Deborah' and her daughter, and Margaret Aritho's lad, John, for his studies in India.

JOHN ARITHO: Oh, my word, it was a huge blessing. It really, really helped me.... a lot with my studies until I graduated in 1975. Got to go and say thank you to Muriel... (Then) I started working in Kenya, then went to South Africa, and was still communicating with her. In 1999 I decided to go to the UK and went to look for her

> in Bournemouth...Her flat was full of artefacts from Kenya, and Audrey's was full of them from India ... It was hilarious spending the whole afternoon with them. We had a great, great time.

In reward for their long, unstinting service and generosity, Muriel and Audrey were each independently honoured by having hospital wards named after them with all due VIP ceremonies to commemorate the event. At Maua Methodist Hospital, a plaque dedicated to Sister Muriel Chalkley directs patients to the Chalkley Ward dedicated to maternity care. The (Audrey) Chalkley Wing at the CSI Ikkadu Hospital leads to a suite of new patient wards.

Upon re-immersion into Britain, the sisters had to find a way to spiritually reconnect, and this was not an easy or obvious undertaking. Muriel in her first two years alone tried to reacquaint herself with Methodism locally. It was very disappointing apparently, for she now found it boring, uninspiring, over-wordy, devoid of spiritual energy, the organ music deadly. She naughtily acting it out to entertain me, playing an 'air' organ with deadly ponderousness: 'DUH....DUH....DONG....DANG!'

Dismayed by the difference between the lively worship in Kenya and this Methodist mausoleum, Muriel never went back. Instead, she cycled around town, trying every church in her circuit: the Anglicans and the United Reform were inspected, the Baptists and the Salvation Army found wanting, Roman Catholics – unimaginable! None would do, until Pat Tuffrey (from Chapter 7) now settled in the Bournemouth Nurses Retirement Home, suggested Cranleigh Chapel, a Charismatic Evangelical Church close to Muriel's home. It took me some time to realise that in fact my 'shamba', a community allotment where with enthusiastic ineptness I grow fruit and veg for the family table, was literally opposite this chapel. It certainly did not look much like a church to me, used to Victorian high gothic. A small, modern, single-storey, pale stucco building it carried no particular distinction at all. But here was where Muriel held witness, preached, spoke in tongues and sang to her heart's content to contemporary hymns accompanied by a portable keyboard, electric guitar, and no doubt, tambourines.

Audrey also found a return to the Methodist Church difficult, after the 'rich' and unique liturgical experience of the CSI. The extraordinary spiritual rewards that came from the deliberate disintegration of denominational identities in the 'catholic' ecumenism of the CSI had been extremely difficult for people back in Britain to understand in the 1960s.

> When, having spoken to a group of Methodists in England and answered their questions for nearly an hour, one of them said indulgently: 'It all sounds very good for India but I am sure you still a Methodist at heart'.
> (Graham, 1980, p. 55)

Some twenty years later, Audrey received a warmer reception than Newbiggin or Graham had found when she carefully suggested introducing the local Methodist minister to some form of CSI worship. An interesting *volte face* was at play, for Muriel had remained so loyal to indigenised Methodism in Kenya, had defected to the Evangelists once back in Britain. Audrey by contrast had willingly relinquished Methodist denominationalism to embrace the CSI's indigenised ecumenicism, and yet dutifully returned to the British Methodist fold again.

In their adjacent flats, Muriel conducted weekly Evangelical fellowship meetings, while Audrey in the spirit of the CSI's anti-sectarianism unity, led a 'Lydia' women's prayer group. Furthermore, Audrey kept up her CSI allegiances through the Methodist Women's Network in Southampton, compiling a book of verses she and Margaret James, a fellow ex-CSI mission worker, had written over the years (all proceeds of any sales to the CSI). A copy of their book, *Reflections*, was sent to me by Susan Dutton. An interestingly ambiguous title, pertaining not to reflection as reflexivity, rather reflection of, rather than on.

Village Women's Classes

Hurry, hurry, don't be late,
Come for the Women's Class at eight!'
The teacher's wife goes to all the huts,
Christians and Hindus, as the suns sets.
The women grow bold, not afraid to share;
To give their witness, or lead a prayer.
Their problems and fears, when shared with others
Are changed to victory in the name of Jesus.
Fifty years ago it all started,
Ikkadu the place, as missionaries chatted;
'Why are the women so silently sitting,
Not even able to join in the singing.

(James and Chalkely, Undated)

It is fair to say that the merit of this little publication lies not in great poetry. However, distinctive insights are yielded into the immersion of women missionaries in the life of communities they worked with, especially in respect to local women. Facilitating women's religious empowerment would inevitably but subtly alter the gendered dynamics of Indian society, an idea that the old zenana mission workers would have recognised (Kent, 1999).

In 1989, Audrey returned for a tour of India and was warmly hosted by the CSI dignitaries she knew well. She was asked to preach in churches for miles around. It was an extraordinarily happy reunion for her: 'Ikkadu was like coming home and the four years I'd been away faded into the background'.[3] She had missed everything about her former life, friends, colleagues, the culture, the food. The latter must have been sorely missed, as the sisters usually ate together and Muriel unsophisticated palate simply could not abide spicy cuisine.

Nunc dimittis

The long retirement the sisters enjoyed together was a very contented and peaceful time. In his lyrical elegy of a Gloucestershire childhood, Laurie Lee (1959) speaks of a great tree planted by a father of one of the ancient, feuding, village 'grannies', at what seemed the beginning of time. I was reminded of it, admiring the big, overgrown garden Muriel looked out over. Oaks of immense stature stood beside the huge, shadowy shrubs, she and Audrey had planted as mere sprigs. 'Young' Susi in her wheel-chair downstairs is probably the last generation of missionaries that this dedicated refuge in Bournemouth will ever see. Audrey, she thought, emu-lated St Francis of Assisi, nature returned her love, for beneath the sun lounger, as Audrey lay singing quiet hymns to herself, a sleep-lulled, wild fox curled, soothed by her lullabies (Figure 10.1).

The sisters spoiled themselves a little, clubbing together with two friends to purchase an old beach hut with some of their remaining inheritance. Beach huts, a national passion (to which I subscribe), these miniature home-from-homes are endearingly ridiculous with their bright paint, print curtains and whistling kettles. There the sisters would spend long days, swimming, sunbathing, making tea and eating sandwiches, regarding themselves as extremely well rewarded for their past labours. By the time Muriel was 88 and Audrey 92, the effort of a short but steep walk to-and-fro was too much to manage and the beach hut had to be given up. It was at this time that Muriel wrote as a postscript to her *Life Story*,

> Now that I am 88 years I feel ready – and even eager to …see Jesus my Lord, but I know Audrey needs me at present, so we await the Lord's timing.

Audrey had in fact become entirely dependent on Muriel for everything, her fine, scholarly mind had become dimmed and confused from the Alzheimer's disease that would lead to her death in a nursing home two years later. Nonetheless, she kept up her usual beatitudes every time she saw Susi with a heartfelt 'Isn't He good to us?'

A photocopy dated 29 April 1985 from the Methodist Mission turns up written for the attention of the 'Central Committee'. It is entitled, 'Thanks

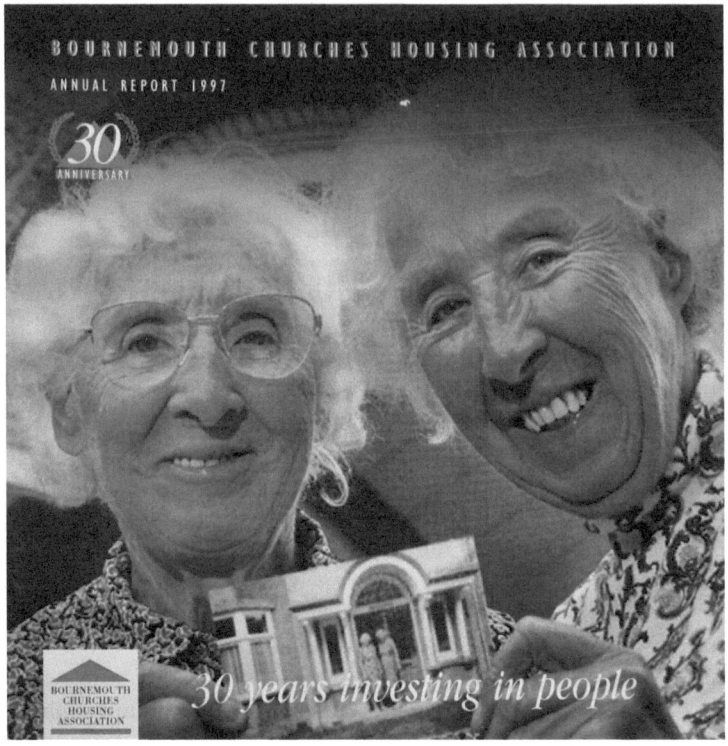

Figure 10.1 Audrey and Muriel in Retirement. Courtesy of Bournemouth Churches Housing Association.

for love-serving missionaries, Miss Audrey Chalkley SRN, SCM, RNT'. Compiled many years before Audrey died in 2013, it would form advance preparation and inspiration for her future obituary, written later by affectionate Susan Dutton, for the *Methodist Recorder* (9 August 2013). Bishop Sundar Clarke's words on Audrey are quoted in this 1985 document and later repeated in her obituary.

> Gentle Audrey, generous Audrey and Godly Audrey....simple, kind and full of the Spirit of God. She radiated her faith in her work. Her love for the poor was so intense and so immense. She was so actively involved in the spiritual renewal in the Diocese and was a live wire in our Spiritual Renewal conferences. She was inspired and she inspired others. She was a woman of Faith, Love and Service. She was one of the finest missionaries we have come across. She was one with the people and she was more Indian than many Indians.

The hardiness of the sisters is attested to by the many years they spent in Asia and Africa submitting to gruelling work regimes without permanent ill health, unlike the earlier missionaries where the combination of tropical disease and overwork proved utterly disabling or fatal, as probably befell Ikkadu's poor Betty Brock. In 2005, in retirement, Muriel developed bowel cancer but pulled through with life-changing surgery, cancer having claimed elder sister Dorothy and her eldest daughter. Eventually, Audrey's dementia led her to start wandering out at nights leading to residential nursing care, dying soon after.

After Audrey's death, Muriel was intensely lonely, her whole life she had cared for others and now there was no one left to care for. Fran's visits to interview her on four separate occasions must have been a distraction at this time of bereavement. Soon afterwards, I met her and adored her cheerful, charismatic, indomitably boisterous spirit.

Despite her early reputation as a dunce', Muriel did creditably in the end. She was awarded an *honoris causa*, Doctorate in Education from Bournemouth University in 2014. Having proposed her in the first place I was given the honour of formally presenting her to the vice-chancellor at the graduation ceremony. Muriel arrived for the ceremony in her wheelchair flanked by nieces, to find that outside the usher, and I were being repeatedly dive-bombed by an evil-minded herring gull, which unable to drive us away from our post, took a final, spiteful revenge by liberally bespattering us with *merde*; a public affront I have had to chastise *aves* before in my writings (Ashencaen Crabtree, 2021, p. 70). Cleaned up and now on stage, pathos was added to bathos, my eyes welling with tears, embarrassingly projected on a huge screen, as, Muriel swathed in the habitual academic gown and velvet-tassled cap, received her doctorate and then proceeded to give the packed stadium a typically Muriel-like 'Praise the Lord' speech of thanks, to awkward public astonishment. One there 'heard' her words, a graduating nurse student receiving her award became inspired to follow in Muriel's footsteps as a missionary nurse.

Muriel was never far from my thoughts although my visits were often irregular and haphazard. A fought for sabbatical in 2014 enabled me and the family to spend seven months researching in Malaysia. I worried about Muriel in the meantime and wrote her long, cheerful letters. A year later, Muriel was delighted when I was formally invited to Israel, treasuring her own memory of a shared pilgrimage taken on the sisters' last furlough.[4] Marvelling, praying and reciting they took in all the holy sites: the Garden of Gethsemane, Mount of Olives, the Sea of Galilee, Bethlehem and so on.

Unlike the sisters' elevating experiencing, mine was depressing and traumatic. Now I was the lonely one. It was Easter-time in Jerusalem. I watched the slow processions of devout Eastern European pilgrims, matronly mostly, wrapped in floral headscarves. They and the scrubbed, fresh-faced American pilgrims, Shaker plain, blocked up the Via Dolorosa in an exasperating devotional, pedestrian traffic jam. Unable to squeeze past this earnest crowd I spent time sitting in a beautiful old courtyard thinking doleful, disillusioned thoughts. A discouraged Canadian Protestant priest asked me to help pray with him. A bent and wizened Catholic nun speaking Latin took me by the hand to show me where the bored Roman soldiers played on the inscribed paving stones. Unlike Muriel and Audrey, I struggled to find God there. So, in some misery of mind and spirit, having heard, seen and learned too much, I boarded the plane back to London with overwhelming relief, and acting entirely out of character, ordered, almost before I had sat down and buckled up, two double measures of gin 'n' tonic, which I downed as though my salvation depended on it. Back in Bournemouth and seeing my dear Christ-besotted, tee-total Muriel eager for my news, I sat down to gaily regale her with happier traveller tales.

The sisters now rest side by side in death, but not in a conventional cemetery with a carved headstone, (stone cherubs would have suited Muriel, with angels for Audrey). The obvious location might have been the local ecumenical necropolis, populated peaceably by Catholics, Muslims, Protestants and Jews of all ethnic backgrounds. Instead, they are interred in a beautiful woodland burial site with living memorials. George Eliot (1871) concludes Middlemarch by referring obliquely to those like virtuous Dorothea who lie in unvisited graves after a life of faithful good intentions. Unlike that fictional do-gooder, ultimately frustrated in enacting her *bona causa* by the stifling gendered conventions of her society, Muriel and Audrey were doers of deeds, fortunate to live in a time and a place that still sufficiently respected women's faith, skills, fortitude, as they stepped forward to do their Lord's work.

Finally, I feel can do no better than to end this story of two remarkable sisters, by quoting Muriel's parting to the unseen reader of her *Life Story*.

As I conclude I just want to witness to the faithfulness of God, and to give Him all the glory. He has helped me through every part of my life and in the words of the old hymn 'I praise him for all that is past and trust Him for all that's to come.

God bless all of you who bother to read all of this!

Muriel

Notes

1 Florence Mutiga, interview with Author. Ibid.
2 Audrey Chalkley, interview with Caroline Ferris. Ibid.
3 Audrey Chalkley, interview with Caroline Ferris. Ibid.
4 Letter to Methodist supporters, 29 September 1979.

References

Ashencaen Crabtree, S. (2021) *Women of Faith and the Quest for Spiritual Authenticity: Comparative Perspectives from Malaysia and Britain*. London/New York: Routledge.

Billington Harper, S. (2000). *In the Shadow of the Mahatma: Bishop V.S. Azariah and the Travails of Christianity in British India*. New York: Wm. B. Eerdmans Publishing Co.

Eliot, G. (1871, 2003) *Middlemarch*. London: Penguin Classics.

Etherington, N. (2012) Social theory and the study of Christians in Africa: A South African case study. *Africa*, 47(1), 31–40.

Graham, C. (1980) *Between Two Worlds*. Madras: Selly Oak College.

James, M. and Chalkley, A. (Undated) *Reflections*. Southampton: Methodist Women's Network.

Kent, E. F. (1999). Tamil Bible women and the zenana mission of colonial South India. *History of Religions*, 39(2), 117–149.

Lee, L. (1959) *Cider with Rosie*. London: Hogarth Press.

Prevost, E. (2008) Married to the mission field: Gender, Christianity and professionalization in Britain and Colonial Africa, 1865–1914. *Journal of British Studies*, 47(4), 796–826.

Prevost, E.E. (2010) *The Communion of Women: Missions and Gender in Colonial Africa and the British Metropole*. Oxford: Oxford University Press.

Pritchard, A.C. (2017) *Sisters in Spirit: Christianity, Affect and Community Building in East Africa, 1860–1970*. East Lansing: Michigan State University Press.

Strayer, R.W. (1978) *The Making of Mission Communities in East Africa: Anglicans and Africans in Colonial Kenya, 1875–1935*. London: Heinemann.

Index

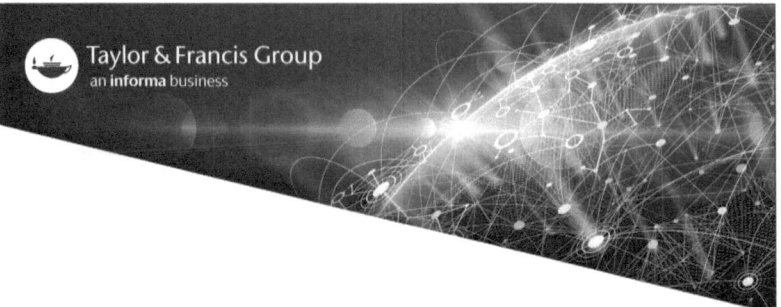
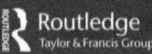
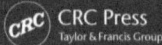